Prescription Privileges for Psychologists:
A Critical Appraisal

Dedicated to

Our students' students.
They will inherit the discipline we create.

Prescription Privileges for Psychologists: A Critical Appraisal

Edited by

Steven C. Hayes
University of Nevada
and
Elaine M. Heiby
University of Hawaii

CONTEXT PRESS
Reno, Nevada

Prescription Privileges for Psychologists: A Critical Appraisal/ edited by Steven C.
Hayes and Elaine M. Heiby.
        p. 282
        Includes bibliographical references
        ISBN 1-878978-30-6 (hardcover)
        1. Clinical Psychologists--Prescription Privileges.
I. Hayes, Steven C.   1948-   II. Heiby, Elaine M. 1952-
RC467.85.P74   1998
616.89' 18--dc21   98-39199
                                                                CIP

© 1998 CONTEXT PRESS
933 Gear Street, Reno, NV 89503-2729

Printed in the United States of America

Preface

Prescription privileges is one of the most controversial topics facing modern psychology. In only a matter of a few years, the proposal that the discipline and profession be changed to a new medical subspecialty has roared onto the central stage of organized American psychology. It gained considerable momentum in 1990 when the U.S. Senates Appropriations Committee recommended that the Department of Defense establish a demonstration prescription training program for psychologists. At about the same time, the American Psychological Association's (APA) Council of Representatives established a Task Force to examine the feasibility of prescription privileges, and to explore curriculum models for training. APA formally went on record supporting the idea in 1995, and has vigorously pursued prescription privileges at federal and state legislative bodies.

The present volume is the result of a conference organized by the American Association of Applied and Preventive Psychology (AAAPP). Over the last several years, AAAPP has recognized the seriousness of the prescription privileges proposal and has begun a systematic effort to evaluate its impact upon the field. In 1993, a survey of the AAAPP membership indicated that a strong majority opposed prescription privileges. The AAAPP Committee Concerned About the Medicalization of Psychology was established in 1994 to evaluate the proposal and issue a report. Based in part on that report, the AAAPP Board in January 1995 endorsed a *Resolution Opposing Prescription Privileges for Psychologists*, becoming the first national scientific psychological society to take a formal position on this issue.

While some pro-prescription advocates thought that change in psychology would come very quickly, the movement has had many recent setbacks, in part due to the rise of an organized opposition within psychology itself. There are good arguments on both sides of the issue, but many leaders in applied scientific psychology felt that such a major change deserved much more critical analysis. AAAPP's Board felt that opposition would, at the very least, slow the pace and allow many of the more controversial issues to be examined.

These issues are complex. Prescription privileges are not arising as an issue in a vacuum. In the era of managed care, the practice of psychology is having a difficult time competing for resources. Many psychologists in the practice community hope to solve this problem by expanding the practice of psychology to include psychoactive medications. Is this a good idea? How would it impact to solve this problem by expanding the practice of psychology to include psychoactive medications. Is this a good idea? How would it impact psychology as a discipline? How would it impact training? Would it solve the problem presented by managed care? Is it the best way to adapt to the present environment?

The AAAPP National Conference on Prescription Privileges for Psychologists was held June 26-28, 1996 at the University of Nevada, Reno to address these and many similar questions. In addition to AAAPP, the conference was supported by the College of Arts and Science and the Department of Psychology at the University of Nevada. Organized by the editors of this volume, the conference was meant to examine the issues carefully and critically. It brought together both pro and con voices, but no effort was made to maintain a balance. Rather, the conference was a kind of critical appraisal of prescription privileges. Our point was neither to have a formal debate, nor a discussion and a vote, but rather to seek out some of the leading experts in the field for each specific area to raise the critical issues that must be addressed regardless of one's position on the issue. Thus, in a way, we think of this volume as a step in a dialogue, aimed at the field eventually reaching some kind of consensus if that is possible. That dialogue should have occurred first, but now that the issue is slowing down, there may still be time for all sides to discuss these issues.

In order to foster that sense of discussion and dialogue, following each major speaker, a discussion leader led an open discussion period with the speakers and the audience. These discussions are in the present volume, though discussion leaders were free to emphasize any issues in their commentaries, not just those raised at the conference.

As the conclusion of the conference, the speakers generally agreed upon the following conclusions:

1. The prescription privileges proposal is polarizing the discipline.
2. Psychology's resources should be focused on advocating the profession to managed care. Doing so will involve the development of treatment standards and the promotion of integrated care.
3. Psychologists wishing to obtain prescription privileges at this time are encouraged to obtain an advanced degree in nursing, a physician's assistant degree, or the like in order to develop more experience with the psychology/prescription privilege hybrid without first having to alter the discipline and its training focus.

In the year following the conference, presenters turned their oral presentations into chapters for the present volume. The chapters and commentaries cover a wide range of issues that are relevant to the prescription privilege debate: its history, the political context, the scientific context, and the professional context. As such, this book presents the first critical appraisal of the prescription privilege issue. Undoubtedly there will be more books, conferences, and arguments. No matter how it turns out, the prescription privilege issue is sure to shape the future of psychology for many years to come, both intellectually and politically.

Steven C. Hayes
Elaine M. Heiby
Spring 1998

Table of Contents

Chapter 1

The Case for Prescription Privileges for Psychologists: An Overview

Morgan T. Sammons, Ph.D.

National Naval Medical Center, Bethesda, MD

Since the early 1950s, the pharmacopoeia for mental disorders has expanded at an astonishing rate. From the time of Delay and Deniker's seminal report on the efficacy of chlorpromazine in psychotic illnesses (1952, cited in Lehmann & Hanrahan, 1954), the number of psychiatric drugs and the number of conditions for which their use has been demonstrated has increased exponentially. The growth of effective pharmacological interventions for mental disorders has revolutionized mental health care and has, without question, led to major clinical advances which have undeniably proven to be of immense benefit to vast numbers of patients. As testimonial to the tremendous boon of modern psychotropics, we need look no further than the precipitous and welcome drop in custodial care which followed the introduction of effective antipsychotic agents. Other grotesque excesses of psychiatric treatment were also tempered by the introduction of drugs providing a measure of behavioral control and symptom relief. It is likely that the mutilatory "treatment" of lobotomy, which represented the most extreme and most ignoble of the excesses of psychiatric practice at midcentury, owed its fortunate demise at least in part to the discovery of effective pharmacological agents (Valenstein, 1986). Yet at the heart of the biological "revolution" lie some interesting paradoxes. Foremost among these is the observation that, in spite of a half-century of intense investigation, no unequivocally curative psychopharmacological agent has yet been developed. All psychiatric drugs, without exception, are more or less palliative. Symptoms may to certain degrees remit with their use, but they rarely, if ever, permanently resolve. Once the patient ceases use of a drug, mental distress will sooner or later recur in the majority of cases. (That the same can be said for most forms of psychological intervention is surely no rationale to tout the advantages of pharmacotherapy.)

The exact extent to which drugs can be said to help patients remains elusive. In part, this is due to the persistence of questionable investigative strategies in psychopharmacology. As Kraemer (1995) has written, statistical methods are often antiquated, psychiatrists are often unconcerned with basic principles of sound research, and much of the current literature focuses on drug efficacy (or the demonstration that a treatment works under ideal situations with ideal subjects), rather than the more telling issue of real world effectiveness. Sample sizes in drug trials are often astonishingly small, making generalizability essentially nil. Open label trials are still commonly encountered, and the literature is clotted with case reports. More fundamentally, the assumptions under which psychopharmacological research is conducted are very often post-hoc, as in the case of monoamine hypotheses of depression. "Rational" drug development is rarely that; Healy (1990) has elegantly described the curious forces of academic fashion and drug industry funding that often dictate which hypotheses are deemed worthy of investigation. In sum, Preskorn's (1996) mordant observation regarding antidepressant treatment, that "the 'placebo' response rate in antidepressant trials is arguably the most reproducible finding in psychiatry" (p. 232), can likely be generalized to much of psychopharmacology today.

Some have argued that because psychiatric drugs are not curative, psychology as a profession should not pursue the adoption of prescriptive authority (Adams & Bieliauskas, 1994). Others hold that the benefits of drug therapies are entirely illusory, and that we expose our patients to far greater harm via their use than any appreciable benefit that might accrue (Breggin, 1991). Still others (Antonuccio, Danton, & DeNelsky, 1995) hold that psychotherapy is the gold standard of treatment for at least the most common form of mental distress, and appear to suggest that psychotherapy trials of eight to sixteen weeks be accomplished before medication is considered. Given the potency of an intervention which psychology already possesses, it is, according to this school, a questionable undertaking to expend the energy and cost associated with the acquisition of prescriptive authority. Finally, a number of psychologists fear that the addition of psychopharmacology to our professional armamentarium will ineluctably change the nature of the discipline, and that graduate psychology education as we know it will fall victim to aggressively invasive "medicalized" curricula (Adams & Bieliauskas, 1994; Hayes, Walser, & Follette, 1995).

Another argument oft employed by those opposed to prescriptive authority deals with the issue of acceptance of prescription privileges by the profession at large. Those opposed to prescriptive authority for psychologists cite the results of opinion surveys to buttress their arguments that the profession is, if not overwhelmingly opposed, then sufficiently divided that it would be perilous to the unity of the profession should some psychologists seek the ability to prescribe. Such authors, (e.g., Dozois & Dobson, 1995) report the results of a number of polls of psychologists suggesting considerable variability in the opinion of respondents on the issue. Although the largest, most scientifically conducted (e.g., randomized) and arguably most representative of these polls (in that it did not simply survey local or professional subsets of psychologists) reported that a clear majority of the 1505 APA members surveyed favored prescriptive authority (APA, 1992), smaller polls with less favorable findings have been conducted. Bypassing the issues of methodology which limit the generalizability of these polls, I submit that, regardless of the findings of opinion surveys, psychologists should not base their collective decision to seek or reject prescription privileges on the basis of public opinion. Decisions with this degree of moment should be based on sound principles of science and practice, and not on opinion, which, as Dozois and Dobson (1995) correctly report, is somewhat fluid on the issue.

It must not be forgotten that the debate surrounding prescriptive authority for psychologists takes place in the context of diminishing psychiatric resources. Although approximately 20% of the American population meets established criteria for a psychiatric or substance abuse diagnosis, (Reiger, Narrow, Rae, Manderschied, Locke, & Goodwin, 1993), the number of trained psychiatrists to meet the needs of these individuals has been steadily shrinking over the past 15 years. In 1994, the proportion of medical graduates entering training in psychiatry (3.2% of all U. S. medical graduates) was less than it was in 1929 (Sierles & Taylor, 1995). Overall numbers of psychiatrists in training programs has remained stable only because of the current policy of supplementing shortfalls in residency matches with international medical graduates. This practice has created large numbers of residents trained in overseas medical schools, a fact which causes some concern among psychiatrist educators. Scully (1995) outlined a proposal to cap residency training programs at 110% of U. S. medical graduates. He noted that doing so would result in a 40% loss in beginning residents nationwide and a 60% loss in the New York area.

Psychotropic drugs are clearly no panacea. Their ability as sole therapeutic modalities to influence positively the course of a mental disorder is, without question, limited. The potency of psychopharmacological treatment in general has been, and continues to be, overstated and its risks minimized. Far too often, drugs are relied on as the bulk of a curative strategy, when effective, low-risk, nonpharmacological interventions are readily at hand. I do not intend to argue that psychologists should rush headlong to embrace psychotropic agents under the current standards which govern their use, nor do I intend to take the opposite view that their use should be entirely abandoned. Both of these views are extreme, and insufficient data exist to support either position. A reasonable middle ground exists, which is that psychoactive medications play a definable role in the treatment of mental distress and that psychologists can use these agents effectively, safely, and without profound threats to professional identity.

Psychoactive agents can and do improve clinical outcome, and are often of considerable benefit to those patients who use them. Their utility is enhanced when they are coupled with effective psychological, behavioral, or environmental interventions. Because of historical biases governing the conduct and funding of clinical investigation in psychiatry, we simply have not amassed an adequate body of data to determine the superiority, if any, of combined treatments over single modality interventions. Nevertheless, some form of combined treatment is often the de facto standard of care, and the additive effects of psycho and pharmacotherapy is one supposition (not entirely without empirical support) which undergirds many of my arguments.

Psychopharmacological agents are not without risk, and such risks are shared by both patient and practitioner. Patients are exposed to potentially severe, even life threatening, side effects and drug interactions. Practitioners are exposed to greater malpractice liability than has customarily been the case for psychologists. Given this climate of increased risk, under what circumstances is it reasonable for psychologists to pursue prescriptive authority? I have argued elsewhere (DeLeon, Sammons, & Fox, 1995), that our collective decision to seek or reject any new technology in psychological practice should be based on the following principles: Enhancement of scope of practice and autonomy for the profession; expansion of range of services and access to care afforded patients; and expansion of the scientific knowledge base and establishment of firmer links between research and practice. Several conditions must be met in order to support the argument that the involvement of psychologists in the development, assessment, and clinical utilization of effective psychoactive compounds to combat mental illness is in keeping with each of these principles.

First, it must be demonstrated that psychopharmacology improves treatment outcome. I will spend much of this paper analyzing the evidence for this, and will demonstrate repeatedly that the degree to which drugs improve treatment outcome has been frequently overstated. Nonetheless, in the final analysis, most psychotropics do improve treatment outcome, at least incrementally, and often substantially. As such, they represent a valuable tool which should not be dismissed from the psychologists' armamentarium.

Second, it should be demonstrated that employing psychopharmacological interventions will serve the common good. Here, available evidence does suggest that a broader range of patients, suffering from a more inclusive spectrum of mental disorders, may be better served by psychologist prescribers. This is especially the case where such individuals now only receive unimodal therapy. Children with externalizing behavior disorders who visit pediatricians are increasingly liable to receive a trial of stimulant medication, generally without the benefit of a comprehensive psychosocial assessment, and almost always without targeted behavioral intervention. Individuals in institutional, inner city, or rural settings may currently have access to pharmacotherapy, but most commonly, psychotropic drugs are dispensed by non-psychiatric physicians or by harried psychiatrists. Such providers often lack the time, training, or inclination to provide comprehensive mental health services (i.e., psychosocial or behavioral treatment in addition to pharmacotherapy). Psychologists who possess the ability to provide both services, I will argue, can and will provide a more comprehensive spectrum of interventions, to the benefit of the public at large.

Finally, to further the development of the profession, direct involvement of psychologists in the provision of psychotropics should increase opportunities for research and further science based practice. I have already alluded to some of the deficits which plague current psychopharmacological research. I hold, as Breggin (1991) has previously asserted, that certain of these deficits exist not because of carelessly applied methodology, but instead are a natural byproduct of the biological culture which has shaped the growth of modern psychiatry. Psychologists bring a different culture and set of skills to psychopharmacological research. The skills which have defined the profession, notably a solid grounding in quantitative methods, research methodology, and techniques of outcome assessment, have already served psychologists well in their roles as basic psychopharmacological researchers. It is argued that these core skills, along with a relativistic and contextual approach to problem solving which is a hallmark of much of graduate psychological education, will produce a provider of pharmacotherapy whose orientation and practice fundamentally differs from current psychiatric practice. By becoming directly involved in the provision of psychotropics, psychologists can positively influence patterns of investigation and practice, to the benefit of patients and profession alike.

History of the Issue

Although the impetus towards prescriptive authority for psychologists has experienced something of a renaissance in the past decade, the concept of blending graduate psychology training with aspects of medicine, (including the prescription of psychoactive agents), has a long history in American mental health. One of the first proposals formally linking psychological training with medical education appeared in the mid-1950s. Lawrence Kubie, the noted psychoanalyst, suggested in a lengthy article in the Texas Reports on Biology and Medicine (Kubie, 1954) that the training of both psychologists and psychiatrists be radically altered by creating a new degree, based on a curriculum combining medicine, psychology, and allied social sciences. The degree was to be called the Doctorate in Medical Psychology. Two primary motivators spurred Kubie to suggest this exceptionally different approach to the integration of the two disciplines. First, he believed that psychologists were insufficiently trained in clinical practice, and lacked appropriate education to handle the medical aspects of their patients' illnesses. Second, he believed that the training of psychiatrists was too exclusively medical and did not give adequate emphasis to training in psychotherapeutic intervention. Kubie based his arguments for the establishment of this new profession on three observations: (a) that psychotherapy was an effective mechanism to combat mental illness; (b) that there existed a shortage of trained psychotherapists to provide such treatment; and (c) that it was impossible to modify adequately the medical school curriculum, with its increasing complexities and even at that time its increasingly biological focus, to train psychotherapists in a timely and efficient manner.

It must be noted that proficiency in psychodiagnostics and psychotherapy, not the ability to prescribe, was Kubie's primary goal. Nevertheless, he believed that Doctors of Medical Psychology should be independent practitioners with hospital admitting privileges. Given the paucity of effective psychopharmacologic agents at the time he conceived this scheme, it is not surprising that he did not address the issue of prescription privileges more fully. In later years, however, he advised against pursuing prescription privileges – not because he felt that psychologists could not be adequately trained, but because he feared this would engender too much opposition from organized medicine (Wanerman, 1992). Kubie's model served as the basis for a large scale program designed to produce practitioners skilled in psychology but versed in basic aspects of medicine, which was brought to life by another psychiatrist, Robert Wallerstein, as the Doctorate in Mental Health (DMH). This program, operating out of the University of California at San Francisco and Langley Porter Institute, was the first program implemented with the explicit goal of training non-physician prescribers of psychotropics.

The intent of the DMH was to produce a hybrid mental health practitioner whose training corrected the overly biological orientation of psychiatrists, while at the same time rectifying the deficiencies in applied medical sciences which prevented psychologists from providing a full range of services to mentally disordered individuals. In addition to lacking certain applied medical skills, the program's designers also believed that research oriented psychology doctoral programs overemphasized quantitative and statistical sciences at the expense of clinical training in psychotherapy (Wallerstein, 1992).

The didactic core of the DMH program was tripartite, consisting of instruction in biological, psychological and social sciences. The biological sequence was largely non-medical school based, but involved courses in anatomy, physiology, biochemistry, microbiology, pathology, pharmacology, neuroanatomy and neuropathology, and epidemiology. The courses were designed to be taken in a two year sequence, of four quarters per year, with an average of two medical courses per quarter in addition to work in other content areas. The following two to three years necessary to complete the program were devoted to clinical work. Prerequisites, aside from a 3.0 grade point average in an accredited baccalaureate program degree (no field of study was specified) were not clearly defined (Wallerstein, 1992).

The DMH produced over 80 graduates but succumbed, after a decade and a half, to political pressures, including an inability to obtain licensure for its graduates. Eventually, the majority of those who completed the degree sought licensure as psychologists, though a few obtained a medical license.

The only program designed specifically to produce doctoral level, psychologist prescribers is the Department of Defense Psychopharmacology Demonstration Project (PDP) which was initiated in 1991 at the Uniformed Services University of the Health Sciences in Bethesda, Maryland. This program has now produced 7 graduates; three more are in training at the time of this writing. The PDP involves over 750 contact hours in a variety of basic and applied medical sciences, including biochemistry, neuroanatomy, pathology and pathophysiology, clinical medicine, health assessment, and pharmacology and psychopharmacology. One year of supervised clinical work, in both inpatient and outpatient settings, is required (see Sammons & Brown, 1997, for a review of the program). The program is based on a fellowship model of training, and is offered only to licensed psychologists who have accumulated postdoctoral experience as clinicians. Its intent is to produce mental health providers who can make informed choices about which treatment (psychotherapy, pharmacotherapy, or both) is the preferred mode of intervention in any particular case, and then provide that treatment.

The PDP has been somewhat limited in scope, inasmuch as only military officers are eligible to enroll. Its curriculum, however, served as a model upon which recommendations for larger-scale training programs were based. In 1995, the Committee for the Advancement of Professional Practice of the APA published these recommendations (APA, 1995), which were adopted, with minor modification, by the APA Council of Representatives in 1996. In brief, these recommendations call for a minimum 300 contact hour didactic curriculum, with exposure to coursework in neurosciences, physiology and pathophysiology, health assessment, laboratory assessment, and pharmacology, psychopharmacology, and clinical psychopharmacology. A minimum of 100 supervised patients treated with psychotropics is the recommended clinical experience. At this point, the APA's recommendations have been have been adopted by at least one accredited school of psychology, which is now enrolling students in a postdoctoral curriculum.

Graduates of the PDP, as well as other non-psychiatric mental health practitioners who have the ability to prescribe (i.e., advanced nurse practitioners) are providing evidence to challenge the notion that exposure to a premedical curriculum, four years of medical school, and a psychiatric residency are mandatory for successful prescription of psychotropics. Nevertheless, a considerable debate continues to focus on the issue of whether or not a medical education is a necessary prerequisite. I will now attempt to summarize the key elements of this debate.

Is a Medical Education Necessary or Desirable in Order to Prescribe?

Although organized psychiatry has labelled the first prescribing psychologists as "public health menaces," a brief examination of history will illustrate that such sobriquets have not been exclusively reserved for those psychologists seeking prescriptive authority. When psychologists were first seeking to establish a foothold in the clinical arena, opposition from psychiatry was strong. Psychologists were deemed unable to diagnose appropriately or clinically manage patients (Adler, 1927). Interestingly, while strong opposition existed to the entrance of psychologists into clinical practice, some such as Adler believed that social workers, who worked far more closely with psychiatrists, would be satisfactory clinicians. Presumably, the subordinate role which social work played at the time vis-a-vis psychiatry may have led to this rather strange judgment.

William Russell, the president of the American Psychiatric Association in 1932, warned against the "mistaken belief" held by psychologists and other "lay workers" that psychiatric problems could be diagnosed and adequately treated without the aid of psychiatrists. He urged the American Psychiatric Association to condemn such practices as "unscientific and dangerous." Additionally, he attempted to dispel the notion that psychiatry and psychology shared common roots. Psychiatry, he argued, is rooted in medicine, whereas psychology grew out of philosophy and metaphysics and thus psychologists lacked the requisite background to be clinicians. (Russell, 1932, cited in Valenstein, 1986).

Those familiar with the debate surrounding prescription privileges will find remarkable parallels between the arguments raised by psychiatrists opposing psychologists as clinicians and those raised by psychiatrists opposing psychologists as prescribers. Pies (1991), for example, argued that the "deep structures" of the two disciplines were sufficiently disparate to preclude psychology from acquiring the ability to prescribe. Pies opined that since psychology is rooted in *logos*, and since psychiatry is rooted in *iatros*, psychologists were, in effect, so hobbled by history that it was impractical for the discipline to seek prescriptive ability. This article was widely cited by psychiatrists (and not a few psychologists) who disagreed with the idea of prescription privileges, in spite of the 100 year record of psychologists as clinical providers of behavioral cures for mental distress. Although Pies admitted that some degree of training in biological sciences was offered in graduate schools, he asserted that the overall paucity of this type of training made it impossible for psychologists to prescribe. To support this argument, he presented the case of an individual with cirrhosis, sleep apnea, and a peptic ulcer and asked if the training of psychologists prepared them to manage such a case. Though the self evident answer to this question is of course negative, three strands of fallacious logic are apparent in Pies' reasoning. It is important to dissect these fallacies, because they are repeatedly used by individuals opposed to prescriptive authority.

The first is that a medical education is required to prescribe safely, and that a psychiatric residency is needed to prescribe psychiatric drugs safely (see also Klein, 1996, for a more recent resurrection of this argument). This we know to be false via the experience of advanced nurse practitioners, dentists, podiatrists, and other non-medical personnel who prescribe systemic drugs (and not a few of these are psychoactive) safely and effectively. We also know that over 80% of all psychiatric drugs are prescribed by non-psychiatrists (Zimmerman & Wienckowski, 1991), and that the issue in the use of these agents is, in almost all cases, one of efficacy rather than safety. Further, examples from the history of psychiatry demonstrate that such stringent criteria were not always employed to produce prescribers of psychotropics. The services of psychiatrists were in such acutely short supply that 80% of all psychiatrists practicing in World War II were physicians who had been given a three month crash course in psychiatry. Far from being dismissed as ill-trained stand-ins after the war, these so-called "90 day wonders" were instrumental in creating many departments of psychiatry after the war (Sierles & Taylor, 1995). One issue which has received little empirical attention is the ability of nonmedical psychotherapists to detect physical conditions masquerading as mental disorders. Though physicians might presume that a medical education is necessary to do so, Sanchez and Kohn (1991) found no difference between medically trained psychotherapists, nonmedically trained psychotherapists, and general physicians in their ability to do this.

The second fallacy in Pies' argument is that the acknowledged shortcomings in biological training in psychology graduate education will not be rectified by fellowship training in psychopharmacology. This is, of course, incorrect. The graduates of the Psychopharmacology Demonstration Project (PDP) at the Uniformed Services

University of the Health Sciences spend an intensive year of coursework in basic and applied biological sciences (see Sammons and Brown, 1997, for a review of this curriculum). The graduates of the Doctorate in Mental Health program were also exposed to an intensive, two year sequence of basic and applied biological sciences (Wallerstein, 1991). Recommendations of the Committee for Advancement of Professional Practice's Task Force on Psychopharmacology (APA, 1995) also called for extensive prerequisite and concurrent training in biological sciences. Although it is too early to determine if such attention to basic biological sciences will continue when prescription training programs become more widespread, early indications suggest this will be the case. A postdoctoral program in clinical psychopharmacology, being offered in 1996 by the Illinois School of Professional Psychology, incorporates 324 hours of classroom contact hours in biochemistry, neuroanatomy, psychopharmacology and pharmacology, pathophysiology, physical assessment, and applied clinical psychopharmacology as well as 750 contact hours of clinical training (Illinois School of Professional Psychology, 1996).

The third fallacy inherent in Pies' argument is that psychologists will be unable to perform the "medical" aspects of prescribing – therapeutic drug monitoring, detection and management of side effects, and recognition of physical conditions which would contraindicate or complicate the use of psychotropic agents. The faulty assumptions underlying this argument are several. First, detection and management of side effects of medication has been, and will continue to be, a central component of psychologists' training in prescribing. All effects of medication are, after all, "side" effects, it is up to the prescriber to detect those which are beneficial (i.e., therapeutic) and those which are detrimental, and maximize the ratio between the two. To illustrate, the recognition of the development of extrapyramidal symptoms in a patient prescribed antipsychotic medication does not require a medical education. Nurses and psychiatric technicians, with appropriate training, routinely recognize and report such symptoms to physicians. Reports of such symptoms, or those dry mouth, blurred vision, or orthostatic hypotension in a patient prescribed a tricyclic antidepressant similarly do not require a physician's interpretation. These adverse side effects can be efficiently detected and managed by those with other than a medical degree, such as prescribing psychologists.

As to the issue of physical examinations, Pies (1991) and others have argued that proficiency in administration of a physical examination is a requisite skill in prescribing. The administration of a complete physical examination, including genital and rectal examinations, is not, however, indicated in the treatment of most outpatients with mental disorders (physical exams are generally required of all patients admitted to hospitals, regardless of the service to which they are admitted). Indeed, Pies found, via an informal survey, that only one of five outpatient psychiatrists surveyed had taken basic vital signs on a patient in the two months prior to his survey! Prescribing psychologists can easily and quickly be trained to take and interpret vital signs, observe for adverse side effects of drugs, and interpret laboratory tests evaluating basic parameters and drug levels. It is neither likely nor desirable that prescribing psychologists will wish to be credentialed in the performance of physical examinations. As we have seen, such examinations are not common in psychiatry (at least past the inpatient residency year), and the requisite skills to perform them atrophy quickly with disuse. The performance of the physical examination is best thought of as a collaborative task, in which the prescribing psychologist relies on the skills of his or her colleagues in general practice or internal medicine. This does not differ from the current practice of psychologists with admitting privileges to hospitals, who rely on their medical colleagues to perform this function.

A further erroneous assumption is that the practice of a psychiatrist and a prescribing psychologist would differ in regards to the management of a patient with concomitant medical illness. Pies admitted that managing the case of multiple organ system failure (i.e., cirrhosis, apnea, and peptic ulcer, as presented above) would "give pause" to even an experienced psychopharmacologist. Indeed it should, and most reasonable psychiatrists would unquestionably consult with their medical confreres on joint management of this patient's needs. So too will prescribing psychologists. Psychiatrists do not manage peptic ulcers, nor will psychologists. Ethical practitioners in both fields will make appropriate consultation when necessary to address all aspects of the patient's needs.

A final fallacy contained in Pies' argument is somewhat more difficult to articulate, but a reasonable approximation would take the following form: Psychopharmacology is an exact science which only exactly trained scientists (psychiatrists) can perform. Pies agreed that other non-physician providers have successfully learned to prescribe, but stated that "it remains to be proved that prescription by any of these disciplines constitutes optimal care" (Pies, 1991, p. 6). I would propose the obverse – that it remains to be proved if psychiatrists provide the optimum care for mental disorders. If we accept the argument proposed by Antonuccio and his colleagues (1995), that nonpharmacological measures are more effective interventions for depression than drug treatments, it can be argued that psychiatrists, who may commonly ignore effective nonpharmacological interventions, risk providing suboptimal care. Additionally, the completion of a residency in psychiatry does not guarantee that the provider will engage in appropriate prescribing practices. Wells and Sturm (1996), in an analysis of cost effectiveness in the provision of mental health services, found that psychiatrists prescribed more minor tranquilizers to patients with depression than did general practitioners. They correctly observed that minor tranquilizers have no demonstrated role in the treatment of major depression, but significantly add to the cost of care. The numerous attempts to develop treatment algorithms that would lead to lesser degrees of variability in provision of psychopharmacology (e.g., Jobson & Potter, 1995) also suggest that many current psychiatric practices are suboptimal. Finally, Platman, Dorgan, and Gerhardt (1976) provided data indicating that the practices of non-physician providers does not deviate from accepted standards of care. Platman, Dorgan, & Gerhardt (1976), conducted an 18 month pilot study in which 33 nurses, social workers, and pyschologists were trained to prescribe psychotropic medications. These 33 clinicians provided a comprehensive range of services to 667 outpatients, including counselling, group treatment, rehabilitation and medication services. Clinicians assumed full responsibility for all aspects of patient care and, although each prescription was countersigned, initiated, maintained and terminated pharmacotherapy for all patients (Over 75% of patients in the study received psychoactive medications). Instruction in psychopharmacology was informal, and consisted of a weekly medication seminar and an orientation course. The authors noted that the program was successful in providing services at non-central clinics and satellites, and that non-physician providers prescribed safely and in a manner consistent with clinical practices of the day.

It seems, then, that the "standards of care" argument is at best an open question, and that psychologists, who are likely to provide behavioral interventions in addition to, or in place of, pharmacological treatments, may actually provide a more positive outcome in a more cost-effective fashion than their physician counterparts. Thus, the argument that psychologists are less able providers of pharmacology on the basis of discipline seems ill-founded in logic, but it is clearly understandable from the point of view of interdisciplinary rivalry. Sixty four years ago, when Dr. Russell rendered his opinion on the suitability of psychologists as general clinicians, no successful somatic treatment for mental distress existed. Thus, psychiatrists of that era attempted to enjoin psychologists from providing the only effective clinical intervention available, which was psychotherapy. Today, when at least partially successful somatic treatments (drugs) exist, psychology is enjoined from providing these treatments, ostensibly due to a collective inability to be trained, but in reality because of guild and economic factors which have led to a monopoly on successful somatic interventions by the medical community. This monopoly is not the exclusive privilege of psychiatry, although psychiatrists have clearly benefitted from it, nor did it evolve from any training particular to physicians. Instead, it grew from a long and successful lobbying effort on the part of the American medical establishment. Because psychology will need to engage in similar political efforts in order to obtain prescriptive authority, the history of the medical monopoly will be briefly sketched.

The Establishment of the Prescriptive Monopoly by Physicians

In modern American health care delivery, the prescription of drugs has been viewed as more or less the exclusive purview of the physician. Although certain other non-physician specialties, such as dentistry, have always had some limited ability to prescribe certain agents, formularies have been limited and prescriptive authority constrained. Scope of practice laws limit the prescriptive authority of such professionals to only those agents commonly used in the treatment of the disorders which they are licensed to treat. Dentists, for example, may prescribe a systemic antibiotic as prophylaxis when certain dental procedures such as extractions are employed; they may not prescribe the identical agent to treat a non-dental abscess or other infection. Likewise, dentists may employ narcotics and other controlled substances for sedation and analgesia for dental procedures, but not for the treatment of other painful conditions or anxiety. No other specialty, with the exception of osteopathy, has acquired the carte blanche for the prescription of any agent, for any condition, which comes with conferral of the medical degree.

It is commonly assumed that non-physician health care professionals have acquired prescriptive ability only recently, and that exclusive prescriptive ability has always been the province of the physician, but a closer examination of the history of allopathy reveals a significantly different picture. Prior to the turn of the 20th century, Americans could procure any drug available simply by visiting a pharmacist. No physicians' order was necessary. According to Harkless (1989), three factors were central in shifting prescriptive authority towards the hands of physicians. First, the quackery of patent medicine vendors, and dangers associated with the use of their products, led journalists and politicians to push for greater regulation of snake-oil remedies. Second, the growing size, political influence, and legal recognition through licensing laws for physicians of the American Medical Association allowed that organization to successfully campaign for greater control over ingredients of and advertising for patent medicines. Third, the manufacturers of drugs, recognizing that physicians were increasingly regarded as experts in the use of medications, began to rely more heavily on doctors to promote their products. Harkless (1989) further noted that moves to place prescriptive authority exclusively in the hands of physicians was expedited by passage of the Pure Food Act of 1906. This act, and subsequent major pieces of regulatory legislation, such as the Federal Food, Drug, and Cosmetic Act of 1938, "embedded the prescription of medications more firmly into the existing medical hierarchy and increased consumer dependence on the physician" (Harkless, 1989, p. 58). Harkless concluded that the dominance of physicians as prescribers was not, therefore, a result of any particular competence exclusive to physicians, but rather a combination of legislative, political and social events which placed decision making power regarding drugs in the hands of the medical profession.

Incremental assaults on physicians' prescriptive monopoly have been waged over the past several decades, and with some success. In part, efforts by organized psychology to gain prescriptive authority have been driven by the successes of other, non physician health care providers in acquiring prescription privileges. Optometrists and nurse practitioners are examples of two such professions. Optometrists have acquired prescriptive ability for diagnostic purposes in 50 states and for therapeutic purposes in over 40. Advanced nurse practitioners now have completely independent prescriptive authority in 11 states (Pearson, 1995), and have more limited authority involving varying, but often minimal degrees of physician oversight in the majority of states (Birkholz & Walker, 1994).

Psychologists have at the time of this writing introduced legislation in California, Missouri, and Montana which would allow for some form of independent prescriptive authority. The California legislation was withdrawn in early 1996 after it became apparent that insufficient votes were present to move it out of legislative committee. The Montana legislation was defeated in committee, after it became apparent that the Montana State Psychological Association, which had not been approached to support this legislation, had significant reservations about the legislative strategy involved. The Missouri legislation is still active. In Indiana, in 1994, the psychology licensing legislation was changed to grant prescriptive authority to psychologists participating in federal demonstration projects. These legislative initiatives have been founded to some degree on the rationale that psychologists may provide a more comprehensive range of services to currently underserved populations. It is extremely unwise to assert that psychologists will prescribe any more effectively than members of other professions, but an examination of current prescribing practices vis-a-vis these special populations may point to areas in which prescribing psychologists can reasonably be expected to use their unique skills to improve service delivery.

Psychopharmacological Practice and Special Populations

The Institutionalized Elderly

Psychologists trained to prescribe can positively alter the treatment regimens of individuals in settings where current psychopharmacological practice has been documented to be suboptimal. Frequently, they will do so not by adding drugs to a treatment regimen, but by using the ability conveyed by prescriptive authority to delete drugs and substitute more appropriate treatments. Consider the example of psychoactive drug use in the institutionalized elderly. Psychoactive agents are commonly inappropriately prescribed for elderly individuals (Willcox, Himmelstein & Woolhandler, 1994), often in excessive doses (Beers et al., 1991) and with poor monitoring (Avorn, Dreyer, Connelly & Soumerai, 1989). Monane, Glynn, and Avorn (1996) found high rates of prescribing of sedative hypnotic compounds to elderly individuals (largely female) residing in nursing homes or similar institutions, as many as 36% of inhabitants were prescribed such compounds. Of those prescribed such agents, 79% demonstrated impaired performance on bedside mental status examinations. Beers, Fingold, Ouslander, Reuben, Morgenstern, and Beck (1993), surveyed the prescribing practices of 306 physicians practicing in 12 Los Angeles area nursing homes. They found not only high rates of prescribing (an average of 7.2 drugs per patient) but also that 40% of the patients being prescribed for received at least one inappropriate prescription. Of interest is their finding that those physicians most likely to write inappropriate prescriptions were least likely to consult with a mental heath specialist (in this case, psychiatrists).

Ray et al. (1993) developed an educational program for physicians to address the problem of high rates of inappropriate use of antipsychotics in nursing homes. They reported that antipsychotics agents are among the most commonly used drugs in nursing homes, and cited estimates suggesting that 20-50% of nursing home residents are prescribed such agents, generally for sedation and behavioral control. In the homes included in their study, approximately 32% of all residents were taking antipsychotic agents when the study began. In those homes where physicians had been instructed in a program of behavioral management techniques, antipsychotic use declined by 72% as compared to 13% in nursing homes where physicians had received no such training. Use of physical restraint in nursing homes also declined as a result of behavioral training, but to a lesser extent.

Avorn and Gurwitz (1995) noted that sedative hypnotics and antipsychotics were among the most commonly employed drugs in nursing home settings (29 and 28 prescriptions per 100 residents, respectively). They observed that use of such agents is apparently greater in the U.S. than in other countries, and that, despite the high rates of use of these agents, alternative approaches (e.g., behavioral management strategies and other psychosocial interventions) have been poorly studied. This is particularly regrettable inasmuch as these are skills which psychologists traditionally have been trained to employ. Psychologists who consult in institutional settings already provide these skills, prescribing psychologists could use behavioral strategies to substitute for or reduce exposure to potentially dangerous drugs. In other words, psychologists may be able to prescribe behavioral treatments and unprescribe pharmacological ones, but only if they are granted prescriptive authority.

Pharmacotherapy in Children and Adolescents

The issue of psychopharmacology in children poses important neurobiological, ethical and emotional concerns. Risk-benefit analyses of the use of psychiatric drugs in this population must take into account the fact that the long term effects of psychoactive medications on developing neural tissues are largely unknown. This is especially significant when the use of medication with demonstrated severe, persistent side effects (i.e., tardive dyskinesia) is considered in a pediatric patient. Ethical issues abound: Are there long term risks involved in having a child rely on a pill rather than self-regulatory processes for behavioral management? Do we predispose children towards reliance on pharmacological agents in place of self-regulatory skills? Since these dilemmas are real, greater circumspection when using drugs in children is warranted.

Unfortunately for clinicians seeking to make informed decisions, the literature supporting the use of pharmacological agents in children and adolescents is, with the possible exception of attention deficit/hyperactivity disorder, inconsistent. Adequate understanding of the efficacy of psychotropics in the treatment of mental disorders in children and adolescents is compounded by the fact that surprisingly few methodologically sound (i.e., double-blinded, placebo controlled investigations with sufficient sample sizes), have been performed. In a comprehensive review, Gadow (1992), summarized the available studies of medication for a number of childhood disorders, with decidedly mixed results. In the instance of childhood and adolescent depression, he reported that no double blinded studies of tricyclic antidepressants (TCAs) in prepubertal children or adolescents had revealed them to be superior to placebo. He cited several studies of particular interest (Geller et al., 1989, 1990, cited in Gadow, 1992), which demonstrated that even when placebo responders were removed from drug trials, the efficacy of TCAs could not be established.

The extreme paucity of well constructed investigations of pharmacological interventions in children complicates the clinical decision making process. Sommers-Flanagan and Sommers-Flanagan (1996) reviewed the literature on use of TCAs in childhood and adolescent depression. They found only five double blind, placebo controlled studies in their review, all reported between 1987 and 1994. In no study was a TCA more effective than placebo. Sommers-Flanagan and Sommers-Flanagan found only one well controlled study of fluoxetine in children and adolescents; in that study, no statistically significant differences between improvement rates on fluoxetine (20-60 mg/day) and placebo were found. The authors estimated specific drug effects for TCAs to be from 8-45%. Placebo efficacy was estimated at 17-68% in the studies reviewed. As a result of the poor performance of psychopharmacologic agents in the studies reviewed, Sommers-Flanagan and Sommers-Flanagan suggested the following criteria be met prior to considering pharmacotherapy for depressed youth: Depression in the absence of environmental determinants, severe depressive symptoms with strong physiological components, no response to 10-15 sessions of psychotherapy, and a clear patient preference for medication.

Rural Populations

Nonavailability of mental health resources may be particularly acute in rural areas, where patient demographics interact with shortages of providers to create special needs. Rural residents tend to be more often unemployed, and are more likely not to have health insurance. They are more likely to be sicker when seeking help, and tend to receive less intensive services which may vary considerably in quality (Shelton & Frank, 1995). Yet the number of psychiatrists employed in rural settings is diminishing, and as much as half of rural mental health care may be provided by general physicians (Shelton & Frank, 1995). Such individuals are quite unlikely to have received adequate training in mental health service provision. A survey of graduate medical education indicated that only five percent of didactic instruction in medical school includes instruction in behavioral sciences of any kind. The third year clerkship in psychiatry, (not mandatory for all students), is the briefest of clerkships of those offered in the third year (Zimmerman & Wienckowski, 1991). Shortages of trained mental health providers are compounded by geographic difficulties in accessing services, allied health care providers may also be in short supply. Inadequate numbers of providers, combined with a populations at disproportionate risk for the development of mental disorders (Wagenfeld, Murray, Mohatt, & DeBruyn, 1994), provides a clear argument for the training of providers who can offer a comprehensive range of mental health services to populations in need.

Treatment of Depression:
Issues in Unimodal and Multimodal Interventions

Pharmacotherapy for Depressive Spectrum Disorders

The efficacy of antidepressants is at this point beyond question, at least in the treatment of major depressive disorder, the condition for which they have been most frequently studied. That said, a number of caveats must be attached. First, the *magnitude* of the effect of antidepressant agents has been questioned (Greenberg & Fisher, 1989). Second, the *comparative efficacy* of antidepressants vis-a-vis other, non-somatic treatments for depression has also been an issue of considerable debate and investigation. The National Institutes of Mental Health Treatment of Depression Collaborative Research Project (Elkin, et al., 1989 and subsequently), is perhaps the best known attempt to reify the potency of these various interventions. Third, the *combined efficacy* of psychological and pharmacological therapies, perhaps the least studied of any of these issues, remains enigmatic, especially for the newer antidepressants (serotonin reuptake inhibitors and others).

The magnitude of response to antidepressant drugs is a subject of intense current debate. Although many studies of antidepressant agents report drug responses on the order of 60-70%, the number of subjects who demonstrate a true drug specific response is considerably lower when placebo responses are factored in. Janicak, David, Preskorn, and Ayd (1993) conducted a meta-analysis of a number of studies involving 2,216 subjects who were treated with either SRIs (fluoxetine, sertraline, paroxetine, or fluvoxamine) or placebo. While 60 to 79% of subjects responded to one of the four drugs, 33 to 48% in all studies also demonstrated a positive response to placebo, yielding drug specific response rates of 25 to 31%. Preskorn (1996), in a comment on these data, noted that while a response rate of this magnitude (25-31%) is not insignificant, it should give pause to those who expect a drug response from two-thirds or more of their depressed patients. Figures such as those cited by Janicak, Davis, Preskorn, & Ayd (1993) are similar to those reported by Greenberg & Fisher (1989) who undertook an exhaustive review of pharmacotherapy outcome studies for depression. They found drug specific effects to be small (an average of 21%), even under good experimental conditions. When the small number of well-designed studies in the literature examining the effects of active placebos were analyzed, evidence for active drug effects diminished even further.

Further evidence that many supposed drug specific effects may actually represent non-specific effects of pharmacotherapy was provided by Greenberg, Bornstein, Greenberg, and Fisher (1992), who conducted a meta-analysis of 22 studies of drug treatment for depression. Their analysis differed from prior efforts in that they specifically examined patient self-report measures, which they believed to be more accurate representations of outcome than clinician observations. Additionally, they selected studies which compared newer antidepressants (trazodone, maprotiline, and amoxapine) to older drugs (the TCAs), and placebo. The effect sizes they reported were quite small, (0.19 for standard antidepressants and 0.25 for newer antidepressants), effect sizes based on clinician's ratings differed significantly from placebo effect sizes, but those based on patient ratings did not. From a methodological point of view, this study is of interest, in that it underscores the importance of assessing patient ratings of improvement. Additionally, it suggests that the Hamilton Rating Scale for Depression may not be the most appropriate outcome measure for clinicians. As has been pointed out elsewhere, Hamilton did not intend for his rating scale to be a research instrument, and many items on the Hamilton have been found to load heavily on factors more specific for anxiety than depression. From a clinical perspective, however, the Greenberg study is compromised by the type of drug examined. None of the "new" antidepressants are actually new. None of the drugs studied were SRIs, and all are associated with significant clinical side effects, many of which may be even more problematic than those associated with the TCAs. The use of amoxapine has always been restricted by its potential association with tardive dyskinesia (it is a phenothiazine derivative). The clinical experience with trazodone, a very sedating antidepressant, has been disappointing, and it is rarely used as a sole treatment for depression. Most clinicians now consider it to be an adjunctive agent, and prescribe it to manage the sleep disruption not infrequently encountered with the use of fluoxetine or sertraline. The authors' findings would have carried greater weight had they used studies of the SRIs in their meta-analysis; their failure to do so is curious inasmuch as such studies were extant at the time they carried out their review.

Indeed, when Greenberg and his colleagues did complete a meta-analysis of fluoxetine outcome (Greenberg, Bornstein, Zborowski, Fisher, & Greenberg, 1994), the combined effect size for fluoxetine treatment (again using both patient and clinician ratings) was substantially higher: 0.40. This effect size was significantly greater than placebo for both groups, and increased to 0.54 when only data on study completers were analyzed. Why this large difference between effect sizes for fluoxetine and older antidepressants should exist is a puzzle, because most studies comparing efficacy of the SRIs and TCAs find no significant differences between the two classes. Also, Greenberg and his colleagues believe that patients often confuse the side effects of drugs with their active effects, and would, presumably, be more inclined to rate those drugs having greater side effects as more effective. But such is not the case with the SRIs. Although by no means devoid of side effects, they are far more benign than the TCAs, and the majority of patients report no adverse side effects with their use. Hence, if the side effects = efficacy hypothesis is correct, the SRIs would be expected to be rated as *less* effective than the TCAs – not twice as effective, as Greenberg and his colleagues reported.

Psychotherapy for Depression

Just as various psychopharmacological therapies for depression tend to have equipotent efficacy, so do the various forms of psychotherapy studied for the condition. Frank, Karp, and Rush (1993) found no true differences in outcome of studies involving cognitive, behavior, and interpersonal psychotherapy; meta-analyses find the response rate to cognitive therapy to range from 46.9% to 58.3% (Depression Guideline Panel, 1993). Overall efficacy of behavior therapy in nine studies was found to be 55.5%. Interpersonal therapy, though less well studied, also appeared to be more effective than cognitive therapy or placebo plus clinical management. Interestingly, all of these forms of therapy have been more advantageous than medication alone, to varying degrees (15.3% for cognitive therapy, 23.9% for behavior therapy, and 12.3% for interpersonal therapy). Similarly, Clarkin, Pilkonis, and Magruder (1996) examined The Depression Guideline Panel's meta-analysis of 22 psychotherapy studies of depression. Cognitive therapy was slightly more effective than medication alone, as was behavior therapy. Interpersonal therapy was found to be as effective as medication alone. Brief dynamic therapy appeared to be less effective than other psychotherapies, but somewhat more than medication alone. They also reviewed several maintenance studies; these studies, while quite limited in number and possessing meth. dological limitations, indicated that cognitive therapy was more effective at maintaining treatment gains than pharmacotherapy: relapse rates for drugs treatment without psychotherapy exceeded 60%, cognitive therapy relapse rates approximated 30%. Other meta-analyses of the efficacy of psychotherapy also suggest that the percentage of patients improved as a result of treatment is equivalent to that in drug studies, if placebo plus active medication effects in the latter studies are combined. That is, around two thirds of treated patients show improvement (see Whiston & Sexton, 1993, for a concise review). This is encouraging news for psychotherapists, especially because verbal interventions are free of the toxicity and medical side effects often associated with psychoactive medications. But the clinician who chooses to view this finding as a blanket endorsement of psychotherapy over medication treatment treads on thin empirical ice. Several cautions must be observed. First, few active components of treatment beyond a supportive therapeutic relationship have been positively identified, even for the best studied and most effective treatments such as CBT (viz. Jacobson & Hollon, 1996; Elkin et al., 1989). A nonspecific effect, similar to the placebo effect in medication studies, may be responsible for the majority of positive change experienced. Second, client variables, such as expectation, may play a dominant role in determining outcome of psychotherapy. Third, the extremely high dropout rate common in most psychotherapy research studies suggests that a number of clients would be underserved if we relied on psychotherapy alone.

Thus, while psychotherapy in randomized clinical trials has been reported by some to be somewhat more effective overall than medication, a problematic issue facing those advocating the sole use of psychotherapy as an effective treatment for depression is the ongoing inability to identify active components of any form of psychotherapy, or to find clear advantages for one form of psychotherapy over another. This the well-known "dodo bird" hypothesis, which posits that all forms of psychotherapy do equally as well; this hypothesis has recently been supported in Seligman's innovative consumer study of therapy (Seligman, 1995a,b). The difficulties posed by the dodo-bird hypothesis are concisely set forth by Jacobson et al. (1996), who conducted a component analysis of cognitive behavioral treatment for depression, using 152 patients with DSM-3-R diagnoses of major depression. Adherence to treatment protocols was closely monitored and therapists, all of whom were skilled in the treatment provided, were judged to have maintained the integrity of each treatment. Treatments consisted of behavioral activation, activation and modification of dysfunctional thoughts, or full cognitive treatment. The authors found no differences between cognitive treatment and either partial treatment, both at posttreatment and six month followup. In the total sample (including dropouts), 39.3% of all subjects showed no response, 60.7% were considered to have responded, and 46.4% were recovered; these numbers did not differ significantly among treatment groups. Six month relapse rates for those rated as either fully recovered or recovered did not differ significantly. In the fully recovered group, relapse rates averaged 13.9% across all therapy conditions.

Do Combined Treatments Improve Outcome?

Although some aver that no greater benefit accrues when psychotherapy and pharmacotherapy are combined to treat depression (i.e., the effects are not additive), this practice is commonplace in clinical settings. Indeed, for all but the most biologically oriented psychiatrists, combined treatments may be considered the norm, in that some form of patient education or supportive treatment is almost always offered patients. Combined treatments are also common amongst psychologists: A recent survey of Washington state psychologists indicated that a significant majority (79%) were at the time of the survey consulting with a psychiatrist regarding medications for their patients (Chiles, Carlin, Benjamine, & Beitman, 1991). Yet the data from well designed studies evaluating this strategy are scant, and there are no science based predictors to guide the clinician in deciding when both strategies should be used (Frank, Karp, & Rush, 1993).

Combined treatment outcome studies are rare, and, at least in the case of the antidepressants, are almost exclusively conducted using agents no longer considered first line treatments for depression (i.e., the TCAs). Some authors nonetheless continue to argue that we may reliably draw the conclusion that the effects of psychological and drug treatments are not additive. To accept this verdict uncritically is a dangerous step. The purity of either intervention is difficult to control for, even in well designed research trials. Also, such trials (upon which the above conclusions are largely drawn) can almost exclusively be said to be tests of the efficacy of combined treatments, rather than the more important question of the *effectiveness* of combined treatments. An interesting paradox, and one which bears further investigation outside the relatively pristine environments of randomized clinical trials, is presented in Seligman's consumer study. While he found that 40% of the individuals in his survey took psychoactive drugs, and that 60% of these individuals reported that the drugs helped "a lot," those who received only psychotherapy improved as much as those receiving psychotherapy plus drugs (Seligman, 1995a, 1995b). Four ancillary findings from Seligman's study bear mention: drugs were more commonly used by family doctors than psychiatrists; only three percent of mental health therapists used drugs as a sole modality; adverse side effects had not been discussed with patients in a significant minority of cases; and use of minor tranquilizers persisted for long periods of time in many patients, despite the lack of scientific support for this practice.

The benefit of combined treatments may be more clear in disorders other than depression. The management of insomnia provides a succinct illustration of a disorder in which psychologists, using primarily behavioral interventions, but having the ability to provide adjunctive pharmacotherapy, can maximize patient care and clinical outcome. Although benzodiazepines are among the most prescribed medications of any class, and are perhaps most frequently prescribed for sleep disorders (among psychotropic agents, only the SRIs are more commonly prescribed), they have no role in the long term treatment of insomnia. Patients habituate to the prohypnotic effects of benzodiazepines. Their efficacy in the treatment of insomnia for longer than 3 months has not been demonstrated; indeed, studies of only two to three weeks in duration have found no difference between benzodiazepine and placebo (Janicak, Davis, Preskorn, & Ayd, 1993). Benzodiazepine use carries the risk of physiological dependence as well as potentially severe discontinuation phenomena (recurrence of the initial disorder or rebound of symptoms; Shader and Greenblatt, 1993). Nevertheless, they are the mainstay of current treatment for insomnia, and continue to be widely used as sole agents for this disorder. Their true benefit, however, may be in their use as short term adjuncts to well conceptualized cognitive or behavioral interventions for insomnia. Morin (1993), for example, noted that benzodiazepines may be of use in short term insomnia due to situational stress, jet lag, and insomnia due to underlying conditions such as involuntary muscle movements or pain. He also noted that even in cases of psychologically mediated insomnia, short term benzodiazepines may be of utility in breaking cycles of sleeplessness and may assist in post-treatment maintenance.

Other examples demonstrating the efficacy of pharmacotherapy as an adjuvant to behavioral regimens are plentiful. Although nicotine polacrilex is no longer a prescription drug, patients who incorporate its use into behavioral cessation strategies may have greater success at quitting smoking. Some research indicates that the most effective regimen in preventing relapse in smoking cessation is a combination of behavioral intervention and nicotine polacrilex. (Fortmann & Killen, 1995). Cinciripini, et al. (1996) found that a combination of behavioral treatment and nicotine patch resulted in lower levels of general distress and higher levels of abstinence at one year followup.

Decision Making in Pharmacotherapy: Towards Science Based Practice in Treating Depression

As I have already stated, the central thesis of those in favor of enabling psychologists to prescribe is that they will use drugs more rationally: That is, pharmacotherapy will be employed as an adjunctive therapy, and psychotherapy will remain the first-line treatment of choice for most conditions. But how will clinicians decide when to use drugs, and at what point in the treatment process will this decision be made? Few data exist to aid the conscientious clinician, those which do exist must be interpreted with great caution due to obvious allegiance biases of the writers. Published treatment algorithms are of little utility. Those which do exist (Janicak, Davis, Preskorn, & Ayd, 1993; Nelson, et al., 1995; Zarate et al, 1995), deal almost exclusively with choices among drugs, with psychotherapy entering late in the decision making process, if at all. Further, the issue has not been studied outside the sterile purview of randomized clinical trials which use stringent diagnostic criteria and generally exclude participants with more than one diagnosis, thereby producing results which may generalize poorly to most clinical settings. Yet a further complication is introduced when allegiance effects in clinical research are examined. Jacobson and Hollon (1996a, 1996b) use as an example the ongoing controversy surrounding the findings of the Treatment of Depression Collaborative Research Project (TDCRP; Elkin, et al., 1989) to limn the difficulties encountered by those seeking to account for allegiance effects and other sources of bias in data interpretation. Although initial findings from this study did not suggest significant differences among psychopharmacological and non drug treatments for depression in mildly to moderately depressed patients, clear differences in favor of drug treatment (imipramine) emerged in the more severely depressed patient subset. But as Jacobson and Hollon observed, CBT in the Collaborative Research Project fared less well than in other studies, leading them to speculate as to whether it had been adequately implemented at all treatment sites. (Parenthetically, Jacobson and Hollon pointed out that there was no difference among any treatment at 18 month followup: Recovery rates ranged from 19% for clinical management plus imipramine to 30% for CBT, a less than splendid showing for all studied treatments). An issue closely related to allegiance (loyalty of therapists to specific treatments) is that of alliance (bonds between patients and therapists). Alliance studies are not new in psychotherapy research, but Krupnick et al., (1996) were able to use TDCRP data to illustrate that alliance is a potent factor in psychopharmacology as well. By employing a standardized scale to measure therapeutic alliance, they discovered that a greater portion of the outcome variance in the TDCRP study was attributable to therapeutic alliance than to treatment method. Of great interest was their observation that therapeutic alliance was a significant outcome factor in both imipramine and placebo conditions. Krupnick et al. speculated that such alliance factors may represent much of the nonspecific effects of drug treatment, and thus may have profound implications for the practice of psychopharmacology. It is quite apparent that allegiance and alliance effects are potent, usually uncontrolled variables in even well designed studies. Their importance is difficult to underestimate, as Jacobson and Hollon (1996a) cautioned:

> We think that proponents of both drugs and psychotherapy have gone beyond the data in drawing inferences about the efficacy (and effectiveness) of their respective interventions, thus transforming the pursuit of knowledge into a debate in which research findings are used selectively and interpreted inappropriately. At one extreme, there are advocates for pharmacotherapy who attempt to invalidate evidence in support of psychosocial treatment and, in doing so, often distort or ignore findings that are inconsistent with their claims. At the other extreme, there are advocates for the psychotherapies who are guilty of a rush to judgment about the worth of the psychosocial interventions. (p. 74)

When such methodological pitfalls abound, how does the clinician proceed in attempting to decide which, or which combinations of treatments to apply? Though many have used the severity of depressive symptoms as a tentative guide, with more severely affected patients receiving drugs, the type rather than the severity of symptoms may be a more sensitive index to differential responding. Patients with significant neurovegetative signs may respond preferentially to drugs, while those with severe cognitive dysfunction may respond more positively to medication (Clarkin, Pilkonis, & Magruder, 1996).

Frank, Karp, and Rush (1993) proposed that psychotherapy alone be considered when it is clearly the patient's preference, when medical contraindications to the use of drugs exist, and when patients present with significant psychosocial difficulties or with personality disorders. In an important exception, Frank and her colleagues specifically cautioned against the use of psychotherapy alone in depression with psychotic or melancholic features.

Preskorn (1996) suggested the following practice implications of the substantial placebo effect in antidepressant treatment as follows: If the goal is to reduce the number of patients unnecessarily exposed to antidepressants, then placebo treatment should be attempted before pharmacotherapy. If, however, the goal is to reduce pain and suffering in the greatest number of individuals, then antidepressant drugs should be given instead of psychotherapy. If the goal is to reduce the cost of treatment, antidepressant drugs should also be used, though this may not hold for patients treated in the long term with antidepressants (If it is true that 50% of all medicated patients respond to something other than active drug effects, it may not make long term economic sense to treat with medication, but this does not consider the cost of relapses, which are significantly higher in placebo treated groups). The cost argument may seem counterintuitive unless one recalls that a placebo condition is not a "no treatment" condition. Patients in placebo conditions are exposed to the same amount of education, provider contact, attention, and support as those in active treatment groups. In the study cited by Preskorn, provider contact time approximated 8-10 hours, an expensive undertaking in any situation. It is conceivable that if these 8-10 hours were spent providing an active, proven treatment for depression, such as cognitive behavioral treatment, that this might indeed prove a more cost effective option, but since the supportive components of CBT treatment have been demonstrated to be as effective as CBT itself (Jacobson & Hollon, 1996) this remains speculation at the current time.

Treatment of Psychotic Disorders

The introduction of effective antipsychotic agents, beginning in the US with chlorpromazine in 1954, proved a tremendous boon to patients with schizophrenia and other psychotic illnesses. Use of traditional antipsychotics, however, has always been limited by their problematic side effect profile as well as the fact that schizophrenics treated with such agents never show a complete response, and a high proportion of schizophrenic patients show no response at all. Hegarty, Baldessarini, Tohen, Waternaux, and Oepen (1994) reviewed clinical outcome studies in schizophrenia for the past century and found that, in global terms, treatment resulted in improvement in only 40.1% after followup averaging 5.6 years. This interesting study bears some examination, not only because of the scope of the review, but also the stringency of inclusional criteria used. The authors required that patients be limited to diagnoses of schizophrenia or dementia praecox. Followup was required, with a minimum period of at least one year and with less than 33% of patients in each study being lost to followup. Numerical outcome data had to be provided and exact treatments specified. A priori selection (on the basis of good or poor outcome) was not permitted. To correct for variability in outcome measures across studies, they converted all outcome data to a ratio scale (number of patients considered improved divided by total number for each cohort).

Their findings revealed that smaller percentages of patients improved in the decades prior to the introduction of pharmacotherapy – 35.4% for the period 1895-1955, as compared to 48.5% for the period 1955-1985. Interestingly, the greatest numbers in terms of percent improved were found between 1960-1985. Since 1986, mean percent improved dropped to 36.4%, equivalent to that found prior to the introduction of antipsychotics. In spite of this, antipsychotic treatment, as compared to convulsive and nonspecific treatments or lobotomy, produced the greatest effect (45.6%). How to account for the overall disappointing showing of antipsychotics, especially in the last decade, when the one qualitatively different antipsychotic (clozapine) has been introduced? Hegarty and his colleagues speculated that the primary reason for the decline in positive outcome has been a refinement of diagnostic criteria, and that the narrowing focus brought about by successive versions of the Diagnostic and Statistical Manual led to the exclusion of psychotic individuals who under broader classification schemes would have been called schizophrenic. There is undoubted merit to this argument, but other explanations may also help elucidate this paradoxical finding. Since the only decades in which modal response to treatment exceeded 50% were the 1960s, 1970s, and the earlier part of the 1980s, it may be necessary to look to trends in mental health treatment occurring during those times for better explanations. Deinstitutionalization, for example, might have been responsible for some spontaneous improvement in patients released from underfunded and understaffed facilities where effective treatment was scarce or nonexistent and conditions astonishingly punitive. A further factor, and one which nicely parallels the improvement curve charted by Hegarty and colleagues, is the rise and subsequent decline of the community mental health movement of the 1960s and 1970s. It is conceivable that more services were available to schizophrenic individuals during these years, and that such services were multifaceted and involved psychosocial support, financial assistance, and consistent followup not available before or since.

Recent clinical successes with atypical antipsychotics, of which clozapine is the prototypical agent, as well as advances in understanding of the neurobiology of psychosis, has given renewed hope to the search for safer, more effective antipsychotic agents (Pickar, 1995). Paradoxically, just as pharmacological researchers are on the verge of introducing a number of new, potentially effective antipsychotics which lack both the short and long term side effects of the typical agents and the risk of agranulocytosis associated with clozapine, there is increasing recognition of a previously unrecognized factor affecting all forms of pharmacological treatment for psychosis. This overlooked phenomenon is the presence of a significant placebo effect. Marder and Meibach (1994) followed positive and negative symptoms in 388 schizophrenic patients who were treated with placebo, risperidone in doses of 2 to 16 mg/day, and haldol, 20 mg/day. A randomized, double blind procedure was employed. While 6 mg/day of risperidone proved superior to other regimens in terms of overall response ratings and prevention of premature termination, and patients treated with risperidone improved at a significantly faster rate than those given placebo. But perhaps the most interesting finding of the Marder and Meibach study, which was neither addressed by the authors nor in an accompanying editorial (Kane, 1994), was that over 50% of all placebo treated subjects were rated "improved" (20% reduction in total positive and negative syndrome scale scores) after 60 days. Kane did acknowledge that haldol did not prove superior to placebo, and that "some doses" of risperidone proved superior to placebo. His comments, however, illuminate a central problem in psychiatric drug studies of schizophrenia. As Kane noted, "Many assume that in schizophrenia there is relatively little chance of placebo response, that a comparison to a standard drug should be sufficient to establish efficacy, and that it is therefore unethical to administer placebo" (page 802). What the Marder and Meibach study clearly demonstrates is that a definite placebo response in schizophrenia exists, and that this effect persists over time (60 days in this case, which approximates the presumptive natural course of an acute episode of psychotic illness). It is essential that the nature of this placebo response be better characterized, and that the nonpharmacological components (e.g., attention, support, or other "artifacts") be examined to determine their own unique potency as treatments for severe mental illness. Fortunately, some have seen a renewed interest in the applications of behavioral and psychological interventions for psychotic disorders (Kane & McGlashan, 1995), the recognition of a significant placebo effect should do much to spur inquiry into this important topic.

Some may use the above findings to buttress the contention that psychiatric treatments for mental distress are fundamentally flawed and should be abandoned. It may be, however, that such studies do not reflect poorer outcome for psychiatric interventions per se, but may be a reasonable reflection of the limits of treatment with any pharmacological agent. Keith and Matthews (1993) noted that the percent of patients improved with single drug treatment for major depression was equal to or greater than the percent of arteriosclerotic patients treated with atherectomy or angioplasty. They also reported data indicating that overall treatment effects for schizophrenia, major depression, panic disorder, bipolar disorder, and obsessive compulsive disorder were greater than any medical treatment for atherosclerosis. Interestingly, the ratio of placebo to specific drug effect responders was higher for psychiatric drugs as compared to other drugs, such as antihypertensives.

Bipolar Disorder

Bipolar disorder is one condition in which polypharmacy is often indicated (Sachs, 1996). In addition to mood stabilizing agents, such as sodium valproate, carbamazepine, or lithium carbonate, antipsychotic agents may be required to manage the symptoms of an acute manic episode. Requirements for antipsychotics, antidepressants, and mood stabilizers will change over the course of treatment of a manic episode, and the clinician must be alert to changes in the clinical picture and respond appropriately. Even with good clinical management, and better characterization of the phases of a manic episode, results with pharmacotherapy alone are not encouraging. Keck & McElroy (1996) reviewed outcome data for mood stabilizers at several points in the illness process (acute mania, acute bipolar depression, and maintenance), and found in addition to a surprisingly few number of well controlled investigations, that improvement rates have often not significantly changed since the introduction of lithium and other mood stabilizers. They noted that before the widespread use of lithium, naturalistic outcome studies suggested that 50-60% of all patients with bipolar illness experienced symptomatic recovery six months to one year following a manic episode. But while lithium treated patients may respond more positively in the short run, with higher rates of remission and longer periods to relapse, long-term maintenance with lithium does not appear to be effective. Probability of relapse in two large studies cited was over 70% after five year followup. Nevertheless, initial response rates are positive for all the mood stabilizers; with a majority of patients showing significantly greater reduction in symptomatology in shorter periods of time than those treated with placebo. Keck and McElroy did not reference studies in which psychological interventions were included as a long term maintenance strategy. Because psychological strategies in bipolar disease are poorly studied, the effects of combined treatment remain unknown.

Treatment of Anxiety Spectrum Disorders

Drugs have demonstrated efficacy in the treatment of panic disorder and associated anxiety disorders. For panic disorder, the antidepressants, both TCAs and SRIs, have been most intensively studied. Among the antidepressants, imipramine is the best studied, and response rates of 70-90% have been reported (Ballenger, 1993). Such figures do not reflect drug specific response at a minimum, the effects of placebo and clinical management should be subtracted from them. The delayed onset of action and the multiple side effects of antidepressants should also be factored into clinical algorithms, Ballenger (1993) reported that one half of patients taking antidepressants experienced significant side effects, weight gain was a problem in one third of these. Ballenger also reported significant improvement with all benzodiazepines, particularly alprazolam, but noted that effective treatment tends to be long term (12-18 months), that medication tapers are required and should be gradual (4-12 weeks) to prevent discontinuation phenomena (rebound, recurrence, and physiological withdrawal), and that a significant proportion (well over 50%) relapse. While the majority of panic disorder patients report initial positive response to medication, long term outcome following pharmacotherapy for panic disorder is not terribly impressive. Katschnig, Amering, Stolk, & Ballenger (1996) found that, of 367 patients interviewed approximately 4 years after completing a medication trial for panic disorder, only 39% remained absolutely free of panic symptoms. Somewhat surprisingly, a significant majority of patients reported that overall functioning and quality of life had substantially improved, in spite of the presence of occasional panic attacks. While these findings are cause for some optimism, the less than impressive ability of drugs to effect long term resolution of panic symptoms must be compared with long term effects of psychotherapy, which may be considerably more robust.

Jenicke (1993) reported on the results of 21 controlled medication trials in the treatment of obsessive compulsive disorder, and noted that in all of these active drug treatment proved superior to placebo, regardless of the class of agent used (TCA, SRI, or MAOI). He noted, however, that in one of the largest of these studies, the Cieba-Geigy collaborative study of clomipramine (Clomipramine Collaborative Group, 1990 cited in Jenicke, 1993), 60% of the 85% reporting improvement improved only moderately.

Ballenger (1993) reported the results of five studies of imipramine and behavioral treatment for panic disorder, in four of these combined treatment was superior to single modality intervention. Another study (Mavissakalian & Michelson, 1986; cited in Ballenger, 1993) found that behavioral treatment was an effective intervention, but those in a drug plus behavior treatment condition were more improved. Ballenger concluded, in spite of admittedly limited evidence, that combinations of antidepressant and behavioral treatment are more effective than either alone. Limited support for this assumption is offered by a recent publication by Wiborg and Dahl (1996), who provided results of an 18 month followup of two groups of panic disorder patients, one of which had been treated with clomipramine and clinical management and the other with a combination of clomipramine and 15 sessions of dynamic psychotherapy. Significant differences in relapse rates were found, with 75% of the medication group relapsing at 18 months as compared to only 20% of the combined treatment group. The study, however, was compromised by a small n (19 completed followups), lack of an attention-placebo for the non-psychotherapy group, and the fact that all psychotherapy was conducted by a single researcher.

Barlow and Lehman (1996) in reviewing current therapies for anxiety disorders, reported that no definitive studies of combined effects of pharmacotherapy and psychotherapy exist. They noted, however, the presence of evidence suggesting that the effects of combined treatment depends logically enough, on the specific effects of each component. For example, imipramine may facilitate exposure based therapy, but alprazolam, with its pronounced anxiolytic effects, likely interferes with learning based treatments. Barlow and Lehman noted that a large, four site combined treatment outcome study is still underway, but that preliminary results show a decided advantage to combined treatments. Nevertheless, the data are far too scant to draw firm conclusions about this form of treatment. As an illustration of the dearth of any kind of investigation into this topic, at the time of this writing, in fact, there is but one published investigation which attempted to compare treatment with SRIs and psychotherapy against three other treatments for panic disorder. deBeurs, van Balkom, Lange, Koele, and van Dyck (1995) assessed the effects of combining in vivo exposure treatment for panic disorder with agoraphobia with three other treatment conditions, one of which involved treatment with the SRI fluvoxamine. In one arm of this study, patients were treated with a traditional 12 session in vivo exposure paradigm. Three other groups of patients were treated with either fluvoxamine, medication placebo, or psychological panic management in lieu of the first six sessions of the 12 session, manualized, exposure model. The authors found all treatments to be effective, however, the effect size of the fluvoxamine-exposure condition was twice as large as effect sizes found for the placebo and psychological intervention conditions. Although this in general well designed study does present some methodological issues (significantly, those who were"pre-treated" with fluvoxamine were allowed to continue this therapy throughout the 12 week trial, others received single modality treatment during the last six weeks; also, use of benzodiazepines and certain other psychoactive medications was permitted), it does present some evidence that combined pharmacological and non-pharmacological treatments may be more potent interventions, at least in the short term, for panic disorder with agoraphobia.

Results of combined treatments for other anxiety disorders other than panic are even more uncertain, according to Barlow and Lehman (1996). Combined treatment for generalized anxiety disorder or for post-traumatic stress disorder has not been studied. Some clear advantages to psychotherapy over pharmacotherapy in the treatment of obsessive compulsive disorder are apparent in early research, but again, this has not been adequately studied. Both medication and psychotherapy may be similarly effective as treatments for social phobia, but in one study cited by Barlow and Lehman neither was superior to placebo plus guided imagery. Jenicke (1993) also reported on the results of a meta-analysis of 38 studies of behavioral treatment for OCD (Christensen, et al., cited in Jenicke, 1993), which found the mean effect side for behavioral treatment to be 1.7 at 80 week followup, a result identical to that of clomipramine at the end of active treatment. No followup data were reported for clomipramine, but Jenicke noted a further study finding a 90% relapse rate upon discontinuation of clomipramine (Pato et al., 1988, cited in Jenicke, 1993). While Jenicke (1993) observed that combined pharmacological and nonpharmacological treatment for OCD was routine clinical practice, only two investigations have studied this question and in one of these there was no evidence that pharmacotherapy interacted with psychotherapy, which was found to be the superior treatment.

In spite of a dearth of research, there is some suggestion, as Jacobson and Hollon (1996b) noted, that CBT may prove a more effective treatment for panic disorder than it does for major depression. Craske and Barlow (1993) reported that concurrent psychopharmacological treatment for panic disorder is not only common (approximately 50%, even among those treated in specialty psychology clinics), but that antidepressant treatment and in vivo exposure may have reciprocal enhancement effects. They cautioned, however, that treatment with some drugs, (alprazolam would be an appropriate example) may interfere with exposure based treatment and may lessen patients' perceptions of self control.

Conclusion

The ability to use psychoactive medication will not fundamentally alter our professional identity. The primary safeguard ensuring this will be maintaining specific training for practice in psychopharmacology at the postdoctoral level. We can maintain allegiance to the core precepts of the discipline while expanding our therapeutic armamentarium with the effective adjunctive use of pharmacological agents. I repeat, however, that this does not relieve educators in psychology of their obligation to modernize graduate training in psychology. The greatest threat to the academic status quo is not additional requirements for prescriptive authority. These requirements, as we have seen, will be postdoctoral, and the curriculum modifications necessary to produce students able to segue into postdoctoral psychopharmacology training *do not differ* from those amendments necessary to produce truly well-rounded generalist practitioners.

The key issue is that educators continue to fail to produce psychologists who can function as true scientist-practitioners in today's health care marketplace. Significant curricular changes must take place if this glaring deficiency is to be rectified. Educators can no longer feign ignorance about the myriad physiological processes affecting psychological functioning. Courses labelled psychophysiology can longer be restricted to the limited purview of special senses and hasty dissections of sheep brains, but must include broad based training in neuroanatomy, neurophysiology, and neuropathology. Psychologists in training must no longer be allowed to dismiss knowledge of Axis III conditions as being outside the scope of knowledge of psychology. Physiological and pathophysiological processes are intimately linked to a broad spectrum of mental disorders, and woe betide the practitioner who cannot adequately assess such conditions in order to provide appropriate, multimodal, intervention. Psychologists who are ignorant of basic physiological processes are marginalized as members of multidisciplinary treatment teams in health care settings. As managed care pushes more of psychological practice into health care settings, where multidisciplinary approaches are common, psychologists risk becoming increasingly marginalized by substandard training. Employers in the not too distant future will ask why they should hire a psychologist, whose training has left her or him bereft of core skills needed to work in health care settings, when another practitioner (say, for example, a nurse with some training in behavioral interventions) can function effectively in both roles. This lack of training is already a critical issue in health psychology, and as I have said, is separate from the prescription privileges debate. More comprehensive science based training is required in graduate programs now, to ensure the survivability of our profession in all applied settings. Enhancement of graduate training in biological sciences cannot come at the expense of training in quantitative measures. Professional psychologists will increasingly be called upon to justify the utility of their interventions, not just in terms of the alleviation of human suffering but in economic terms as well. Some may cavil at the inequity of this situation, but we delude ourselves if we believe that we can return to an earlier, simpler era where clinicians were given free rein in implementing any form of treatment they wished for whatever period of time. We must accept the fact that this glorious era is more a romantic notion than reality. Cost and service delivery concerns have always molded treatment, and while the current health care delivery climate is aggressively pecuniary in focus, we will inevitably be called upon to demonstrate efficacy and cost-efficiency of psychological services. The quantitative bases of psychology provide the core skills which allows us to do this uniquely well vis-a-vis other mental health providers, as is the intensive training in behavioral assessment and outcome which is a hallmark of superior graduate training in psychology.

We must accept the verdict of over 20 years of psychotherapy outcome research which has conclusively demonstrated that doctoral training is not a requisite condition for the provision of psychotherapy. Psychotherapy is an effective but nonspecific intervention which can be administered by individuals exposed to far less intensive training than that given to doctoral level practitioners. If we continue to insist that the role of doctoral level clinicians be largely limited to provision of verbal or behavioral therapy, we create a recipe for obsolescence. To ensure the survival of psychology as a clinical discipline, we must expand our roles well beyond traditionally defined boundaries. Such roles might include psychologists as trainers. If our pursuit of the grail of defining the specific effects of psychotherapy is successful, (and there is some reason for optimism here), psychologists will be needed to train less intensively educated mental health providers in new, specific therapies. Another new role for psychologists will be as assessors of outcome, but on a nomothetic scale, rather than the idiographic perspective which has characterized our endeavors in the past. While assessing individual response to treatment will remain important, and development and application of psychometrically sound individual outcome measures will remain an essential function of doctoral providers, we must be able to develop equally stringent measures to apply to systems. The cost effectiveness of psychological interventions must be measured according to increasingly complex multifactorial algorithms. The statistical grounding of our discipline makes psychologists the professional group of choice to perform such complex outcomes assessments. This portion of our heritage must be maintained.

It has become clear that rational psychopharmacology has remained an elusive goal. The heritage of the allopathic tradition has not given rise to the development of effective means of assessing the outcome of drug intervention, and, where such means exist, their existence has had little effect on clinical practice. Psychologists are uniquely qualified to remedy this situation. The ability to combine well founded quantitative methods of behavioral analysis with expertise in both psychopharmacology and behavioral interventions is a skill almost exclusively limited to doctoral level psychologists. We cannot fully realize this capability if we remain unable to prescribe psychoactive drugs in addition to behavioral interventions. Acquiring prescriptive authority will allow us to adopt a central role in service delivery and have a direct influence on the provision of rationally conceptualized, science based mental health interventions. This will open up tremendous opportunities in all sectors of psychology. Basic science researchers will benefit, with expanded roles in new drug development, new models for assessing efficacy. Academicians will benefit, in that subject areas previously regarded as ancillary will become central to the training of scientist practitioners, opening new opportunities for teaching, clinical supervision, and interdisciplinary efforts to integrate psychology into all areas of training for health care delivery. Clinicians will benefit from an expanded, science based therapeutic armamentarium which will allow them to treat a broader range of patients with disorders once thought untreatable by standard psychological interventions. We must do so while keeping in mind one essential fact: The potency of psychological interventions and the absolute necessity of combining these to provide effective treatment. As Benowitz (1992) has written:

> . . . there is true pathos in the clinician who feels that there is no treatment
> but that found in the use of drugs, devices, or procedures. This is especially
> poignant when nonmedical structures have provided the proof that non-
> pharmacologic alternatives work. (p. 775)

The ultimate beneficiaries of rationally designed, combined interventions will be individuals with mental distress, whose treatment will no longer be based on artificial limits imposed by traditional within discipline prejudices or interdisciplinary turf battles, but by empirically validated formulae which will include, when appropriate, the judicious use of psychoactive agents. In sum, it is my belief that rational psychopharmacology is a science based practice; and that allowing psychologists to prescribe will establish greater links between science and clinical practice. It will provide an expanded armamentarium to treat a broader range of patients with a greater range of mental disorders. The expansion of doctoral and post doctoral curricula to allow psychologists to prescribe will strengthen, not weaken, the discipline and bring us closer to a global understanding of the multifactorial causes of mental distress. It is for these reasons that I embrace the notion of prescriptive authority for appropriately trained psychologists. For these same reasons, the entire profession, basic scientists, academicians, and clinicians all, should unite behind the effort to create a unique, and uniquely valuable mental health clinician: The psychologist prescriber.

References

Adams, K. M., & Bieliauskas, L. A. (1994). On perhaps becoming what you had previously despised: Psychologists as prescribers of medication. *Journal of Clinical Psychology in Medical Settings, 1,* 189-197.

Adler, H. A. (1927). The relationship between psychiatry and the social sciences. *American Journal of Psychiatry, 147,* 428-430.

Antonuccio, D O., Danton, W. G., & DeNelsky, G Y. (1995) Psychotherapy versus medication for depression: Challenging the conventional wisdom with data. *Professional Psychology: Research and Practice, 26,* 574-585.

American Psychological Association (1995). Report of the CAPP Task Force on Prescription Privileges. Washington: Author.

Avorn, J., Dreyer, P., Connelly, K. and Soumerai, S. B. (1989). Use of psychoactive medications and the quality of care in rest homes. Findings and policy implications of a statewide study. *New England Journal of Medicine, 321,* pp. 54-55.

Avorn, J., & Gurwitz, J. H. (1995). Drug use in the nursing home. *Annals of Internal Medicine, 123,* 195-204.

Ballenger, J. C. (1993). Panic Disorder: Efficacy of current treatments. *Psychopharmacology Bulletin, 29,* 477-486.

Barlow, D. H., & Lehman, C. L. (1996). Advances in the psychosocial treatment of anxiety disorders. *Archives of General Psychiatry, 53,* 727-735.

Beers, M. H., Fingold, S. F., Ouslander, J. G., Reuben, D. B., Morgenstern, H., & Beck, J. C. (1993). Characteristics and quality of prescribing by doctors practicing in nursing homes. *Journal of the American Geriatrics Society, 41,* 802-807.

Beers, M. H., Ouslander, J. G., Rollingher, I., Reuben, D. B., Brooks, J., and Beck, J. C. (1991). Explicit criteria for determining inappropriate medical use in nursing home residents. *Archives of Internal Medicine, 151,* 1825-1831.

Bennett, B. (1994). Personal communication.

Benowitz, N. L. (1992). Substance abuse, dependence, and treatment. In Melmon, K. E., Morelli, H. F., Hoffman, B. B., & Nierenberg, D. W. (Eds.) *Melmon and Morelli's Clinical Pharmacology and Therapeutics (Third Edition)* (pp. 763-787). New York: McGraw-Hill.

Birkholz, G., & Walker, D. (1994). Strategies for state statutory language changes granting fully independent nurse practitioner practice. *Nurse Practitioner, 19,* 54-58.

Breggin, P. R. (1991). *Toxic Psychiatry.* New York: St. Martins.

Broskowski, A. T. (1995). The evolution of health care: Implications for the training and careers of psychologists. *Professional Psychology: Research and Practice, 26,* 139-146.

Chiles, J. A., Carlin, A. S., Benjamine, G. A. H., & Beitman, B. D. (1991). A physician, a nonmedical psychotherapist, and a patient: The pharmacotherapy-psychotherapy triangle. In Beitman, B. D., & Klerman, G. L. (Eds.). *Integrating pharmacotherapy and psychotherapy* (pp. 105-120). Washington: American Psychiatric Press.

Christensen, J., Hadzi-Pavlovic, D., Andrews, G., & Mattick, R. (1987) Behavior therapy and tricyclic medication in the treatment of obsessive-compulsive disorder: A quantitative review. *Journal of Consulting and Clinical Psychology, 55,* 701-711.

Cinciripini, P. M., Cinciripini, L. G., Wallfisch, A., Haque, W., & Van Vunakis, H. (1996). Behavioral therapy and the transdermal nicotine patch: Effects on cessation outcome, affect, and coping. *Journal of Consulting and Clinical Psychology, 64,* 314-323.

Clarkin, J. F., Pilkonis, P. A., & Magruder, K. M. (1996). Psychotherapy of depression. *Archives of General Psychiatry, 53,* 717-723.

Clomipramine Collaborative Group (1991). Clomipramine in the treatment of patients with obsessive-compulsive disorder. *Archives of General Psychiatry, 48,* 730-738.

Craske. M. G., & Barlow, D. H. (1993) Panic disorder and agoraphobia. In Barlow, D. H. (Ed.). *Clinical Handbook of Psychological Disorders (2nd Edition)*. New York: Guilford.

de Beurs, E., van Balkom, A. J. L. M., Lange, A., Koele, P., & van Dyck, R. (1995). Treatment of panic disorder with agoraphobia: Comparison of fluvoxamine, placebo and psychological panic management combined with exposure and of exposure in vivo alone. *American Journal of Psychiatry, 152*, 683-691.

DeLay, J., & Deniker, P. (1952). *Reactions biologuiques observees au cours du traitement par le chlorhydrate de dimethylaminopropyl-N-chlorophenothiazine* (4560 R.P.) Congres des psychiatres de langue francaise, Luxembourg, July 22-26, 1952.

DeLeon, P. H., Sammons, M. T., & Fox, R. E. (1995). A commentary: Canada is not that far north. *Canadian Psychologist, 36*, 320-326.

Depression Guideline Panel (1993). *Depression in Primary Care: Volume 2. Treatment of Major Depression. Clinical Practice Guideline Number 5*. Rockville, MD: U. S. Department of Health and Human Services, Public Health Service, Agency for Health Care Policy and Research, AHCPR Publication No. 93-0551.

Dozois, D. A., & Dobson, K. S. (1995). Should Canadian psychologists follow the APA trend and seek prescription privileges?: A reexamination of the (R)evolution. *Canadian Psychologist, 36*, 289-304.

Elkin, I., Shea, M. T., Watkins, J. T., Imber, S. D., Stosky, S. M., Collins, J. F., Glass, D. R., Pilkonis, P. A., Leber, W. R., Doherty, J. P, Fiester, S. J., & Parloff, M. B. (1989). NIMH Treatment of depression collaborative research program I: General effectiveness of treatments. *Archives of General Psychiatry, 46*, 971-982.

Fortmann, S. P., & Killen, J. D. (1995). Nicotine gum and self -help behavioral intervention for smoking relapse prevention: Results from a trial using population-based recruitment. *Journal of Consulting and Clinical Psychology, 63*, 460-468.

Frank, E., Karp, J. F., & Rush, A. J. (1993). Efficacy of treatments for major depression. *Psychopharmacology Bulletin, 29*, 457-475.

Gadow, K. D. (1992). Pediatric psychopharmacotherapy: A review of recent research. *Journal of Child Psychology and Psychiatry, 33*, 153-195.

Geller, B., Cooper, T. B., Graham, D. L., Marsteller, F. A., & Bryant, D. M. (1990). Double-blind placebo-controlled study of nortriptyline in depressed adolescent using a "fixed plasma level" design. *Psychopharmacology Bulletin, 26*, 85-90.

Geller, B., Cooper, T. B., McCombs, H. G., Graham, D., & Wells, J. (1989). Double-blind placebo-controlled study of nortriptyline in depressed adolescents using a "fixed plasma level" design. *Psychopharmacology Bulletin, 25*, 101-108.

Greenberg, R. P., Bornstein, R. F., Greenberg, M. D., & Fisher, S. (1992). A meta-analysis of antidepressant outcome under "blinder" conditions. *Journal of Consulting and Clinical Psychology, 60*, 664-669.

Greenberg, R. P., Bornstein, R. F., Zborowski, M. J., Fisher, S., & Greenberg, M. D. (1994). A meta-analysis of fluoxetine outcome in the treatment of depression. *Journal of Nervous and Mental Diseases, 182*, 547-551.

Greenberg, R. P. & Fisher, S. (1989) Examining antidepressant effectiveness: Findings, ambiguities and some vexing puzzles. In Fisher, S., & Greenberg, R. P.(Eds). *The limits of biological treatment for mental distress: Comparisons with psychotherapy and placebo.* (pp. 1-37). Hillsdale, NJ: Erlbaum.

Hayes, S. C., Walser, R. D., & Follette, V. M. (1995). Psychology and the temptation of prescription privileges. *Canadian Psychology, 36,* 313-320.

Harkless, G. E. (1989). Prescriptive authority: Debunking common assumptions. *Nurse Practitioner, 14,* 57-61.

Healy, D. T. (1990). The psychopharmacological era: Notes toward a history. *Journal of Psychopharmacology, 43,* 152-167.

Hegarty, J. D., Baldessarini, R. J., Tohen, M., Waternaux, C., & Oepen, G. (1994). One hundred years of schizophrenia: A meta analysis of the outcome literature. *American Journal of Psychiatry, 151,* 1409-1416.

Jacobson, N. S., Dobson, K. S., Truax, P. A., Addis, M. E., Koerner, K., Gollan, J. K., Gortner, E., & Prince, S. E. (1996). A component analysis of cognitive-behavioral treatment for depression. *Journal of Consulting and Clinical Psychology, 64,* 295-304.

Jacobson, N. S., & Hollon, S. D. (1996a). Cognitive behavior therapy versus pharmacotherapy: Now that the jury's returned its verdict, its time to present the rest of the evidence. *Journal of Consulting and Clinical Psychology, 64,* 74-80.

Jacobson, N. S., & Hollon, S. D. (1996b). Prospects for future comparisons between drugs and psychotherapy: Lessons from the CBT-versus-pharmacotherapy exchange. *Journal of Consulting and Clinical Psychology, 64,* 104-108.

Janicak, P. G., David, J. M., Preskorn, S. H., & Ayd, F. J. (1993). *Principles and Practice of Psychopharmacotherapy.* Baltimore: Williams and Wilkins.

Jenicke, M. A. (1993) Obsessive-compulsive disorder: Efficacy of specific treatments as assessed by controlled trials. *Psychopharmacology Bulletin, 29,* 487-499.

Jobson, K. O., & Potter, M. D. (1995). International psychopharmacology algorithm project report. *Psychopharmacology Bulletin, 31,* 459-459.

Kane, J. M. (1994). Risperidone. *American Journal of Psychiatry, 151,* 802-803.

Kane, J. M. & McGlashan, T. H. (1995). Treatment of schizophrenia. *The Lancet, 346,* pp. 820-825.

Katschnig, H., Amering, M., Stolk, J. M., & Ballenger, J. C. (1996). Predictors of quality of life in a long-term followup study in panic disorder patients after a clinical drug trial. *Psychopharmacology Bulletin, 32,* 149-155.

Keck, P. E., & McElroy, S. L. (1996). Outcome in the pharmacologic management of bipolar disorder. *Journal of Clinical Psychopharmacology, 16,* 15S-23S.

Keith, S. J., & Matthews, S. M. (1993). The value of psychiatric treatment: Its efficacy in severe mental disorders. *Psychopharmacology Bulletin, 29,* 427-430.

Klein, R. G. (1996). Comments on expanding the clinical role of psychologists. *American Psychologist, 51,* 216-218.

Kraemer, H. C. (1995). Methodological and statistical progress in psychiatric clinical research. In Bloom, F. E., & Kupfer, D. J. (Eds.) *Psychopharmacology: The Fourth Generation of Progress.* (pp. 1849-1860). New York: Raven.

Krupnick,J.L.,Sotsky,S.M.,Simmens,S.,Moyer,J.,ElkinI.,Watkins,J.,&Pilkonis, P A. (1996). The role of the therapeutic alliance in psychotherapy and pharmacotherapy outcome: Findings in the National Institute of Mental Health Treatment of Depression Collaborative Research Program. *Journal of Consulting and Clinical Psychology, 64,* 532-539.

Kubie, L. S. (1954). The pros and cons of a new profession: A doctorate in medical psychology. *Texas Reports on Biology and Medicine, 12,* pp. 692-737.

Lehmann, H . E., & Hanrahan, G. E. (1954). Chlorpromazine. New inhibiting agent for psychomotor excitement and manic states. *American Medical Association Archives of Neurology and Psychiatry,* 227-237.

Marder, S. R., and Meibach, R. C. (1994). Risperidone in the treatment of schizophrenia. *American Journal of Psychiatry, 151,* 825-835.

Mavissakalian, M., & Michelson, L. (1986). Agoraphobia: Relative and combined effectiveness of therapist-assisted in vivo exposure and imipramine. *Journal of Clinical Psychiatry, 47,* 117-122.

Nelson,J. C.,Doherty,J. P.,Henschen, G. M.,Kasper, S.,Nierenberg, A. A.,& Ward, N. G. (1995) Algorithms for the treatment of subtypes of unipolar major depression. *Psychopharmacology Bulletin, 31,* 475-482.

Monane, M., Glynn, R. J., & Avorn, J. (1996). The impact of sedative-hypnotic use of sleep symptoms in elderly nursing home residents. *Clinical Pharmacology and Therapeutics, 59,* 83-92.

Morin, C. M. (1993). *Insomnia: Psychological Assessment and Management.* New York: Guilford Press.

Pato, M. T., Sohar, 0., Kadouch, R., Sohar, J., & Murphy, D. L. (1988). Return of symptoms after discontinuation of clomipramine in patients with obsessive compulsive disorder. *American Journal of Psychiatry, 145,* 1521-1525.

Pearson, L. J. (1995) Annual update of how each state stands on legislative issues affective advanced nursing practice. *The Nurse Practitioner, 20,* 13-51.

Pickar, D. (1995). Prospects for pharmacotherapy of schizophrenia. *The Lancet, 345,* 557-561.

Pies, R. W. (1991). The "deep structure" of clinical medicine and prescribing privileges for psychologists. *Journal of Clinical Psychiatry, 52,* 4-8.

Platman, S. R., Dorgan, R., & Gerhardt, R. J. (1976a). Psychiatric medication: The role of the non-physician. *International Journal of Social Psychiatry, 22,* 56-60.

Platman, S. R., Dorgan, R., & Gerhardt, R. J. (1976b). Some social and political ramifications of utilizing non-physicians as chemotherapists. *International Journal of Social Psychiatry, 22,* 65-69.

Preskorn, S. H. (1996). A dangerous idea. *Journal of Practical Psychiatry and Behavioral Health, 1,* 231-234.

Ray, W. A., Taylor, J. A., Meador, K. G., Lichtensten, M. J., Griffin, M. R., Fought, R., Adams, M. L. & Blazer, D. G. (1993). Reducing antipsychotic use in nursing homes: A controlled trial of provider education. *Archives of Internal Medicine, 153,* 713-721.

Reiger, D. A., Narrow, W. E., Rae, D. S., Locke, B. Z., & Goodwin, F. K. (1993). The de factor US mental and addictive disorders service system: Epidemiologic Catchment Area prospective one year prevalence rates of disorders and services. *Archives of General Psychiatry, 50*, 85-94.

Russell, W. L. (1932). The presidential address: The place of the American Psychiatric Association in modern psychiatric organization and progress. *American Journal of Psychiatry, 12*, 1-18.

Sachs, G. S. (1996). Bipolar mood disorder: Practical treatment strategies for acute and maintenance phase treatment. *Journal of Clinical Psychopharmacology, 16*, 32S-40S.

Sammons, M. T. (1994). Prescription privileges and psychology: A reply to Adams and Bieliauskas. *Journal of Clinical Psychology in Medical Settings, 1*, 199-207.

Sammons, M. T., & Brown, A. B. (in press). The Department of Defense Psychopharmacology Demonstration Project: An evolving experiment in postdoctoral education for psychologists.

Sammons, M. T., Sexton, J. L., & Meredith, J. M. (1996). Basic science training in psychopharmacology: How much is enough? *American Psychologist, 51*, 230-234.

Sanchez, P.N., & Kohn, M. (1991). Differentiated medical from psychological disorders: How do medical and nonmedically trained clinicians compare? *Professional Psychology: Research and Practice, 22*, (2), 124-126.

Scully, J. H. (1995) Why be concerned about recruitment? *American Journal of Psychiatry, 152*, 1413-1414.

Seligman, M. E. P. (1995a). Mental health: Does therapy help? *Consumer Reports*; November, 1995, 734-739.

Seligman, M. E. P (1995b). The effectiveness of psychotherapy: The consumer reports study. *American Psychologist, 50*, 965-974.

Sierles, F. S., & Taylor, M. A. (1995). Decline of U. S. medical student career choice of psychiatry and what to do about it. *American Journal of Psychiatry, 152*, 1416-1426.

Shader, R. I., & Greenblatt, D. J. (1993). Use of benzodiazepines in anxiety disorders. *New England Journal of Medicine, 328*, 1398-1405.

Shelton, D. A., & Frank, R. (1995). Rural mental health coverage under health care reform. *Community Mental Health Journal, 31*, 539-552.

Sommers-Flanagan, J., & Sommers-Flanagan, R. (1996). Efficacy of antidepressant medication with depressed youth: What psychologists should know. *Professional Psychology: Research and Practice, 27*, 145-153.

Valenstein, E. S. (1986). *Great and Desperate Cures: The rise and decline of psychosurgery and other radical treatments for mental illness.* New York: Basic Books.

Wagenfeld, M. O., Murray, J. D., Mohatt, D. F., & DeBruyn, J. C. (1994). *Mental Health and Rural America: 1980-1993.* Rockville (MD): Office of Rural Health Policy, National Institutes of Mental Health.

Wallerstein, R. S. (Ed.) (1992). *The Doctorate in Mental Health: An Experiment in Mental Health Professional Education.* Lanham, University Press of America.

Wanerman, L. (1992). The early years: Launching the program, 1971-1975. In Wallerstein, R. S. (Ed.), *The Doctorate in Mental Health: An Experiment in Mental Health Professional Education* (pp. 21-40). Lanham, MD: University Press of America.

Wells, K. B., & Sturm, R. (1996). Informing the policy process: From efficacy to effectiveness data on pharmacotherapy. *Journal of Consulting and Clinical Psychology, 64,* 638-645.

Whiston, S. C., & Sexton, T. L. (1993). An overview of psychotherapy outcome research: Implications for practice. *Professional Psychology: Research and Practice, 24,* 43-51.

Wiborg, I. M., & Dahl, A. A. (1996). Does brief dynamic psychotherapy reduce the relapse rate of panic disorder? *Archives of General Psychiatry, 53,* 689-694.

Willcox, S. M., Himmelstein, M. D. and Woolhandler, S. (1994). Inappropriate drug prescribing for the community-dwelling elderly. *Journal of the American Medical Association, 272,* (4), 292-296.

Zarate, C. A., Daniel, D. G., Kinon, B. J., Litman, R. E., Naber, D., Pickar, D., & Sato, M. (1995). Algorithms for the treatment of schizophrenia. *Psychopharmacology Bulletin, 31,* 461-468.

Zimmerman, M A., & Wienckowski, L. A. (1991). Revisiting health and mental health linkages: A policy whose time has come. . .again. *Journal of Public Health Policy, Winter,* 1991, pp. 510-524.

The opinions expressed in this chapter are solely those of the author and do not in any way represent the official opinions of the U.S. Navy or the Department of Defense.

Discussion of Sammons

Arguments for the Use of Prescription Authority

Blake H. Tearnan, Ph.D.
Healthsouth Rehabilitation Hospital of Reno

Prescriptive authority for psychologists has been debated by the psychological profession for a number of years, but it is only since 1991, with the initiation of the Department of Defense Fund Psychopharmacology Demonstration Project (PDP), that so much attention has been directed to this controversial topic. This is reflected in various publications and recent legislative proposals. The curriculum of various graduate programs has also begun to reflect the general acceptance of the importance of the biological basis of human behavior and the inevitable move toward prescription privileges for psychologists.

The AAAPP National Conference On Prescription Privileges For Psychologists also signals the growing interest in the topic of prescription privileges for psychologists. In the "Case for Prescription Privileges for Psychologists: An Overview," Dr. Morgan Sammons presents arguments for the use of prescriptive authority. In this balanced presentation, he discusses numerous arguments that have been raised by detractors of prescription authority and proponents for prescription privileges. He presents these arguments within the context of a profession struggling to assimilate evolving models of human behavior and faced with the economic realities of managed care.

One argument Dr. Sammons addresses in his chapter that is often put forth by academic psychologists, is that the push toward prescription privileges represents a crisis of identity within professional psychology. Opponents of this view assert that psychology is threatened by the forces of managed care and that recent developments in psychology and the attractiveness of legislation sanctioning prescription authority is economically driven. Sammons and others counter that prescription authority is a natural extension of the responsibilities of psychologists, which have increased steadily over the years. This is due in part to the failure of psychiatry to reach adequate numbers of patients, the expansion of psychology into non-traditional areas, and the growth of applied psychology.

A related issue is the question of whether prescription privileges belongs within the discipline of psychology. Some have argued, including Steven C. Hayes, that psychology is defined by a level of analysis that is distinct from other fields. A move to prescribe drugs by psychologists will require that psychologists study various organ systems. This is biology, it is argued, not psychological knowledge. Sammons rightly points out that psychology is concerned with all aspects of human behavior and the mechanisms that affect that behavior. A critical role of the discipline of psychology is to develop powerful and effective interventions that influence behavior at all levels, including possible pharmacological treatments of behavior.

Psychologists against prescription authority also argue prescription privileges would fundamentally change psychology and cause an irreversible qualitative shift leading to the betrayal of psychology's traditional psychological models in favor of the biomedical model. However, Sammons contends that prescription privileges and the inclusion of biological factors as explanatory mechanisms of behavior is a reflection of the general acceptance of the biopsychosocial model of behavior. Graduate psychology curriculums have already recognized this fact, and have introduced courses on the organic basis of behavior, pharmacology and the new discipline of medical psychology. As far back as the late 1970s, the University of Georgia's clinical program encouraged its clinical graduate students to take courses in organic psychopathology, recognizing the psychiatric manifestations of physical illness; Sammons points out that the core of psychological training would remain intact with the existing knowledge base supplemented. To reassure psychologists convinced that the introduction of biological factors and pharmacology would fundamentally change the discipline of psychology, courses on pharmacology would only be offered at the post-doctoral level. However, graduate curriculum would offer courses on the biological basis of human behavior to help better prepare students interested in pursuing prescription privileges.

Another popular argument against prescription privileges that is discussed by Sammons is that the medicalization of psychology will cause the discipline to abandon its psychotherapeutic origins in favor a strict biomedical model of behavior. These proponents catastrophize that psychology will come under the influence of the pharmaceutical companies and federal funding for research related to drugs. However, there is no basis for the fear that psychology would abandon its scientific and behavioral origins. Psychology has become more biologically based because it recognizes the inadequacies of early psychological models, including psychodynamic theory. Simply because medical explanations of behavior are thought by most biological psychiatrists to lend credibility to the practice of psychiatry, especially to their medical brethren, does not mean psychologists will behave similarly and abandon their historical roots. Psychologists are better trained in research, as argued by Sammons, and can more critically examine the psychological literature. There is no evidence to suggest they will flock to drug based interventions, especially since at this stage the efficacy of drug therapy has not been clearly demonstrated.

Many have suggested that professional psychology is turning its attention to prescription authority to rescue it from the economic lows caused by managed care. They see prescription privileges as a flight of fancy, since psychology needs to emphasize its traditional roles and strengths as a unique discipline with strong and principled roots. It is argued that psychology offers interventions that are important to the changing needs of the health care system, and should spend more time educating people about the strengths of its discipline instead of responding to a crisis that is economically driven. Sammons ends his chapter with the observation that the right to prescribe medications by psychologists expands their authority to offer treatment interventions that they are currently denied. This is in part economically driven, given the nature of the health care delivery system. Psychologists need to recognize the realities of a health care system that may, in the end, see no need for doctoral level psychologists whose care is restricted and practiced more cheaply by less expensive providers. Medication privileges open the full range of mental health therapies to psychologists and politically positions them more favorably to negotiate with a health care system who cares little for the sanctity of psychological tradition. Prescription privileges would allow psychologists to treat other populations and offer medications to patients who currently seek help from their family doctors or from psychiatrists. Psychologists would be seen as more essential to manage care since their range of treatments would be greater and physicians might refer to *psychologists* with privileges more often

Sammons' core thesis is the expansion of doctoral and post doctoral curriculum to allow psychologists to prescribe will strengthen, not weaken the discipline and help psychology better recognize the multi dimensional nature of behavior and open up possibilities of practice denied in the past. Because psychiatry has been seduced by drug companies and practiced pharmacology, often without adequate scientific basis, does not mean psychology will bend in its reach and abandon the traditions which define it as a unique discipline committed to the scientific basis of human behavior.

Chapter 2

The Case Against Prescription Privileges for Psychologists: An Overview

Elaine M. Heiby, Ph.D.
University of Hawaii

A British psychology journal recently published an article entitled "George Albee: Founder of true community care" (1995). Albee is quoted as follows:

> I regard with horror the current political effort on the part of clinical psychology to obtain prescription privileges. The biggest issue today confronting American psychology is a fight for the right to prescribe drugs by clinicians. I see this as surrendering to the medical model. There are other pressures—the enormous pharmaceutical companies in the United States are supporting psychologists' quests for drug privileges. They are more interested in having 100,000 psychologists prescribing drugs than preventing social ills. (p. 511)

I personally became horrified by the proposal that psychologists be trained to independently prescribe psychotropic medication in 1990 when the Hawaii Psychological Association invited me to present the "con" side in a debate. I was puzzled by the adversarial way the issue was to be discussed. How could prescription privileges be so polarized when it was such a new idea? I asked for time to review the literature before deciding whether to participate in a debate.

I was startled to learn prescription privileges legislation was already underway in Hawaii (DeLeon, 1990, Summer). No formal discussions about prescription privileges had taken place in the Department of Psychology at the University of Hawaii. The conventional protocol for doctoral program development was being bypassed. Prescription privileges was not a national trend that my colleagues had irresponsibly failed to follow. No other state had licensed prescription privileges, and no other major university psychology department had undertaken medical training. At least I understood why prescription privileges was to be debated rather than critically analyzed. Legislation requires psychologists to take a position for or against this issue.

My literature search was also disturbing. I found about a dozen articles and presentations on prescription privileges, a preponderance of which claimed that society needs more psychotropic drugs and psychologists ought to prescribe them (Barron, 1989; DeLeon, 1990, April; Burns, DeLeon, Chemtob, Welch, & Samuels, 1988; Fox, 1988a, 1988b; Graham, 1990; Jennings, 1988). Some articles involved unsubstantiated and uncollegial critiques of psychiatry and medicine (cf., Raphael,

1990, Winter) and had a propaganda-like tone (cf., Sorotzkin, 1991). While objections from psychiatrists may be duly noted, valid concerns raised by psychologists (DeNelsky, 1990, August; Piotrowski, 1989-1990, Winter) seemed to be completely ignored. At the same time, the American Psychological Association (Board of Professional Affairs, 1989; Youngstrom, 1990, June) was pursuing privileges before the issue had been discussed throughout the membership.

I realized the very nature of the discipline was prematurely going to change by legislative fiat if more psychologists did not become involved. My university would be one of the first to be affected if the faculty and administration abrogated its rights and responsibilities to guild organizations and politicians. So I felt obliged to take the "con" position along with J. Tom Greene in the Hawaii Psychological Association's debate (Prescription privileges for psychologists debate, 1990, July). We refuted that prescription privileges training and responsibilities were minor extensions of psychology. We argued that psychologists who wish to prescribe should obtain a medical degree to maintain current ethical standards and protect the domain of psychology. We concluded that medical mental health treatment can be provided more cost-effectively by collaboration between physicians and psychologists. We asked the proponents to assume a more respectful attitude toward medical colleagues and disciplinary boundaries. We were confident of our objections, but felt out on a limb.

In the past several years there has been a more balanced literature published and broader organizational and grass root's involvement in the prescription privileges debate. By 1995, at least three national associations studied and formally opposed prescription privileges (Hayes & Heiby, 1996). These include the American Association of Applied and Preventive Psychology, the Council of University Directors of Clinical Psychology Programs, and the Society for a Science of Clinical Psychology (Section III of Division 12 [Clinical] of the American Psychological Association). The opposition by organizations is supported by numerous critical reviews of the prescription privileges issue (Committee recommends, 1995, March; DeNelsky, 1990, August, 1996; Evans, 1991, November; Hayes, Walser, & Follette, 1996; Heiby & Hayes, 1996; Kardelnig, 1995, August; Karon, 1994, Fall; Kingsbury, 1992a; McColskey, 1993, Winter; Moldawsky, 1991, Fall, 1995 [in DeLeon, 1995, Winter]; Piotrowski, 1989-1990, Winter; Saeman, 1995; Sanua, 1992, 1993a, August, 1995; Sorotzkin, 1991).

But just as academic and scientist-practitioner organizations have come to formally consider the desirability and feasibility of prescription privileges, the American Psychological Association (Martin, 1995, September; Prescription privileges, 1995, Fall) and some state psychological associations chose in 1996 to pursue legislation in at least three states (Missouri, California, and Hawaii). Just as the collegial dialogue over prescription privileges had begun to more broadly represent the interests of the discipline, this collegiality was strained by the need to address prescription privileges in the adversarial legislative context. None of the 1996, or subsequent, legislation passed, so there is still a chance that further debate of this issue can take place in a more collegial fashion than in the past.

Some proponents continue to construe the divisiveness over prescription privileges as a simple turf issue between psychology and psychiatry while they ignore or disparage (DeLeon, 1996, Winter; Graham, 1990) most objections of their colleagues. Some proponents of prescription privileges have chosen to bypass resolving this issue within the field by directly lobbying legislators to force training in prescription privileges by judicial means and some of this activity is covert (Clipson & Hammell, 1994, September). This adversarial attitude has already created a rift in psychology. I have been in the boxing ring with my colleagues at the Hawaii State Legislature and it is not the type of interaction I find constructive. It left wounds with psychologists, physicians, consumer groups, and legislators.

Soon after prescription privileges was being proposed, Piotrowski (1989-1990, Winter) predicted that the issue would be more divisive within psychology than between psychology and medicine. More recently, Lorion (1996) calls for a collegial rather than adversarial approach to prescription privileges in saying "if we simply pause and reflect on the substantive aspect of the debate over prescription privileges, we may recognize an opportunity for psychologists to converge rather than fractionate . . . this controversy does not affect only psychologists involved in clinical sciences and services; all of psychology, it's basic as well as applied fields, will be affected by the manner in which these issues are deliberated and ultimately resolved." (p.219.).

I believe there are at least five somewhat overlapping reasons why prescription privileges would be detrimental to the science and profession of psychology and to the public. These five reasons underscore why this divisive topic should be resolved within the discipline and not at state legislatures. Some reasons necessarily acknowledge that the drive for prescription privileges by guild organizations is an ill-directed attempt to solve real problems facing applied psychology (Hayes & Heiby, 1996). Some psychologists are clearly looking for more and different work. Opposing prescription privileges can be effective only if this dissatisfaction is also addressed.

Five Reasons To Oppose Prescription Privileges

Reason One: Prescription Privileges Would Undermine Training in Psychological Science

The desirability of the effect of prescription privileges upon the discipline is largely determined by the nature of the necessary training. The cost of training is especially relevant in this age of educational budget cutbacks. Some have proposed that training to prescribe independently would be a minor undertaking, requiring only about 100 hours (Burns et al., 1988; DeLeon, 1992, August; DeLeon, 1993, September; DeLeon, Sammons, & Sexton, 1995; Folen, 1994; Graham, 1990; Wiggins, 1995, Winter). If such were the case, however, there would be far less controversy. Most agree adequate training in the practice of invasive medicine would be extensive, and substantially change psychology curricula at the under-graduate, graduate, and post-doctoral levels (American Psychological Association [APA], 1992a; Butz, 1994; Bruner, 1995; Chamberlain, 1994; DeLeon, 1995,

Winter; DeLeon, Fox & Graham, 1991; DeNelsky, 1990, August; Fox, 1988a; Garfield, 1995, July; Greene, 1995, September; Hayes & Heiby, 1996; Hayes, et al., 1996; Karbelnig, 1995, August; Karon, 1994, Fall; Kingsbury, 1992a, 1992b; Klein, 1996; Lorion, 1996; May & Belsky, 1992; McColskey, 1991, September; McNamara, 1991; Moldawsky, 1991, Fall, 1992, November; Pachman, 1996; Resolution Opposing Prescription Privileges, 1995; Sanua, 1993a, 1993b, 1993c, August, 1994; Soucer, 1991, Fall; Sterling, 1992; Tabin, 1992; Wade, 1992, Winter).

A common thread among most who argue prescription privileges would involve extensive medical training is a respect for the standards of the M.D. and a concern about the safety of the consumer. The serious nature of prescribing highly toxic and poorly understood psychotropic drugs (e.g., Sanua, 1992, August) would require medicalizing the psychology curricula. Prescribing psychologists would be held liable for a person's entire health status. Current curricula include very little premedical undergraduate and medical graduate training, and few psychologists are prepared to teach these courses (APA, 1992; Lorion, 1996). Throughout the history of applied psychology, research, training, and practice have been limited to situational, verbal, and noninvasive physical procedures. The use of interventions that invade the human cavity has been done in collaboration with physicians. With such disciplinary boundaries, psychological science provides a rich and rapidly growing knowledge base for applied psychology. For example, doctoral training in clinical psychology readily takes six or seven years. The domain specific to clinical psychology is so complex that respecialization programs designed for experimental psychologists usually take three years. Surely, adequate training in the discipline of medicine would take longer than respecializing within the same discipline of psychology.

Training proposals for prescription privileges are under development (DeLeon & Wiggins, 1996) and one of the more extensive ones would take two to three years (APA, 1992). This program has been critiqued for focusing too narrowly on psychopharmacology and failing to include medical domains necessary to be responsible for the effect of medication upon organ systems (Klein, 1996). Prescribing medication is practicing medicine. Medical school curricula have not been dismantled. Medical students cannot prescribe independently after completing the pharmacology components of training. In addition, Klein points out that no medical training program for psychologists can be designed until national academic standards for applied psychologists have been developed. Current standards vary widely and most states certify psychologists in title, not in the performance of particular procedures such as administering psychotropic medication. In order to evaluate whether medical training for a Ph.D. in psychology can be less than an M.D., the definition of a licensed psychologist must be standardized.

It is not likely that the training in medicalized psychology would involve the time and resources required for a Ph.D.-M.D., so that the standards historically held by psychology and medicine are retained. It is more likely that the standards of both disciplines would be compromised, with psychology taking the hardest hit (Chamberlain, 1994; DeNelsky, 1990, August, 1996; Karbelnig, 1995, August; Sanua,

1993a, August). This is not because psychology has less to offer. This is because medical practice and continuing education needs are more formalized, and medical malpractice is more lethal and objectively defined. It is no accident that malpractice liability cases are far more common for psychiatry than psychology (Deardorff, Cross, & Hupprich, 1984). Whatever form training took, regulatory standards for prescription authority would have immediate major effects upon psychology programs and the priority of resources. Prescription privileges would direct resources away from psychological science as more faculty positions are dedicated to medical training. Similarly, students drawn to a medicalized psychology would have less interest in psychological principles than those in the past. The growth of psychological science and practice would be impeded from the bottom up and from the top down. Some proponents of prescription privileges acknowledge these effects on psychology training (Buie, 1988; Fox, 1988a; Fox, Schwelitz, & Barclay, 1992) but have yet to provide arguments about their desirability and economic feasibility. What is to be eliminated from the psychology curriculum, and why? Who would pay for additional training?

There may be a day when psychology has advanced its missions so that the domain of the field comes to include medical science and practice beyond what is needed to collaborate. Right now, psychology's plate is full (Karbelnig, 1995, August; Moldawsky, 1992, November). Graduate and post-doctoral curricula are already overloaded. The need for research and training in empirically-supported and cost-effective psychological procedures is far from satisfied, precluding inherent forces that the field's domain must expand to cross disciplinary boundaries with medicine. If a need for prescription privileges evolves from a reciprocal influence between science and practice, academic and applied psychologists will be in agreement. However, the divisiveness of prescription privileges indicates medical training is not a natural outgrowth of precedents as some proponents purport. Three commonly cited precedents for training in prescription privileges include that psychologists: 1) appreciate the biological level of analysis of behavior (Brentar & McNamara, 1991; Fox, 1988a, 1988b); 2) have collaborated with physicians (DeLeon, 1990-1991, Winter); and 3) are comparable to allied physical health professionals, such as optometry, who have earned limited prescription authority in some states (Burns, et al., 1988; DeLeon & Wiggins, 1996). Upon close inspection, these precedents are not convincing causal factors for medicalizing psychology training.

Biological bases as a precedent

It has long been acknowledged in psychology that there exists a biological substrate to human behavior and experience, making it specious to suggest that the field has overlooked the importance of the effects of drugs upon behavior and must medicalize to do so. Psychologists have commonly used noninvasive physical methods, such as biofeedback (Jansen & Barron, 1988). Many psychologists use invasive physical methods independently with infrahumans and in collaboration with physicians when studying humans. Collaboration has resulted in important contributions to basic psychology and areas where applied psychology and medicine overlap, such as neuropsychology and health psychology. In those instances where psychologists independently employ invasive physical procedures in research with animals, both their training and work are narrowly focused. Psychologists who have been working with animals for years are not seeking privileges to practice veterinary medicine. So appreciation of the role of biology in behavior does not mean that the training of applied psychologists is positioned to include medicine any more than appreciation of forensic factors in behavior is a precedent for psychology programs to train lawyers.

Professional collaboration as a precedent

One pro-prescription privileges argument suggests once a professional collaborates with someone in another discipline, the need to be trained in that other discipline has somehow been demonstrated. Proponents of prescription privileges cite collaboration between psychologists and physicians in the U.S. Indian Health Service (DeLeon, 1990-1991, Winter) and in the military during the Desert Storm war (DeLeon, 1992, August). Surveys have indicated that such collaboration is generally common (Barkley, 1991, Spring; DeAngelis, 1995, October; DeLeon, 1991, Fall; Egli, 1991, Fall; Jennings, 1988, December). Psychologists also consult with school teachers, social workers, lawyers, parole officers, and many others. So far, this pro-prescription argument has not been extended to these other professions, nor is it offered in its logical reverse, less everyone who consults with a psychologist may be evolving into one.

Other professions provide a precedent

Some argue that because doctoral level nonphysician health professions, such as podiatry and optometry, have acquired independent prescription authority in most or all states, training in psychology must head in the same direction (Bernay, 1994, Fall; Burns et al., 1988; DeLeon, 1991-1992, Winter; DeLeon, 1992, August; Forman, 1992-1993, Fall; Wiggins, 1995, Winter). It is also pointed out that most states permit supervised prescription privileges for nurses and physician assistants, so doctoral training in psychology must be more than sufficient. The vast differences between training in the discipline of psychology and the physical health professions make this allusion unwarranted. One distinguishing characteristic of the training of psychologists is that it is based upon the singular discipline of psychological science. The training of allied health professionals is multidisciplinary and already premedical and medical in nature. Obtaining prescription privileges did not overhaul the training for those professions and presumably the quest for prescription privileges was not as internally divisive as it is within psychology.

In summary, there is no inherent need for training in psychology to medicalize for the science and profession to thrive. Adequate training in independent prescription privileges would reallocate resources away from psychological science (Chamberlain, 1994) to duplicate what already exists in medical and allied physical health training programs. Training in psychological science does not have to be sacrificed because there are psychologists who wish to seek medical training. Those who wish to independently practice medicine have the opportunity to do so now. The traditional way is to obtain an M.D. (e.g., Kingsbury 1992a, 1992b) but alternative options are developing. As mentioned, in several states nursing programs train for licensed independent prescription authority (DeLeon, 1991-1992, Winter). In addition, the U.S. Department of Defense is evaluating a two year physicians assistant program as medical training for psychologists (DeLeon, 1993, Winter), although this and other physician assistant programs are designed for supervised practice (DeLeon, 1991, April) and the graduates must have medication prescriptions co-signed (DeLeon, 1994, March). The $300,000 per year (Sleek, 1996, February) program will be evaluated by the American College of Neuropsychopharmacology after its termination in July 1997 (DeLeon, 1995). Given the supervisory nature of the training, however, it is not clear if the results would generalize to the independent practice sought by pro-prescription privileges psychologists.

Reason Two: Prescription Privileges Would Undermine Psychological Services

Many who assert that training for prescription privileges would be minimal also assert that the practice of medicine would not detract from the practice of psychology even though, at the same time, the prescribing psychologist presumably would be a "complete provider" (Alne, 1996, January; Burns et al, 1988; Brentar & McNamara, 1991; DeLeon, 1993, April). Those proposing more extensive training have concluded that the practice of psychology would change substantially (APA, 1992; Lorion, 1996). One perspective by Kingsbury (1992a, 1992b), who has an M.D. and Ph.D. in psychology, provides a testimonial of the responsibilities of an independent "prescribing psychologist." He finds that the demand of practicing medicine and keeping up with the psychopharmacology literature precludes dedicating much time to psychotherapy or keeping up to date in psychology. The medicalized psychologist would be responsible for the entire health status of the client and subsequently engaged in highly time-consuming tasks. The time required for continuing education, medical histories, physicals, and consultations with physicians involved with the client would force the prescribing psychologist to dedicate most professional time to medical responsibilities. Another testimonial concerning the demands of medical practice comes from Tim Adams when he was a student in the U.S. Department of Defense Psychopharmacology Demonstration Program mentioned earlier. He states training "emphasizes recognition of what are normal physical findings with an understanding of normal organ functioning. This included using the medical tools and laboratory finding that assist in differentiating pathological vs. normal states of being . . . I am responsible for recognition of physical and psychological pathology, consultation, and appropriate treatment for my patients. . . as a psychologist prescribing medications and being responsible for the physical well-being of a patient, the role is not different from the psychiatrist . . . I spend considerably more time each day being concerned about basic bodily functions than I ever imagined" (DeLeon, 1995, Winter, p.30).

DeNelsky (1990, August) provides evidence that psychiatrists have engaged in less psychotherapy since biological treatments came to be dominant about twenty years ago, and psychiatrists tend to agree that this trend has undermined their profession (McIntyre, 1994, January; Sanua, 1991a, 1991b, 1992; Shapiro, 1991, August). DeNelsky and others argue that the time-efficient intervention of prescribing and the possible quick acting effect of drugs create contingencies that will modify the behavior of psychologists to act more like psychiatrists (DeNelsky, 1990, August, 1996; Soucer, 1991, Fall; Sterling, 1992; Tabin, 1992; Wade, 1992, Winter). As a consequence, the mental health consumer would have fewer opportunities to acquire psychotherapy derived from psychological science. Similarly, other services applied psychologists now provide would also be compromised, such as assessment, supervision, prevention, program evaluation, treatment evaluation, and consultation. The reciprocal nature of psychological science and practice would be interrupted to the demise of both. This abandonment of applied psychology would take place when the field is making great strides in developing effective and cost-efficient interventions (e.g., Fisher & Greenberg, 1995, September/October; Greenberg & Fisher, 1990, January; Sanua, 1995, 1995, April)) and standards of treatment (Hayes, et al., 1995). The prescription privileges advocates have yet to address the rationale for a change in practice when there is strong empirical support and a societal need for psychological strategies.

With applied psychologists medicalized, consumers seeking nonmedical mental health services would need to seek alternatives, such as from social workers (Cantor, 1991, Fall; Moldawsky, 1991, Fall; Sanua, 1993a, 1993c) . However, that option for nonmedical treatment may be short lived. Leaders of the prescription privileges movement for psychologists support the same extension of medical authority to social work (DeLeon, 1991, April; 1991, Fall; Jancin, 1989, June; Sanua, 1993c; Should psychologists prescribe certain drugs?, 1991; Wiggins, 1995, Winter).

While medication is sometimes indicated for psychological problems, applied psychology is not outmoded or stagnant. Many comparative outcome studies conclude that psychotherapy is the treatment of choice (Antonuccio, Danton, & DeNelsky; 1995; Fisher & Greenberg, 1995, September/October; Greenberg & Fisher, 1990, January; Sanua, 1995). Psychology has a secure position in the health professions and will continue to make important contributions to society unless we ourselves choose to abandon the discipline. It has taken decades for the public to appreciate the characteristics that distinguish the practice of psychology from other professions such as psychiatry and social work. Medicalizing psychology would obfuscate the field's unique contributions. The prescription privileges proponents by definition are dissatisfied with the practice of psychology without using chemical interventions. As mentioned earlier, these psychologists may find job satisfaction by going to medical or nursing school. They might find it rewarding to increase collaboration with physicians. However, the pro-prescription privileges literature has not provided convincing evidence or arguments to suggest that collaboration is impossible, or that the practice of psychology has become less valuable and needs replacing. The proponents who assert that the practice of medicine would not detract from the practice of psychology clearly underestimate the nature of medical practice.

Quality comprehensive care cannot be provided by one professional in the mental health field when such care includes situational factors (e.g., housing), psychological factors (e.g., mood regulation skills), and biological factors (e.g., diabetes). Multidisciplinary teams are required for continuity of comprehensive care including social workers, psychologists, and physicians (Center for Alternative Dispute Resolution, 1990; Evans, 1991, November; Kingsbury, 1992b).

Reason Three: There Is Not a Societal Need for Prescription Privileges

Some have argued that it is the obligation of psychologists to obtain authority to prescribe psychotropic medication because there are many consumers who need these drugs and they cannot get them (Burns et al., 1988;DeLeon, Sammons, & Sexton, 1995). Underserved medical mental health consumers are said to include children, the elderly, those living in rural areas, and people with chronic disorders (Board of Professional Affairs, 1989). Proponents of prescription privileges claim there is a shortage of psychiatrists and other physicians adequately trained to prescribe psychotropic medication. It is noted that about 70% of these medications are prescribed by nonpsychiatric physicians (DeLeon, 1992, January), although no evidence of malpractice or lack of collaboration with mental health specialists is presented. Collaboration with physicians is viewed as not viable because of a perceived interruption in the continuity of care (Brentar & McNamara, 1991). Proponents of prescription privileges conclude that psychologists trained to prescribe would alleviate the shortage of physicians by practicing in rural areas and public institutions. It has been argued that prescription privileges for other nonmedical mental health professions, including social work, could also alleviate such shortages (DeLeon, 1991, Fall). However, a shortage of physicians has not been established (Barkley, 1991, Spring), malpractice or difficulty with collegial collaboration have not been demonstrated, and it has yet to be shown that consumers are clamoring for more drugs.

Surveys indicate that the United States does not have a shortage of physicians and the geographic distribution of psychologists and physicians is similar, but there is some geographic maldistribution of most professionals, including psychiatrists and psychologists (Public Health Service, 1995; Shellow & Coleman, 1991). One survey reports that 20% of applied psychologists practice in rural settings (Egli, 1991, Fall), but the adequacy of this distribution was not evaluated. Another survey reported that only 10% of psychologists would be willing to volunteer time to serve the chronically mentally ill, one of the underserved populations (APA, 1990). Applied psychologists are licensed to practice in rural areas and public mental health institutions but have not been shown to do so more than psychiatrists (May & Belsky, 1992). Clearly, claims that psychologists are more altruistic than physicians are unfounded.

Possible shortage problems must be resolved so that incentives are provided for all health professionals to serve the underserved (Evans, 1991, November; Korbelnig, 1995, August). Such incentives include policies that encourage and reimburse multidisciplinary treatment (Center for Alternative Dispute Resolution, 1990; Heiby, 1992). Prescription privileges for nonmedical mental health professionals, such as psychologists and social workers, would not resolve the geographic maldistribution problem.

Claims that psychologists (and, perhaps, social workers) would do a better job prescribing psychotropic medication than physicians and other medical health professionals (APA, 1990; DeLeon, 1993, Winter) are simply not substantiated. Such attacks upon medicine reflect poorly upon the discipline of psychology and suggest an uncollegial attitude (Raphael, 1990, Winter). Collegiality with medicine is essential for collaboration in research and training and in the provision of comprehensive care for the mental health consumer.

Such collaboration is dictated by psychology's professional ethics and is commonly practiced (Cavaliere, 1995, July; Committee concerned about , 1995, November; DeLeon, 1991, Fall). One survey reported that 85% of applied psychologists regularly consult with a physician and 78% have regularly been consulted by one (Barkley, 1991, Spring). Thus, collaboration among mental health professionals already exists and can address societal needs for comprehensive care (Heiby, 1994).

Collaboration might be enhanced by a Committee on Interprofessional Affairs including state and national organizations representing mental health service providers, supervisors, policy makers, and academicians (Heiby, 1992). One pilot program has demonstrated that brief training can increase the rate of collaboration between psychologists and physicians and improve the quality of treatment in rural areas (Bray & Rogers, 1995, Fall). There is also evidence that psychologists can effectively collaborate as equal members in primary health care teams, and guidelines to facilitate this transition have been developed (DeAngelis, 1995, October). Therefore, continuity of care concerns of the proponents of prescription privileges could be addressed by integrated care that is being encouraged by the health care industry. In fact, the organizational structure of some managed care companies requires collaboration. For example, some policies reimburse for prescriptions only if they are written by the primary care physician who often does so at the direct recommendation of a specialist. Prescription authority for psychologists would be irrelevant under such circumstances.

Maintaining disciplinary boundaries may be the preference of the mental health consumer. A survey of the general adult population found that the preferred solution to solving a mental health problem was psychotherapy for 63% and medication for 15% of the respondents (APA, 1992). Other general public surveys have found that about 75% are more comfortable seeking services of psychologists than psychiatrists who are viewed as too ready to prescribe medication (Sanua, 1993b, August; 1994, August; 1995).

It would also reduce health care costs if providers collaborate rather than train in each other's specialties. As mentioned earlier, there is no question that the inherent expense of prescription privileges for psychologists would increase the cost of service delivery. Taxpayers and consumers would eventually pay for the more expensive training, regulation, malpractice, and continuing education. Whether or not medication may seem indicated, the prescribing psychologist may have to routinely refer clients to a physician if prescription privileges training is anything short of a medical degree, also adding to the expense of psychological practice.

In conclusion, the rationale that prescription privileges are needed to responsibly address societal needs has not been supported. There is not a national shortage of physicians but some geographic maldistribution of all health professionals. Collaboration among psychologists and physicians can provide continuity of care for underserved populations and reduce overall health care costs.

Reason Four: Financial Gain Is Not A Valid Argument

All health professionals are facing reduced incomes and adjusting to cost containment policies and psychologists are no exception (Hayes & Heiby, 1996). Managed care has reduced the income of those accustomed to working in a private practice without capitation of services. Managed care industries also hire subdoctoral level mental health professionals to provide psychotherapy, reducing the market for those psychologists who do not provide diversified services (Hayes & Heiby, 1996; Humphreys, 1996). To exacerbate matters, there may be an oversupply of psychologists (Moses, 1992, March). The response of some applied psychologists is to make more money as psychotherapists who prescribe. Some proponents of prescription privileges make it clear that this financial motive justifies medicalizing psychology (Clark, 1994, Spring;DeLeon, 1993, Summer; Litwin & Goswell, 1989, August; Samuels, 1994, Fall; Wiggins, 1995, Winter). Critics have suggested that it is the primary motive and an unfitting reason for any professional activity (Bruner, 1995; Roberson, 1995, September).

Some proponents of prescription privileges argue that if psychologists could practice medicine, they would be more competitive with physicians and social workers in the health care market. (DeLeon, 1994, Fall; Forman, 1992-1993, Fall; Fox, 1988a; Minke, 1994, Fall). Financial resources for prescribing psychologists are paraded. It is noted that in 1991 psychotherapeutic drugs was a $1.3 billion industry with 135,896,000 prescriptions written (DeLeon, 1992, January). It is suggested that psychologists should be able to recoup more of their educational financial investment, noting psychologists recoup three times and psychiatrists six times the investment (DeLeon, 1993, Fall). DeNelsky (1990, August; 1996) also concludes that pro-prescription privileges psychologists are more likely to prescribe medication than conduct psychotherapy because they are clearly responding to financial motives that more quickly and more handsomely reinforce writing prescriptions than the hard work of psychotherapy. Karon (1994, Fall) agrees, pointing out that psychologists who support prescription privileges would elect to make more money giving drugs (up to $300,000 per year) than conducting psychotherapy (up to $100,000 per year).

The reduced incomes and oversupply of psychologists are problems facing the discipline that call for solutions that consider what is best for the science, profession, and consumer (Karbelnig, 1995, August).   There are many ways to address the marketability of applied psychology. Psychologists must respond to the changing contingencies of the health care industry, as do all health care professionals. One response is to acknowledge that applied psychologists can no longer rely upon the provision of psychotherapy as the only marketable skill (Humphreys, 1996; Hayes & Heiby, 1996). While there is still a need for doctoral psychotherapy providers, some studies have demonstrated that subdoctoral providers can be effective and cost-efficient (Berman & Norton, 1985; Christensen & Jacobson, 1994). Psychology still offers unique services that go far beyond individual psychotherapy and does not have to duplicate psychiatry to be viable in the health care market (Committee concerned about, 1995, November).

Applied psychologists are trained to provide scientifically-derived and thus cost-effective services that are wanted by the health care industry (Hayes, 1995, Spring). Managed care organizations expect efficacious treatment which psychologists have been trained to provide and supervise (Hayes & Heiby, 1996). In addition, psychologists are also trained to conduct treatment outcome evaluations, consultation with management, consumer satisfaction surveys, inservice training, policy evaluations, quality assurance, forensic work, divorce mediation, prevention services, child custody evaluations, career counseling, administration (Levy, 1995, Fall), health policy analysis, needs assessment, cost-benefit analyses, and multidisciplinary team work (Humphreys, 1996; Murray, 1995, April). Psychologists can promote how psychological treatment can prevent physical illness by reducing disease-promoting behavior and by enhancing compliance to medical regimens (Humphreys, 1996; Yates, 1994). As already noted, psychologists can become equal members of primary health care teams (DeAngelis, 1995, October).

The quest to practice medicine instead of advocating psychology suggests that there are some psychologists lacking self-confidence, pride, and perhaps the competence to practice effective, and thus marketable, services (Greene, 1995, September, 1995, Fall; Evans, 1993). The economic relevance of applied psychology can be retained by providing continuing education for those who need to learn and advocate these well-established services to society.

If there is an oversupply of psychologists as one estimate suggests (Moses, 1992, March), then training programs must also reduce the number of graduates in applied psychology. Some have argued there is a need for 1 psychologist per 100,000 people while the national average is currently 23 per 100,000 with only four states with fewer than the average (Moses). There are 65,000 licensed doctoral psychologists in the United States, which creates a mental health services market unlike any other country where subdoctoral training is more common (Peterson, 1996). An extensive supply of applied psychologists may be one reason pharmaceutical companies have been supportive of prescription privileges (Egli, 1991, Summer; Egli, 1994, Fall; Sanua, 1994).

Prescription privileges would not resolve concerns about an oversupply of applied psychologists or a reduction in income that is also experienced by physicians. The excess number of applied psychologists will be resolved by market factors. Prescription privileges' possible increase in practice opportunities and income would be fleeting (DeNelsky, 1990, August, 1996; Hayes & Heiby, 1996). Prescription privileges for psychologists would set the precedent for other nonmedical providers, such as social workers and counselors (DeLeon, 1991, Fall; Jancin, 1989, June). The authority to prescribe would not secure psychology a place in the health care market when both medical and nonmedical as well as doctoral and subdoctoral providers are licensed to prescribe (Hayes & Heiby, 1996).

Reason Five: Prescription Privileges Involve an Erosion of Ethics and Standards

As the finanical motive illustrates, one of the more troubling aspects of the prescription privileges movement is the implications for the field's code of ethics and standards of professional conduct. One of the early proponents of prescription privileges acknowledged that practicing medicine violated ethical standards and suggested that these standards be revised to accommodate what previously had been deemed unacceptable (Fox, 1988a). The American Psychological Association's standards for practice (Board of Professional Affairs, 1987) indicate that psychologists are obligated to collaborate with physicians and those who wish to practice medicine should meet society's standards for practice, not create new ones. Specifically, the Board asserts "Psychologists who change or add a specialty meet the same requirements with respect to subject matter and professional skills that apply to *doctoral* education, training, and experience in the new specialty" (p.715; emphasis added) and "In the best interest of the users, providers of psychological services endeavor to consult and collaborate with professional colleagues in the planning and delivery of services when such consultation is deemed appropriate" (p. 716).

Erosion of ethical standards became apparent in the most recent ethical code of conduct (APA, 1992b) which omits standards from the earlier version (Ethical principles, 1981). Of relevance to the prescription privileges movement, the current code omits forbidding provision of duplicate services by other professionals. The 1981 code stated in Principle 7b "If a person is receiving similar services from another professional, psychologists do not offer their own services directly to such a person" (p.636). It seems the stage had been set for psychologists to compete with psychiatrists for patients.

Proponents of prescription privileges seem to reject some of the American Psychological Association's (Board of Professional Affairs 1987) standards out of hand. Collaboration is declared inadequate or unnecessary (DeLeon, 1991, Fall). Proposals for training programs do not even come close to a doctoral degree in medicine, sometimes requiring only 100 hours (Folen, 1994) and some have argued this is too extensive (Prescribing psychologists' register, 1995, August/September). Training programs in prescription privileges that do not exist have been advertised

(DeLeon, 1991, August; DeLeon, 1993, January). Several proponents of prescription privileges proudly admit that many psychologists currently practice medicine without a license to do so (Clipson & Hamell, 1994, September). This malpractice is not seen as troubling to proponents and is seemingly justified by DeLeon who stated "prescribing is a little function which is really no big deal – except for turf reasons" (Jancin, 1989, June; p.1) and "prescription privileges is no big deal. It's like learning how to use a desk-top computer" (DeLeon, Sept. 7, 1993, p. E6) and "everyone says this medication works" (Youngstrom, 1990, June; p. 13). Similarly, Minke (1995, Spring) claims learning to prescribe is not a complex skill, and others (Fox, 1988b; Rodgers,1995, May-June) assert psychotropic drugs are not harmful. Documentation of the toxic and sometimes lethal effects of psychotropic medication (e.g., Antonuccio et al., 1995; Breggin & Tinauer, 1992, November; Sanua, 1992, August; 1993a, 1993c, August) is summarily ignored.

Many of the motives for prescription privileges described by some proponents also do not fit the discipline's historical standards for quality service but instead appear downright self-serving (Evans, 1991, November; 1993; Greene, 1992, June, 1995, September, 1995, Fall). These explicitly stated motives include not only financial gain (Brentar & McNamara; Clark, 1994, Spring;DeLeon, 1993, Summer; Litwin & Goswell, 1989, August; Forman, 1992-1993, Fall; Minke, 1994, Fall; Samuels, 1994, Fall; Wiggins, 1995, Winter) but also greater professional self-esteem (Brentar & McNamara, 1991; Forman, 1992-1993, Fall; Rodgers, 1995, May-June) and an explicit desire to destroy the profession of psychiatry along with unsubstantiated critiques of the quality of medical practice (DeLeon, 1993, Winter).

Evans (1993) has suggested ethics have become eroded over prescription privileges because this idea evolved from politics rather than scholarship. He wonders if pro-prescription privileges psychologists are insecure in their ability to implement effective psychotherapy, and thus are seeking alternative routes to "gain wealth, prestige, personal power, etc., rather than a desire to help patients" (Evans, 1991, November, p.4). Greene (1995, September; 1995, Fall) agrees with Evans' points and adds that the pro-prescription privileges literature reflects poorly on the profession by suggesting not altruism as claimed, but a naiveté' and disrespect toward medicine and psychiatry, difficulty accepting limitations of competence, and an inability to accept the ambiguities of the profession.

Psychology has been authorized by licensing as an autonomous profession because it introduced empirically-supported psychological interventions in treatment and prevention settings. These advances of the discipline have been science-driven and based upon the highest of ethical and professional standards. The current prescription privileges proposals did not develop from a reciprocal influence between practice and research, but seemingly derive from precipitous guild concerns of practitioners. The adoption of minimal and substandard medical procedures by applied psychologists grossly erodes the ethics and standards that have been distinguishing characteristics of psychology. This erosion of ethical standards also seems hypocritical. On the one hand, pro-prescription privileges psychologists argue that the field can easily acquire the expertise necessary to encroach heavily on the domain of medicine. One the other hand, the American Psychological Association insists that other mental health professionals (e.g., social workers) could not possibly perform functions that psychology has abrogated to itself (Sleek, 1995, January).

The need to adopt stronger standards for psychology fortunately has been recognized (e.g., Dawes, 1994; McFall, 1996). The American Association of Applied and Preventive Psychology (AAAPP) has responded to this need and is in the process of developing scientific and ethical standards for applied psychology (Hayes et al., 1995). While AAAPP has been at the forefront in denouncing the prescription privileges movement (Resolution opposing prescription privileges, 1995), it has done so responsibly by offering honorable alternatives for psychologists to adapt to the climate of the health care market without losing its very soul (Hayes et al., 1995).

Conclusion

Despite these five concerns, the recent legislative drive for prescription privileges is partly justified by some surveys that have indicated that there is a significant interest in prescription privileges (e.g., APA, 1990, 1992c; DeLeon, 1994, Fall; Prescription privileges survey, 1995). However, this interest may be only skin deep. Surveys cited by pro-prescription psychologists do not constitute a mandate or consensus on this issue. Other surveys report that a majority opposes prescription privileges (Litwin & Goswell, 1989, August; Piotrowski & Lubin, 1989; *The Scientist Practitioner*, 1993). In addition, surveys concluding support for prescription privileges have been critiqued on sampling, generalizability, and the use of biased and incomplete questions designed to elicit positive responses (Braun, 1992, Fall; Moldawsky, 1991, Fall). Even among those psychologists who support prescription privileges, not many of them are willing to pursue additional training for such privileges (DeLeon, 1990-1991, Winter), suggesting that respondents' support for medicalizing psychology may be quite weak. Recently, Piotrowski (1996) found that only nine percent of 500 respondents would be interested in completing a one to two year training program for prescription privileges. Perhaps the previously noted negative effects of prescription privileges upon training, service, consumers, marketability, and ethics have been persuasive. After all, the majority of the articles opposing prescription privileges has been published since most surveys indicating support of prescription privileges were conducted.

So why are some psychologists seeking legislation to obtain prescription privileges without a preponderance of support? Why does the American Psychological Association ignore the opponents of prescription privileges (McColskey, 1993, Winter)? As mentioned earlier, in 1996 legislation was introduced in California, Missouri, and Hawaii. Given the divisiveness of this issue within psychology, it is no surprise that all bills failed or were withdrawn. However, more than a loss of a particular prescription privileges bill has resulted. Psychology has many agenda items at state legislatures and may appear less persuasive on other issues if it presents as a divided house on any one of them. It is premature to seek prescription privileges at state legislatures, and doing so can damage the discipline's relationship with policy makers. The damage within the science and profession is far more serious. Those who support prescription privileges need to address the reasons others oppose it in a collegial, rather than adversarial and judicial manner. Finally, those who oppose prescription privileges need to work toward solving the underlying problems, including an oversupply of psychologists, a need to train for the changing health care market and multidisciplinary teamwork, and an erosion of the discipline's ethics and standards of practice. I hope this AAAPP conference will encourage our colleagues to debate, not legislate.

References

Alne, D. J. (1996, January). Prescription privileges: The time is now. *NYS Psychologist*, 18.

American Psychological Association (1990). *Survey of American Psychological Association members*. Washington, D.C.

American Psychological Association (1992a). *Report of the ad hoc task force on psychopharmacology of the American Psychological Association*. Washington, D.C.

American Psychological Association (1992b). Ethical principles of psychologists and code of conduct. *American Psychologist, 47*, 1597-1611.

American Psychological Association (1992c). *Survey of general population of the United States on prescription privileges for psychologists*. Washington, D.C.

Antonuccio, D. O., Danton, W. G., & DeNelsky, G. Y. (1995). Psychotherapy versus medication for depression: Challenging the conventional wisdom with data. *Professional Psychology: Research and Practice, 26*, 574-585.

Barkley, R. A. (1991, Spring). Health services committee: Prescribing privileges for health psychologists: Implications from the clinical child psychology task force. *The Health Psychologist, 13* (1), 2.

Barron, J. (1989). Prescription rights: Pro and con: Should psychologists seek the same skills and responsibilities as psychiatrists? *The Psychotherapy Bulletin, 24* (3), 22-24.

Berman, J. S. & Norton, N. C. (1985). Does professional training make a therapist more effective? *Psychotherapy Bulletin, 98*, 401-407.

Bernay, T. (1994, Fall). Prescribing privileges are good for psychology, including psychoanalysis. *Psychologist-Psychoanalyst, 14* (4), 14-16.

Board of Professional Affairs (1987). General guidelines for providers of psychological services. *American Psychologist, 42*, 712-723.

Board of Professional Affairs (Nov. 9-12, 1989). *Resolution regarding prescription privileges for psychologists*. Unpublished manuscript.

Braun, J. A. (1992, Fall). Letter to the editor. *The Independent Practitioner, 12* (4), 186.

Bray, J. H. & Rogers, J. C. (1995, Fall). Linking psychologists and family physicians for collaborative practice. *The Independent Practitioner, 15* (4), 178-179.

Breggin, P. R. & Tinauer, L. (1992, November). Letter to the editor. *Monitor, 23* (1), 3.

Brentar, J. & McNamara, J. R. (1991). The right to prescribe medication: Considerations for professional psychology. *Professional Psychology: Research and Practice, 22,* 179-187.

Bruner, R. L. (1995). Letter to the editor. *The Independent Practitioner, 15*(3), 145-146.

Buie, J. (1989, July). Psychiatry loses edge on market new study shows. *APA Monitor,* p.30.

Burns, S. M., DeLeon, P. H., Chemtob, C. M., Welch, B. L. & Samuels, R. M. (1988). *Psychotherapy, 25,* 508-515.

Butz, M. R. (1994). Psychopharmacology: Psychology's Jurassic Park? *Psychotherapy, 31,* 692-697.

Cantor, D. W. (1991, Fall). The prescription privilege debate: Not now, maybe never. *The Independent Practitioner, 11* (4), 13-14.

Cavaliere, F. (1995, July). Psychologists as medication advisors. *APA Monitor, 26* (7), 40.

Center for Alternative Dispute Resolution (1990). *Improving treatment and services for people with serious mental illnesses: A report from the Mental Health Roundtable submitted to the 15th legislature in response to senate resolution 77.* Hawaii State Legislature, Honolulu, HI.

Chamberlain, L. (1994). Psychopharmacology: Further adventures in psychology's Jurassic Park. *Psychotherapy, 29,* 47-50.

Christensen, A. & Jacobson, N. S. (1994). Who (or what) can do psychotherapy: The status and challenge of nonprofessional therapies. *Psychological Science, 5,* 8-14.

Clark, J. H. (1994, Spring). Prescription privileges? Not for everyone. *AAP Advance, 10,* 21.

Clipson, C. R. & Hammell, B. F. (1994, September). The privilege of prescribing. *San Diego Psychologist, 3* (8), 1-3.

Committee concerned about the medicalization of psychology formed (1995, November). *The Scientist-Practitioner, 5* (1), 3,5.

Committee recommends stand to be taken against prescription privileges. (1995, March). *The Scientist-Practitioner, 4,* 8 -10.

Dawes, R. M. (1994). *House of cards: Psychology and psychotherapy built on myth.* New York: The Free Press.

DeAngelis, T. (1995, October) Primary-care collaborations growing. *APA Monitor, 26* (10), 22.

Deardorff, W. W., Cross, H. J., & Hupprich, W. R. (1984). Malpractice liability in psychotherapy: Client and practitioner perspectives. *Professional Psychology: Research and Practice, 15,* 590-600.

DeLeon, P. H. (1990, April). Psychoactive medications: The debate reaches Hawaii's legislature. *Register Report, 16* (2), 9-10.

DeLeon, P. H. (1990, Summer). Washington Scene. *The Psychotherapy Bulletin, 25* (2), 7-10.

DeLeon, P. H. (1990-1991, Winter). Prescription privileges—the APA governance. *The Psychotherapy Bulletin, 25* (4), 8-11.

DeLeon, P. H. (1991, April). The Department of Defense prescription project—doing fine. *Register Report, 17* (1), 12-14.

DeLeon, P. H. (1991, August). Prescription privileges: A training and "scope of practice" issue. *Register Report, 17* (2), 4-6.

DeLeon, P. H. (1991, Fall). Prescription privileges-A gradually maturing concept. *The Psychotherapy Bulletin, 26* (3), 6-10.

DeLeon, P. H. (1991-1992, Winter). Prescription privileges-the evolution continues. *The Psychotherapy Bulletin, 26* (4), 7-9.

DeLeon, P. H. (1992, January). National health insurance-alive and doing well. *Register Report, 18* (1), 4-6.

DeLeon, P. H. (1992, August). Prescription privileges: Continuing progress "scope of practice" issue. *Register Report, 18* (3), 4,15-16.

DeLeon, P. H. (1993, January). PASARR-a nice success story. *Register Report, 19* (1), 17-19.

DeLeon, P. H. (1993, September). Untitled. *Los Angeles Times*, Sept. 7, p. E6.

DeLeon, P. H. (1993, Winter). Prescription privileges debate continues. *Hawaii Psychologist, 15* (1), 11.

DeLeon, P. H. (1993, April). Prescription privileges-evolution within APA governance. *Register Report, 19* (2), 12-13.

DeLeon, P. H. (1993, Spring). Prescription privileges-evolving progress. *The Psychotherapy Bulletin, 28* (1), 7-10.

DeLeon, P. H. (1993, Summer). The Clinton-Gore national health reform movement. *The Psychotherapy Bulletin, 28* (2), 6-10.

DeLeon, P. H. (1993, Fall). Prescription privileges-a qualitative difference. *The Psychotherapy Bulletin, 28* (3), 10-13.

DeLeon, P. H. (1993, Winter). Prescription privileges-some interesting observations. *The Independent Practitioner, 13* (1), 38-40.

DeLeon, P. H. (1994, March). The maturation of the prescription privilege evolution within the APA governance. *Register Report, 20* (1), 16-18.

DeLeon, P. H. (1994, Fall). The prescription privilege agenda: Developments at the state level. *The Independent Practitioner, 14* (5), 239-241.

DeLeon, P. H. (1995, Fall). The DoD project: Perilous but interesting times. *The Independent Practitioner, 15* (4) 169-171.

DeLeon, P. H. (1995, Winter). Prescription privileges: Exciting federal developments. *The Independent Practitioner, 15* (1), 30-31.

DeLeon, P. H. (1995). Progress on prescription privileges. *The Independent Practitioner, 15* (3), 122-123.

DeLeon, P. H. (1996, Winter). Prescription privileges: Beyond the navy experience. *The Independent Practitioner, 16* (1), 15-17.

DeLeon, P. H., Fox, R. E., & Graham, S. R. (1991). Prescription privileges: Psychology's next frontier? *American Psychologist, 46*, 384-393.

DeLeon, P. H., Sammons, M. T., & Sexton, J. L. (1995). Focusing on society's real needs: Responsibility and prescription privileges. *American Psychologist, 50*, 1022-1032.

DeLeon, P. H. & Wiggins, J. G. (1996). Prescription privileges for psychologists. *American Psychologist, 51,* 225-229.

DeNelsky, G. Y. (1990, August). *The case against prescription privileges for psychologists.* Paper presented at the 1990 convention of the American Psychological Association, August, Boston, MS.

DeNelsky, G. Y. (1996). The case against prescription privileges for psychologists. *American Psychologist, 51,* 207-212.

Egli, D. (1991, Summer). Expanded psychological practice committee (EPPC) report. *The Independent Practitioner, 22* (3), 15-16.

Egli, D. (1991, Fall). Expanded psychological practice committee (EPPC). *The Independent Practitioner, 11* (4), 21-23.

Egli, D. (1994, Fall). Psychopharmacology in independent practice: Prescription privileges. *The Independent Practitioner, 14* (5),218-219.

Ethical Principles of Psychologists. (1981). *American Psychologist, 36,* 633-638.

Evans, I. M. (1991, November). *Values in behavior therapy: Implications for training clinical students from the "me" generation.* Paper presentation at the panel entitled "Prescription privileges, for example. . . ," Steven Hayes, Chair, at the annual meeting of the Association for Advancement of Behavior Therapy, November 22, New York, New York.

Evans, I. M. (1993). Prescription privileges for psychologists: A crisis of self-confidence and leadership. *The Scientist-Practitioner, 3* (1), 18-21.

Fisher, S. & Greenberg, R. P. (1995, September/October). Prescriptions for Happiness? *Psychology Today.* 32-37.

Folen, R. (1994). Letter to the editor. *Hawaii Psychologist, 17,* 6.

Forman, B. D. (1992-1993, Fall). Prescription privileges: The marketing view. *The Psychotherapy Bulletin, 27* (3),14.

Fox, R. E. (1988a). Prescription privileges: Their implications for the practice of psychology. *Psychotherapy, 25,* 501-507.

Fox. R. E. (1988b). Some practical and legal objections to prescription privileges for psychologists. *Psychotherapy in Private Practice, 6,* 23-30.

Fox, R. E., Schwelitz, F. D. & Barclay, A. G. (1992). A proposed curriculum for psychopharmacology training for professional psychologists. *Professional Psychology: Research and Practice, 23,* 216-219.

Garfield, S. L. (1995). Letter to the editor. *APA Monitor, 26* (7). Letters to the editor, 3.

George Albee: Founder of true community care (1995, November). *The Psychologist,* 510-511.

Graham, S. (1990). APA President Stanley Graham addresses HPA-OPA conference. *Hawaii Psychologist, 13* (2), 4-5.

Greenberg, R. P. & Fisher, S. (1990, January). To prescribe or not to prescribe. *National Register, 16* (1), 5, 10-11.

Greene, J. T. (1992, June). Letter to the editor. *APA Monitor, 23* (6), 3.

Greene, J. T. (1995, September). Letter to the editor. *The National Psychologist, 4* (5)

Greene, J. T. (1995, Fall). Letter to the editor. *The Independent Practitioner, 15* (4), 193.

Hayes, S. C. (1995, Spring). Using behavioral science to control guild excesses. *The Clinical Behavior Analyst*, pp. 1 & 17.

Hayes, S. C., Follette, V. M., Dawes, R. M., & Grady, K. E. (1995). *Scientific standards of psychological practice: Issues and recommendations*. Reno, NV: Context Press.

Hayes, S. C. & Heiby, E. M. (1996). Psychology's drug problem: Do we need a fix or should we just say no? *American Psychologist ,51*, 198 - 206.

Hayes, S. C., Walser, R. D., & Follette, V. M. (1996). Psychology and the temptation of prescription privileges. *Canadian Psychology/Psychologie canadienne, 36*, 313-320.

Heiby, E. M. (1992). *Some questions and concerns regarding psychologists prescribing medication.* Paper presentation at the meeting of the American Psychiatric Association's Joint State Legislative and Public Affairs Institute, Miami, February 28-March 1, 1992.

Heiby, E. M. (1994, Fall). A rejoinder to Minke's "Prescription privileges revisited". *Hawaii Psychologist, 17* (3), 3-4.

Humphreys, K. (1996). Clinical psychologists as psychotherapists. *American Psychologist, 51*, 190-197.

Jancin, B. (1989, June). Says psychologists will win prescribing privileges fight. *Psychiatry News ,1*.

Jansen, M. & Barron, J. (1988). Introduction and overview: Psychologists use of physical interventions. *Psychotherapy, 25*, 487-491.

Jennings, F. L. (1988, December). *Psychologists and prescription privileges*. Unpublished manuscript.

Karbelnig, A. (1995, August). Prescription privileges: An iatrogenic disease for psychology. *The California Psychologist, 28* (8), 22-23.

Karon, B. P. (1994, Fall). The Prescription Privilege Initiative and Division 39. *Psychologist-Psychoanalyst, 14* (4), 16-18.

Kingsbury, S. J.(1992a). Some effects of prescribing privileges. *American Psychologist, 47*, 426-427.

Kingsbury, S. J. (1992b). Some effects of prescribing privileges. *Professional Psychology: Research and Practice, 23*, 3-5.

Klein, R. G. (1996). Comments on expanding the clinical role of psychologists. *American Psychologist, 51*, 216-218.

Levy, A. (1995, Fall). Whither psychologists? The role of psychologists in the near future. *The Independent Practitioner, 15* (4), 183-184.

Litwin, W. J. & Goswell, D. L. (1989, August). *Limited prescription privileges for psychologists: Is there a consensus?* Paper presentation at the annual convention of the American Psychological Association, New Orleans, LA.

Lorion, R. P. (1996). Applying our medicine to the psychopharmacology debate. *American Psychologist, 51*, 219-224.

Martin, S. (1995, September). APA to pursue prescription privileges. *APA Monitor*, p.6.

May, W. T. & Belsky, J. (1992). Response to "Prescription privileges: Psychology's next frontier?" or the siren call: Should psychologists medicate?. *American Psychologist, 47,* 427.

McColskey, A. S. (1991, September). Letter to the editor. *The Independent Practitioner, 11* (3).

McColskey, A. S. (1993, Winter). Letter to the editor. *The Independent Practitioner, 13* (1), 57.

McFall, R. M. (1996). Making psychology incorruptible. *Applied & Preventive Psychology, 5,* 9-15.

McIntyre, J. (1994, January). Don't throw the couch out. *Psychiatric News, 24* (2), 3.

McNamara, J. R. (1991). Some unresolved challenges facing psychology's entrance into the health care field. *Professional Psychology, 12,* 391-399.

Minke, K. A. (1994, Fall). Prescription privileges revisited. *Hawaii Psychologists, 17* (3) , 2,4.

Minke, K. A. (1995, Spring). HPA President Minke shares thoughts on prescriptions. *Hawaii Psychologist, 18* (2), 6-7.

Moldawsky, S. (1991, Fall). Say no to drugs. *The Independent Practitioner, 11* (4) 14-17.

Moldawsky, S. (1992, November). Letter to the editor. *Monitor, 23* (1), 3-4.

Moses. S. (1992, March). Too many clinicians? Articles debate issue. *Monitor, 23* (3), 44-45.

Murray, B. (1995, April). Legal issues, managed care top educators' priorities. *APA Monitor ,26* (4), 45-46.

Pachman, J. S. (1996). The dawn of a revolution in mental health. *American Psychologist, 51,* 213-215.

Peterson, D. R. (1996). Making psychology indispensable. *Applied & Preventive Psychology, 5,* 1 - 8.

Piotrowski, C. (1989-1990, Winter). Prescription privileges: A time for some serious thought. *The Psychotherapy Bulletin,* 16-18.

Piotrowski, C. & Keller, J. W. (1996, March). *Do psychologists want to be retrained for prescription privileges?* Paper presentation at the Southeastern Psychological Association, Norfolk, VA.

Piotrowski, C. & Keller, J.W. (1996). Prescription privileges and training issues for practicing psychologists. *Psychological Reports, 78,* 445-446.

Piotrowski, C. & Lubin, B. (1989). Prescription privileges: A view from health psychologists. *The Clinical Psychologist, 42* (3), 83-84.

Karon, B. P. (1994, Fall). The Prescription Privilege Initiative and Division 39. *Psychologist-Psychoanalyst, 14* (4), 16-18.

Prescribing Psychologists' Register Inc. Memorandum (August/September, 1995). Unpublished manuscript.

Prescription privilege for psychologists: APA takes historic action (1995, Fall). *AAP Advance,* 1, 12.

Prescription privileges for psychologists debate at the Hawaii Psychological Association Meeting (1990, July 5). Honolulu, HI.

Prescription privileges survey. (1995). *Hawaii Psychologist, 18* (1), 2.

Public Health Service, Division of Shortage Designation, Bureau of Primary Health Care, HRSA (September 30, 1995). Selected Statistics on Health Professional Shortage Areas as of September 30, 1995. Rockville, MD.

Raphael, S. (1990, Winter). Great satan strikes again. *Newsletter of the New York Society of Clinical Psychologists, Inc., 23* (2), 1,5.

Resolution opposing prescription privileges for psychologists.(1995). *The Scientist Practitioner, 4,*4.

Roberson, K. (1995, September). Letter to the editor. *California Psychologist, 28* (9).

Rodgers, D.A. (1995, May-June). *The National Psychologist,* 14.

Saeman, H. (1995). Science group deplores 'medicalizing psychology, plans guerrilla war' against prescription privileges. *The National Psychologist, 4* (2), 3.

Samuels, R. (1994, Fall). Expanded independent practice: The early years. *The Independent Practitioner, 14* (5) 217-218.

Sanua. V. D. (1991a, Summer). An Overview: A history of "miracle" cures in the treatment of mental disorders. *The Rights Tenet, 6,*11.

Sanua, V. D. (1991b, May). Undue emphasis on organic etiology of mental disorders? *International Psychologist, 7*877.

Sanua, V. D. (1992). To prescribe or not to prescribe? That's not the question! *The New York State Psychologist, 13* (1), 27,51.

Sanua, V. D. (1992, August). *Psychotropic drugs: Prescription for disaster: A review of the literature on the side-effects of psychiatric drugs.* Paper presentation at the annual convention of the American Psychological Association, Washington, D.C.

Sanua, V. D. (1993a, August). *Prescription privileges versus psychologists' authority! Why I am against the use of psychotropic drugs.* Paper presented at the annual convention of the American Psychological Association, Toronto, Ontario.

Sanua, V. D. (1993b, August). *Perceptions of psychologists and psychiatrists.* Paper presented at the annual convention of the American Psychological Association, Toronto, Ontario.

Sanua, V. D. (1993c, August). *A critical appraisal of DeLeon's columns on prescription privileges which appeared in the "National Register": Written from the bottom of the hill!.* Paper presented at the annual convention of the American Psychological Association, Toronto, Ontario.

Sanua, V. D. (1994). Quo vadis APA? Inroads of the medical model. *The Humanistic Psychologist, 22,* 3-27.

Sanua, V. D. (1995, April). Prescription privileges: A response. *NYSPA Notebook, 7(4).*

Sanua, V. D. (1995). "Prescription privileges" vs. psychologists' authority: Psychologists do better without drugs. *The Humanist Psychologist, 23,* 187-212.

The Scientist Practitioner (1993, December; vol 3(4)).

Shapiro, L. E. (1991, August). APA and drug companies: Too close for comfort. *Psychiatric News, 14,*20.

Shellow, R. A. & Coleman, P. (1991). *Prescribing privileges for psychologists: Should only "medicine men" control the medicine cabinet?* Unpublished manuscript.

Should psychologist prescribe certain drugs? (anonymous, 1991, January). *Health Letter, 7* (1), 1-2.

Sleek, S. (1995, January). Managed care sharpens master's-degree debate. *Monitor, 26* (1), 8-9.

Sleek, S. (1996, February). Congress grants extension to prescription privileges. *Monitor, 27* (2), 34.

Sorotzkin, B. (1991). Letter to the editor. *The Psychotherapy Bulletin, 26,* 6.

Soucar, E. (1991, Fall). A bitter pill. *The Independent Practitioner, 11* (4), 12-13.

Sterling, M. E. (1982). Must psychology lose its soul?. *Professional Psychology, 13,* 789-796.

Tabin, J. K. (1992, Fall). Letter to the editor. *The Independent Practitioner, 12* (4) 187.

Wade, T. C. (1992, Winter). Tranmorgrification of psychology: Prescription "privileges" for us? *Hawaii Psychologist, 15* (1), 12-14.

Wiggins, J. G. (1995, Winter). Psychopharmacotherapy: How much training is necessary? *The Independent Practitioner, 15* (1)32-34.

Yates, B. T. (1984). How psychology can improve effectiveness and reduce costs of health services. *Psychotherapy, 21,* 439-451.

Youngstrom, N. (1990, June). On privileges issue, field is tilting to 'yes'. *Monitor, 21* (6), 12-13.

Footnotes

Portions of this article were drawn from the American Association of Applied and Preventive Psychology's (AAAPP) report of the Committee on Prescription Privileges as well as from AAAPP's Committee Concerned About Medicalizing Psychology's legislative testimony and report "Arguments and counter arguments: Prescription privileges for psychologists." These documents are available from AAAPP, 1010 Vermont Avenue, N.W., Suite 1100, Washington, DC 20005-4907.

Discussion of Heiby

The Case Against Prescription Privileges for Psychologists: Issues and Implications

Alan E. Fruzzetti, Ph.D.

University of Nevada

Arguments for or against psychologists prescribing psychoactive medications may usefully be divided into three sets: 1) those pertaining to assumptions, goals or values; 2) hypotheses about the impact of large numbers of prescribing psychologists on the science and practice of psychology; and 3) those that consider practical issues in training *if* we assume prescription privileges for psychologists is desirable. The practical issues in training are best left to those medical professionals who have already created training and knowledge standards for prescribing privileges. Thus, let us consider in this commentary only the first two sets of issues and arguments, beginning with those concerning assumptions and values.

At the assumptive (preanalytic) level, the prescription privilege movement, by its very existence, implies that consumers currently have inadequate access to competent prescribing providers. Dr. Elaine Heiby has argued that consumer need for increased prescriptions has not been established. In fact, there is considerable evidence that psychoactive medications are already overly prescribed (Jacobs, 1995). Heiby notes that within the prescription privilege movement there is no direct or implied mechanism to increase services to those that are currently underserved in their general mental health needs (primarily poor people). In fact, on the contrary, trying to improve financial conditions for psychologists is often cited as an important factor among those advocating that psychologists gain prescription privileges. Treating poor people is not their agenda. Finally, there is not currently, nor is there projected to be, a shortage of physicians (including psychiatrists), psychiatric nurse practitioners, or other professionals who already prescribe psychoactive medications.

The prescription privilege movement also assumes or implies that psychoactive medications are safe and effective in general and preferable to existing alternatives (e.g., empirically supported treatments). What is important here is not to debate again the drugs versus psychotherapy issue, but to note that there are ample credible data available to question medication efficacy and/or safety (e.g., Antonuccio, this volume; Greenberg, Bornstein, Greenberg, & Fisher, 1992; Jacobs, 1995; Jacobson & Hollon, 1996) and the models upon which they are founded (e.g., Ross & Pam,

1995), and thus to render the status of drug safety and efficacy a question, position or assumption, as opposed to a fact.

Erosion of Ethical Standards

Dr. Heiby also raises another issue that is essentially about values: The introduction of special procedures leading to prescription privileges for psychologists may erode our ethics and standards. Firsts, she is correct in noting that psychologists can already prescribe medications if they follow existing routes to achieve competence in this skill (physician's assistant, nurse practitioner, medical school, etc.). Consequently, any psychologist wanting prescribing authority is not currently precluded from seeking such training and expertise without eroding the standards and foundations of training for psychologists that currently exist. The principle is simply that medical professionals have already established standards and procedures for training in prescribing medications, and that psychologists (and anyone else, especially those from non-medical professions) should simply adhere to existing standards. Enacting differential (lower) standards for psychologists may violate ethical principles pertaining to standards of care.

The additional value issue, the proposition that psychologists' financial gain is sufficient to merit prescribing authority, also raises ethical questions, although not necessarily within the ethical guidelines of the American Psychological Association (1992a, 1992b). Rather, an ethical issue facing all health care, including mental health care, providers is providing the best services available to those in need. Although pro bono work is not required by APA guidelines per se (APA, 1992a), it is common among health care professions to view balancing immediate personal financial self-interest with the needs of those who cannot afford established fees. Thus, if psychologists were arguing that they want prescription privileges in order to make drug treatments available to those who at present do not have such access, they might be arguing from a strong ethical vantage point (providing services to those in need). Arguing to provide drug treatments because the *providers* are in financial need instead raises ethical problems.

Turning to the impact of enacting special procedures for psychologists to gain prescribing authority, Dr. Heiby notes that there would likely be negative consequences for training in psychological science and for the delivery of psychological services. In addition, I think there would also be a negative impact on research (basic psychological research, psychopathology research, and treatment development). Let us consider these three areas separately.

Undermining Training in Psychological Science

The logic Dr. Heiby employs to predict deleterious consequences for training in psychological science is sound: The amount of time required to provide adequate biological and chemical science foundations, plus pharmacology itself, is substantial. Thus, in order to provide this training, *either* the costs would be excessive (adding years to training) *or* shortcuts would be made and the ultimate quality of training in psychological science would be compromised to make room for biology, chemistry, and pharmacology. The only alternative would be diminished standards of training in pharmacology, again raising ethical issues concerning standards of practice (see above).

Just as relevant as time in the curriculum for coursework and practica are the indirect influences of prescription privileges on training in psychological science. For example, faculty must be hired to teach these courses, taking faculty lines away from those researching and teaching in basic or applied psychology. Maybe drug companies would fund some positions, as they do in medical schools (directly through endowments or indirectly through research grants). However, such funding mechanisms only further erode the centrality of behavioral science in psychology. Again, for psychologists wishing to prescribe, they already have that option by training in nursing, as a physician's assistant, in medical school, and other programs that lead to existing certification.

Undermining the Delivery of Psychological Services

Again, Dr. Heiby's points are clear and precise: There is a natural response cost to psychological services when providers also must learn and maintain skills in psychopharmacology. Would practitioners continue to receive the same continuing education in psychological theory, assessment and treatment and *add* CE training in psychopharmacology? Or, would they engage in less of the former in order to satisfy the latter? The history of psychiatry over the past 40 years may be instructive: The contingencies of medication management and reimbursement have moved psychiatry training and practice away from mixed psychological and medical treatments almost exclusively to the domain of psychopharmacology (with notable exceptions, of course). If financial gain for providers is one of the more compelling determinants of the prescription privilege movement, all the more reason to believe it will operate effectively to diminish the provision of effective psychological treatments and increase the dispensation of medical treatments.

Chilling Effect on Basic Psychological Research and Treatment Development

We need look no further than the medicalization of psychological disorders through the widespread adoption of the DSM system (American Psychiatric Association, 1994) to realize the enormous negative effect that large numbers of psychologists gaining prescription privileges would have on psychological research. It is already nearly impossible to receive federal grant funding without using DSM-defined categories of disorders. The complete hegemony of this system, despite its general lack of construct or treatment validity (Fruzzetti, 1996) clearly demonstrates the triumph of politics (and reimbursement) over science. Further extending drug treatments would be another step down this path. Prescription privileges for psychologists would invite pharmaceutical company funding of research, with their well-known policies of restricting publication of outcomes unfavorable to them. There are a limited number of researchers in basic psychology and psychopathology, with even more limited financial support for often expensive research. Again, contingencies of funding would steer more intellectual resources toward biomedical and pharmaceutical research within psychology, away from our roots and strengths in psychology as a behavioral and cognitive science.

In addition, the development and testing of new psychological treatments is a laborious and expensive process. In contrast, pharmaceutical companies regularly underwrite treatment development and testing of new drugs (and new drug combinations), making research in this area more fundable, faster, more quickly publishable, and so on. All of these consequences could not help but pull excellent psychological researchers toward pharmacological, rather than purely psychological, treatment development. I am not arguing that work in psychopharmacology should not be undertaken. On the contrary, medical and pharmacological scientists should and do conduct such research. At present, there is considerably more funding overall for medical/pharmacological treatment research in mental health (it is impossible to know the exact ratio because much drug research is privately funded) than for psychological treatments. I am simply suggesting that prescription privileges for psychologists will exacerbate this existing difference, resulting in an even greater imbalance. Given the accomplishments of the past decade of newer psychological treatments, retarding these efforts would be extremely unfortunate, with deleterious effects on psychological and psychopathology research, and especially on psychological treatment development.

In summary, it seems that the psychologist prescription privilege movement is predicated on faulty assumptions and questionable values, and would likely significantly erode the products of psychological science in terms of research, training, and the delivery of psychological services to those in need. This is a prescription for a disastrous future.

References

American Psychiatric Association (1994). *Diagnostic and statistical manual of mental disorders* (4th ed.). Washington, DC: Author.

American Psychological Association (1992). Ethical principles of psychologists and code of conduct. *American Psychologist, 47,*1597-1611.

American Psychological Association (1992). Rules and procedures. *American Psychologist, 47,* 1612-1628.

Fruzzetti, A. E. (1996). Causes and consequences: Individual distress in the context of couple interactions. . *Journal of Consulting and Clinical Psychology, 64,* 1192-1201.

Greenberg, R. P., Bornstein, R. F., Greenberg, M. D., & Fisher, S. (1992). A Meta-analysis of antidepressant outcome under "blinder" conditions. *Journal of Consulting and Clinical Psychology, 60,* 664-669.

Jacobs, D. H. (1995). Psychiatric drugging: Forty years of pseudo-science, self-interest, and indifference to harm. *Journal of Mind and Behavior, 16,* 421-470.

Jacobson, N. S., & Hollon, S. D. (1996). Cognitive-behavior therapy versus pharmacotherapy: Now that the jury's returned its verdict, it's time to present the rest of the evidence. *Journal of Consulting and Clinical Psychology, 64,* 74-80.

Ross, C. A., & Pam, A. (1995). Pseudoscience in biological psychiatry. New York: John Wiley.

Chapter 3

The Political History of the Prescription Privilege Movement Within the American Psychological Association

Victor D. Sanua, Ph.D.
St. John's University

On August 10, 1995, prior to the Convention of the American Psychological Association in New York, the APA Council of Representatives were presented with the following issue: "Since California and other states are gearing up for a legislative battle for prescription privileges (California already has Senate Bill 777), the Council of Representatives needs to make it totally clear that it supports prescription privileges for those psychologists whose training and experience qualify them to provide such physical intervention." (APA Agenda, 1995, p. 245)

The main motion in 1995 was that the Council of Representatives should reaffirm as policy its 1986 acceptance of the following resolution: "The practice of psychology encompasses the observations, assessment, or the alteration of behavior and/or concomitant physiological functioning through behavioral procedures. The techniques available to effect such alterations include both physical as well as purely psychological interventions applied by psychologists operating within the limits of individual training and experience." (APA Agenda, 1995, p.245)

The purpose of this chapter is to review the history that led to this vote and to subsequent actions to strengthen this position by the leading association in organized American psychology. There are a number of vectors that might explain this final decision. Some of these vectors are very clear, such as:

1. The pushing for prescription privileges by well-placed psychologists within the APA administration, particularly the leadership of Divisions 12 and 42 (the influence of these divisions will be discussed later).

2. The influence of the drug companies who have provided these psychologists with financial backing. The drug companies are developing future markets for the use of their drugs. While there are about 30,000 psychiatrists in the American Psychiatric Association (which most psychologists call "small APA" or ApA), there are upwards of 100,000 psychologists who are potential prescribers of psychotropic drugs (which is why this organization is often called "big APA").

3. Economics in an era of managed care. Psychotherapy is a very costly treatment. Insurance companies and managed care are likely to encourage a quick fix

through medication and weaken the use of psychotherapy for which the psychologists have been trained.

Sources of Support

Many leaders in the practice community have taken the position that chemotherapeutic (prescriptive) interventions have become a significant aspect of the treatment/management of mental health problems and psychologists must not be denied them. For example, Rogers H. Wright former president of the California Psychological Association has said that "restricting psychology's scope of practice to purely psychological intervention would preclude or severely limit psychological practice." (Wright, 1995). Similarly, the former president of American Psychological Association Ronald Fox (1988) stated, "as psychology has grown in knowledge and sophistication, its practitioners have felt increasingly hampered by several constraints that make the full use of their knowledge and skills difficult to exercise." (p. 501).

These views have moved from individual opinion to organization policy over many years. In 1981 the American Psychological Association Board of Professional Affairs (BPA) appointed the Psychologists' Use of Physical Intervention (PUPI) committee, which considered prescriptive privileges as part of psychology's legitimate need for physical interventions. The Committee provided the following recommendations:

1. B.P.A. should review the contributions psychologists can make in the field of chemotherapeutic interventions.
2. Psychologists' role in the use of controlled substances must first be dictated by consumer interest; and
3. Psychologists should seek routine participation in the use of controlled substances at present by establishing psychobehavioral assessment and compliance procedures to evaluate the efficacy of such substances.

The PUPI's Report, completed in 1981 and revised again five years later (BPA, 1986) was adopted in 1986 by the Board of Directors of the Division of Clinical Psychology (12), which instructed its Council Representatives to seek acceptance of the report as APA policy. Division 22 (Rehabilitation) joined forces with Division 12 to push for the resolution outlined above, which was passed.

While prescriptive privileges were not specifically referenced in the resolution, they were specifically referenced in the original report which dealt at length with the necessity of psychologists being able to apply physical interventions of all kinds, including controlled substances (i.e. medication)(APA Agenda, 1995, p. 246). Until very recently, however, the official position stated by the APA Chief Executive Officer was that, "APA has no position for or against prescription privileges for psychologists"(Fowler, 1995 p. 3). This official neutrality angered pro-prescription advocates in APA, such as Wright (1995) who called Fowler's stance "grossly incorrect." "If indeed APA's role to date in the issue of prescriptive privilege is, in effect, to take 'no stand' on the issue, one can surmise that it will continue to raise the question for the broad spectrum of American psychologists, 'what is APA's relevance to the development of psychology?'" (Wright, 1995, p. 4). The charade of APA's disinterest evaporated in 1996 when the APA Council of Representatives formally endorsed prescription privileges for psychologists, albeit in an odd manner to be described shortly.

Disinterest Despite the Support

This final step in the process of adopting prescription privileges as an official goal of APA has occurred in the context of a relatively low level of interest among rank and file psychologists measured in a number of ways. For a number of years, APA has been appointing committees, providing funds, having retreats, offering its pages to the prescription privileges-seeking psychologists, and promoting drug-financed workshops and symposia at APA conventions. Yet the rank and file of the membership still shows little interest. At APA conventions, most drug-related sessions have been poorly attended. For example, the mid-winter clinical APA conventions in Scottsdale, Arizona, only 4 people attending a session given in prime-time, Sunday at 10 A.M., chaired by a presidential candidate for one of the divisions, and two physicians.

A national APA videoconference workshop on psychopharmacology and depression in December 1995 provides another example. In spite of wide promotion, the workshop videoconference had to be canceled because of too few registrants. Further evidence of this lack of interest among the membership is evident in the circular mailed to State Psychological Association by Marlyne Kilbey, Chair of the APA Board of Educational Affairs Working Group, and Edward Bourg, Senior Consultant. The first paragraph reads as follows:

> In a memorandum dated May 19, 1995, we invited State Psychological Association to provide feedback on a draft model curriculum for Level 1 training in psychopharmacology developed by the BEA Working Group on Psychopharmacology. Unfortunately, we did not receive any written response to this memorandum. Furthermore, an open forum held at the APA Convention, which provided another opportunity for discussion of this work, was not attended by many representatives of State Psychological Association. Accordingly, we are making an extra effort to seek your important feedback... (p.1)

Manipulating Political Action

In an unusual chain of events revealing how politically manipulated the process had become, there was no official vote. Jerry H. Clark, a former president of the California Psychological Association, who was trying to persuade them to vote positively for prescription privileges, contacted members of the council by phone. Clark was the mover of the motion submitted to the Council under agenda no. 26. His basic argument was that APA would aid in the passing of a bill submitted to the legislature advocating prescription privileges should show support for their efforts so that they could state that APA was formally behind the bill.

The National Psychologist carried the following headline (Saeman, 1995) in connection with the Council vote, "APA Council ponders prescription privileges, then endorses issue with a one-sided votes" (p. 1). In fact, however, there was no vote. The list of those who, according to Clark, accepted the argument appeared in the agenda list. There was a note at the end of the list that indicated that there were a number of additional yes votes from representatives who had asked to not have their names published. There was some opposition during the Council discussion in New York, but in view of the overwhelming number of names on that list for prescription privileges, a regular vote was felt to be useless, and therefore the motion was passed without a vote. The minutes of the meeting stated simply, "Council voted to adopt the following resolution (see above) on prescription privileges." However, there was no information about the details of the vote.

The newsletter of the Association for the Advancement of Psychology (AAP) which is the national advocacy group for psychology and is chaired by Jerry H. Clark and Rogers Wright, described the process in some detail. The following summary of the AAP article was taken from an annotated bibliography prepared (Prescription Privileges...,1995) by AAAPP's Committee Concerned about the Medicalization of Psychology:

Reports the August 1995 vote of the APA's Council of Representatives to "reaffirm" a policy of physical interventions with specific reference to prescription privileges. Council instructed Education, Practice and Science Directorate and its Boards of Professional Affairs, Educational Affairs, and Scientific Affairs to develop a model curriculum and legislation in support of this policy. Of 119 members, 77 (2/3rds) cosponsored the policy and were supported by an additional 10 -15 members (ed. note: exact vote not reported. Notes APA became involved in prescription privileges formally in 1979 when its Board of Professional Affairs established the Psychologists' Use of Physical Interventions committee. The BPA accepted the recommendations in 1981 and the APA in 1986. The recommendation states the scope of practice includes a wide range of physical interventions (including chemotherapeutic) but makes no specific mention of prescription privileges Council adoption of prescription privileges spearheaded by Jerry Clark (former president of California Psychological Association) and Roger Wright (AAP Executive Officer and former President of CPA and Div. 12). Argues Council's motion will increase chances to pass legislation in planning for California, Hawaii, Montana, etc. and expects 5-10 more states to pursue prescription privileges in near future. Claims most psychologists find it "intolerable" to limit services to partial care. Concerned with overmedication of the elderly and that over 50% of mental health claims were submitted by general care physicians. (p. 5)

Support in the Context of Controversy

This historic change in association policy was by no means unanimous. *The National Psychologist* provided a sampling of views expressed during the debate. To demonstrate the contentious nature of this issue, if not the final and unusual political process, I shall give primarily those of well-known opponents of the motion:

Arthur Kovacs

Kovacs, a longtime California psychologist, began by noting that the current debate over prescription rights has nothing to do with science, "It has to do with economics. If psychologists thought their income would not go down, we wouldn't be talking about it. But I don't think it's a good survival tactic."

Stanley Moldawsky

"Psychology's image will change. We will be in greater demand, but for the wrong reasons."

Bert Karon

"A psychologist doing only psychotherapy can't hope to earn more than $100,000 a year. Someone who limits his/her practice to medication and evaluation, can easily earn $300,000. I don't think psychologists are genetically more moral than psychiatrists and given a chance to be medicating, we will be as corrupted as they were, and our patients will be corrupted. That's why most psychologists outside APA governance are against it."

Gary Denelsky

"Writing prescriptions will not simply add a tool to our toolbox. Instead, we are adding a tool that will take over the toolbox. Twenty years ago, psychiatry decided to go in that direction. What has happened? They don't do psychotherapy. Why? Because they are so preoccupied, so consumed, and so driven by the propaganda of the pharmaceutical industry. The same thing can happen to psychology through the skillful marketing of a multibillion-dollar pharmaceutical industry. There is no multibillion dollar psychotherapy industry promoting the proven benefits of psychological interventions."

Patrick DeLeon

In contrast to these views, supporters saw the APA vote as a victory and a vindication. DeLeon said "I see it as a public service. I think psychologists can do it well, and improve the quality of life of children and the elderly. I think it's good for society and therefore good for psychology. Prescribing should be for those who want it, and have the appropriate training."

Disinterest, Controversy, and the Immediate Impact of the APA Vote

The positive vote at APA was not very helpful to those who were pushing the California bill. The bill was pulled from the hearing calendar once it was evident that since it would demise rather swiftly if a vote would have been taken (Saeman, 1996). Once again, the issue did not seem to receive strong support from rank and file psychologists (Saeman, 1996). Surveys in San Diego and Los Angeles showed that 50% of psychologists favored the bill, 18% opposed it and 32% remained indifferent.

These results are not surprising since they reflect national trends even within practice dominated associations. For example, in 1995, there was a general survey of 1700 APA members (Kohout, Wicherski, and Grocer) asking them about prescription privileges. It was found that 16% "strongly agree," and 39.2% "agree" (altogether, 55.21) that "Appropriately trained psychologists should prescribe medication." Note, however, that this was despite the use of the word "appropriately" which tends to demand a supportive response.

According to Pietrowski (1989), the conflict is not so much between psychologists versus psychiatrists, but between psychologists versus psychologists. Pietrowski and Killer (1996) found that 49% gave a "yes" answer and 43% gave a "somewhat" answer when asked if the prescription privileges move "will change the identity of the profession of psychology." Pietrowski (1989) categorized psychologists' opinions into three types:

1. "If psychologists are not granted prescription privileges, they will become third class citizens in the mental health delivery system."
2. "If APA pushes for the issue, I will personally testify against it in the strongest terms to congressional committees."
3. "I assume that the next thing psychology will want is the right to perform surgery."

Following the unusual and overwhelming acceptance of the pro-prescription motion by the APA Council, a variety of writers worried in print about its possible negative effects, both at the level of process and content. This included some who had been at least somewhat in support of prescription privileges in the past. For example, Shore (1996), sent a circular letter to all the members of the APA Council, posing the question, "We must ask: How closely does Council reflect the thinking of the membership, and how democratic are our procedures?"

Regarding voting procedures and communication with the membership, she made the following points:

1. Membership should know what issues will be on Council's agenda.
2. As a result of the lack of communication before Council discussions and voting, membership has little or no opportunity to discuss issues with their Representatives and Representatives may not know how strongly some of their constituents feel about some issues.
3. The *APA Monitor* is sometimes prohibited from informing membership about controversial agenda items before the vote, which is of grave concern.
4. Membership is not informed about how their Representatives voted on issues.

Regarding prescription privileges for psychologists, Shore argued that APA should not seek prescription privileges for psychologists, especially at this time for the following reasons:

1. The most important issue facing our profession is the threat of being eliminated or made irrelevant by managed care. All our available resources should be

going to save the profession by working to expose, regulate, and replace managed care with a more pro-patient medical and mental health system.

2. Though obtaining prescription privileges may help some psychologists survive in the short run, it will hasten the professional end for those psychologists who want to be psychotherapists.

3. By seeking prescription privileges, we will be participating in the "de-professionalization" of all the professions, thus helping managed care achieve this goal.

4. We weaken our own arguments about the superiority of doctoral level training.

5. This is the worst possible time to seek prescription privileges. Now more than ever, we must work with psychiatry, medicine and all professions to free professionals and consumers alike from the control of managed care. Seeking prescription privileges will force psychiatry and medicine to oppose us, causing us both to divert our monies from the major battle and fight each other. This is exactly what the industry wants. We should not oblige.

6. Prescription privileges and a new focus on medication will dilute and diminish psychology's focus on psychological treatment and psychotherapy.

7. Again, the general membership was unaware that the general seeking of prescription privileges was to be voted by the Council. This is such an important topic, with potential consequences, that it should be discussed openly and at some length with membership.

Similarly, Sleek (May, 1996), who has written pro-prescribing articles in the past, raised concerns as to the problems that might develop with prescription privileges, such as side effects. Further, he writes, "As a result, psychology may develop fewer psychotherapeutic techniques for psychosocial problems because of time constraint." The latter fear has always been expressed by the anti-drug psychologists. Sleek quoted the views of Bonnie Strickland who "worries that prescription privileges could lead psychologists to medicate particularly difficult patients, especially those from a culture they don't fully understand. Is it possible that the pendulum is swinging back after the recent excesses on prescription privileges efforts."

Reflecting a process of polarization, other opinions became or remained strongly supportive. Some who were once lukewarm to the idea, now climbed on board (e.g. compare Cantor, 1991, with her vote on the resolution). Despite indications of disinterest and controversy, it is probably fair to say that most supporters have been buoyed by the changes in APA policy. Robert Resnick, past president of APA, in one of his columns (1995) in the *APA Monitor* reflected on the vote taken in New York on prescription privileges, stating that this was another "milestone in the continuing evolution of the practice of psychology." (p. 2) In a previous column (1995), he wrote that "the lack of plentiful research on the effectiveness of psychotherapeutic intervention has hampered our ability to thrive in the changing health care system" (p.

2). This is somewhat surprising since given the large body of research on psycho-therapy which indicates its general superiority over drugs, particularly in light of the serious side effects drugs can produce.

The Form and Nature of the Pro-Prescription Argument

I shall now examine some of the writings of those who have been espousing prescription privileges for psychologists, to delineate how the pro-prescription position has been advanced in print, since the form and substance of the arguments are revealing. Perhaps the most dominant person in this movement is Patrick DeLeon. As an assistant to Senator Inouye, former Chairman of the Army Appro-priations Committee, as a person active in APA governance, he has been able to wield great influence on the development of the prescription privileges movement. As a recording Secretary, DeLeon had a lot of clout with the Council of Represen-tatives and staff of APA. For many years, he was a favorite luncheon speaker at various clinical conferences where he was given an opportunity to propound the idea that prescription privileges is "the logical evolution of professional practice" (DeLeon, Folen, Jennings, Willis et al., 1991). He has regularly written on the topic in a column in the *Register Report* as well as through frequent articles in the newsletter of Division 42, *Psychologists in Independent Practice* , in the *Clinical Psychologist* (Div.12 of APA), *Psychotherapy Bulletin* and in the pages of the *American Psychologist.*.

What is interesting about this body of written material is its relative lack of intellectual engagement with the issues. Prescription privileges in DeLeon's hands is a political, not an intellectual or scientific issue. I will list several examples.

Disengagement from the Intellectual Issue

Greenberg and Fisher (1990) raised a number of criticisms of the drug literature in general and DeLeon's position in particular. These included the dangers of the drugs, the absence of blind controls, the fact that "active placebos" generally do as well as real drugs, and the superiority of psychotherapy in reducing relapse rate. In his response, DeLeon simply did not address himself to these issues raised by Greenberg and Fisher. Similarly, in the July issue (1990) of the *Register Report*, a letter to the editor by Pies expressed concern about psychologists getting prescription privileges. At the end of the letter, the editor noted "Response: DeLeon declined to respond."

The range of important issues that are avoided is impressive. For example, in none of his writing has DeLeon dealt with the important question of side effects. There is no mention anywhere of tardive dyskinesia and other neurological problems that occur with the use of some types of drugs. Similarly, one of the argument which is often used by DeLeon is that if psychologists get prescription privileges, they can also stop medication. Yet nowhere does DeLeon discuss how this is going to work out in a practical manner when psychologists go counter the decisions of those who are the first to prescribe the medication.

Do Not Cite Scientific Data, Cite Your Friends' Opinions

References to the scientific literature about the information he provides is virtually absent in most of DeLeon's writings. He often suggests the reader get in touch with the psychologists he mentions. He repeatedly refers to "our President" Jack Wiggins or Stanley Graham, as if to provide a type of moral authority to his efforts. So far as I am aware neither Wiggins or Graham have written anything scientific about drugs. Their writings, like DeLeon's, have been position pieces arguing that prescription is good for psychologists.

This expanding network of references in opinion pieces to other opinion pieces is characteristic of the pro-prescription literature. DeLeon calls upon a number of psychologists like Fox and Resnick, both former APA presidents, for support; and Egli, who was Chairman of the Expanded Psychological Practice Committee. Fox (1988) refers to Adams' article in the *Georgia Psychologist* to strenghen his argument about prescription privileges. All these authors are known for being ardent advocates for prescription privileges, and none of these articles are scholarly intellectual arguments.

Inevitability and Bravado

Another tactic in pro-prescription privilege writings is to argue that great progress is being made and that the change in inevitable. For example, DeLeon described the Department of Defense training project in glowing terms over many years, saying it was "doing fine," (1991, April), "a gradually maturing concept," (1991, Fall), that "the evolution continues," (1991-1992 Winter), that it is "alive and doing well," (1992, January), has made "significant progress," (1992, Spring), and represents "an evolving consensus," (1992, Fall), and a "nice success story," (1993, January). Yet in FY 1996, the Defense Authorization Act signed by the President on February 10, 1996 ended the Project in June of 1997. Even in the face of failure, while ApA described the termination of the project, APA focused on details that seemed to avoid this fact, such as that three psychologists will continue to prescribe and seven will continue with their course work.

Minimization

Another approach is to minimize the whole issue, as if there were much ado about nothing. For example, while the Department of Defense's model is for a two-year period of didactic courses, and one year of supervised experience, DeLeon suggests a period of 6-8 weeks. He often states that learning to prescribe is not a "big deal," saying another time that "It is like learning how to use the computer."

Familiarity

DeLeon has the tendency to shorten the first names of his supporters such as Mich, Bob, Ron, Ray, Sam, Stan, Joe, Charlie, Pat, Doug, and so on. The effect is to make pro-prescription advocates and their arguments friendly, supportive, and rather chummy. Sessions to discuss prescription privileges among psychologists are called "retreats," as if the matter were personal and soulful, not empirical and evidentiary. This approach does not fit the picture of the scientific deliberations usually expected of psychologists, since only people sympathetic to the cause are invited.

Feel Free to Abandon "Psychology"

It is revealing that, despite the argument that prescription privileges are based in the history of psychology, the advocates of prescription privileges seem to be moving away from psychology as a term. For example, in the 1994 issue of *The Independent Practitioner*, Egli informed his readers that the "Expanded Psychological Practice Committee" had been renamed the "Psychopharmacology in Independent Practice" committee. In the Fall 1994 (5) issue of the *Independent Psychologist*, Egli provided the reason: "to maintain liaisons actively with the pharmaceutical industry." This will help him to provide *quality* psychopharmaceutical education as part of his goal "to offer continuing education opportunities for psychologists who are interested in developing this knowledge and skill base" (p. 218). Egli in a number of articles has tried to document his ability to get funds from drug companies. In the Fall 1994 issue of the Independent Psychologist, he noted that the APA Division 42 had obtained grants from numerous pharmaceutical companies, statement repeated in the 1994 Winter issue. In the Spring issue of 1994, he described specifically the workshops that were supported by Bristol-Myers Squibb.

False Comparisons

DeLeon often refers to the fact that optometrists, dentists podiatrists, nurses, physicians' assistants, pharmacists, etc. in many instances, after a long struggle with the establishment, are able sometimes to prescribe. Unlike these professions, however, psychology is a non-medical field that is quite divided in its thinking about prescription privileges. The lack of consensus makes it very difficult for legislators to pass bills, since they are reluctant to become involved in turf battles. Substantively, Ph.D. training in psychology hardly has any dealings with physical problems per se.

Forced Fit with Psychological Terminology

Burns, DeLeon, Chemtob, Welch, and Samuels (1988) provided a rationale for introducing prescription privileges that shows another way advocates argue for change: to fit psychopharmacological interventions into the language of psychology. They argue that in the early years of psychology, very little was known about the biological correlates of behavior and emotions. They argue that we would now consider medication as a stimulus, and psychopharmacological interventions as another tool for psychologists to use like behavior modification and biofeedback. Thus these chemicals would be considered as independent variables, while their behavioral effects would be viewed as dependent variables. The similarity in terminology is forced and superficial. While behavior modification and biofeedback are grounded on a strong theoretical and experimental basis within psychology, any effects of psychotropic drugs are based in another field.

Social Appeals

One of the strongest statement on prescription privileges by DeLeon appeared in the *American Psychologist* (1995). He is joined by the two navy psychologists, Sexton and Sammons, who had received citations during the opening sessions of APA in 1995 in New York. The conclusions are grand social appeals, as if those who oppose prescription privilege oppose society at large.

1. "Psychology has a societal responsibility to 'give back' to our nation that which we have received." (p. 1022)
2. "We gradually come to appreciate that only by systematically addressing society's need [giving psychotropic drugs, my remarks], will our profession ultimately be well served by our nation's public policy officials." (p.1023)
3. "...one must expect that the day will soon arrive when every clinician will be able to readily call up on his or her desktop computer suggested pharmacology profiles based upon evolving research protocols." (p.1030)

It Is Happening Anyway and No One Has Been Hurt

In the *American Psychologist,* DeLeon and Wiggins (1996) address the maturity of psychology to use other modes of treatments. They point out that "a very significant number of our professional colleagues have been 'functionally prescribing' for years, often without any documented training, having learned, for example, of the psychoactive effects of medications their patients have received for cardiac, diabetic, thyroid or other health conditions. And we have come to appreciate that, not surprisingly, they have not had any 'quality of care' problems." (p. 227). In other words, we are already doing it and no one is being harmed, so we might as well continue. Despite extensive evidence that psychotropic drugs are difficult to prescribe and have serious complications (Sharif & Rao, 1995), Wiggins and DeLeon (1996) conclude:

In all candor, we have very little respect for the validity of the public hazard allegations that have been made by those external to psychology and would merely suggest that those opposed should carefully review the available literature. (p. 228)

Survival

In 1993, APA President Jack Wiggins delivered his presidential address in Toronto. He indicated that 70% of the membership of APA derive some portion of their income from health care services. These people, he argued, are being battered in the health care market by managed care. His solution was to reposition psychology in the marketplace. The most effective way to do that was for psychologists to prepare themselves to prescribe psychotropic medication. He stated that by "combining biomedical and psychosocial treatment, we can serve the public better." (p. 491). His argument, however, is more financial than intellectual. He refers to a study by Mora (1993, Aug. 16) showing that psychiatrists who limit themselves exclusively to individual psychotherapy make "only" $105,000 to $120,000 per year. The general public, however, does not view drug prescribing psychiatrists more favorably than psychologists (Sanua, 1993).

The Rise of Drug Company Money

These many changes in the attitudes and arguments of psychologists have not occurred in a vacuum. Drug company funds are gradually becoming a significant source of revenue to organized American psychology, but without the protections that have evolved in medically-oriented groups.

The American Psychiatric Association is very strict about including in the programs and publications the names of the drug companies that are financing them. The following is the ApA credo:

Disclosure

Each speaker is required to disclose the existence of any financial interest and/or other relationship(s) (e.g., employee, consultant, speaker's bureau, grant recipient, research support) he/she might have with a) the manufacturer(s) of any commercial product(s) to be discussed during his/her presentation and/or b) the commercial contributor(s) of the activity. (Taken from a brochure sent out by Columbia University announcing a conference on schizophrenia in 1996)

The American Psychological Association does not require similar ethical standards of psychologists. As a result of this looseness of standards, it is difficult to know to what extent any activity with drug content is financially supported by a drug company.

Drug company sponsored programs are often elaborately presented, especially as compared to psychology standards. For example, prior to the 1991 APA convention in San Francisco, APA members were encouraged by mail brochures to attend a symposium, "Anxiety: A cooperative approach," sponsored by Division 42 and supported by Upjohn Company. The advance brochure read: "When a psychologist reaches out to the medical community and develops relationships with physicians, the ultimate effect is better patient care ... We hope you will join us at this exciting event. The enclosed brochure provides a description of the program and information on our faculty." At the session there were two young ladies at the door encouraging passers-by to attend the symposium. A 16-page brochure was placed on each chair in a large room. It had the pictures of all participants, summaries of their presentations, references of their major work and suggested readings. All speakers had at their disposal unusually elaborate color slides and transparencies to enhance their presentations.

In 1992, a large number of elaborate color posters advertised drug workshops, four of them to be given by Ciba–Geigy. One poster had a dark background and the face of an attractive woman with a somewhat anxious look. Spread on her face, there were circles showing hands under a tap and seeming to wash. One day as I was looking at a poster, a young lady approached me and encouraged me to attend the workshop and showed an attractive binder of the Ciba-Geigy Corporation which I would receive if I attended the workshop. To promote these same workshops, the company slipped under each of our hotel doors during the night a brochure with the same picture of the sad-looking woman. Prior to the convention, I had received through the mail a brochure inviting me to attend these same workshops.

Interestingly, the same workshops, with virtually the same speakers, were also presented at the convention of the American Psychiatric Association. They were advertised with the same colorful posters. In other words, psychologists were receiving the same fare as psychiatrists, marketed in identical ways. The exhibit for Ciba-Geigy Corporation at APA had a three-booth exhibit with 5 people encouraging attendance at these workshops.

The effect of drug company money in organized American psychology has continued to be more and more obvious. In 1994 in Los Angeles, there was an open bar during the social hour of one of the clinical divisions which was financed by a drug company. Eli Lilly, manufacturers of Prozac, gave nice pens and brochures about the drug, which indicated that besides their use with depression they could also be used for obsessive-compulsive disorders. Divisions 50, 12, and 28 joined forces with Dupont Pharma Company to sponsor a symposium on the use of drugs (specifically Trexan–naltrexone HCL–which they manufacture) to treat alcoholism. Beautiful color brochures with the summary of presentations were placed on each chair, and bountiful trays of food and drink were available in the back of the room. Altogether, there were 23 sessions at the 1994 APA meeting on psychotropic drugs. In 1995 the level of drug company involvement racheted up yet again. In addition to the now customary booths, support for symposia or educational workshops, distribution of pens and other gifts, they added an elaborate breakfast for 600 psychologists, and pre-convention institutes complete with elaborate refreshments, brochures, and presentation materials.

ApA has already traveled this same road. In 1994, ApA received $2,000,000 in support from drug companies, not counting honoraria and travel expenses for psychiatrists (*Psychiatric News*, September 1995). According to Public Citizen, about 25% of the money received was not acknowledged in program brochures.

As if to justify this new openness to drug company money, psychology organizations now regularly promote a biological model more generally. For example, at the 1993 APA convention in Toronto, Antonio Puente, also a member of the APA Ad Hoc Task Force on Psychopharmacology, introduced the APA Topical Miniconvention program of workshops under the heading of "The Biological Revolution" with the following remarks:

> Psychology is becoming more biological. Numerous reasons for this trend *include recent discoveries concerning the genetic and biological origin of several major mental disorders* (italics added) [See Sanua's papers critical of such statements, 1996, 1996a] and advances in neuroscience notably neuroimaging, that allow for increasingly sophisticated neuropsychological research . . .
> From the practical standpoint, the desire of many psychologists to prescribe medication necessitates increased biological knowledge. (p.xxvi)

Similarly, *The Prescribing Psychologists' Register* (PPR), which has had a booth at the more recent APA conventions, sent out a brochure stating: "With the new psychoactive medications becoming so advanced and beneficial, how long can we keep running to the 'G.P. or other M.D.' to help us get our own patients the appropriate medication?" (p. 3). In other words, the possibility of prescription privileges is leading to the active promotion of a biological model and overstatement of its benefits as compared to the results of scientific studies. PRI sells correspondence courses that purportedly prepare psychologists to prescribe drugs. At their booth at the exhibit hall of the convention, their representative was busy trying to persuade more psychologists to join the program.

Thus, we are seeing both a major increase in drug company money in psychology and a rise in the rhetoric supportive of the biological model. Some of the logic behind the move toward prescription privileges has been criticized even within the APA structure, particularly by scientific constituencies. For example, the report of the APA Task Force on Psychopharmacology, was criticized in several areas by the APA Board of Scientific Affairs. Here are a few excerpts of their criticisms:

> The Board of Scientific Affairs has already expressed its serious reservation about the Report of the Ad Hoc Task Force on Psychopharmacology . . . It is our view that the Task Force which prepared the report was insufficiently representative of psychologists who have considerable expertise in many areas covered by the Report. [Their inclusion] would have given the Report more credibility. More generally, a wider range of people with expertise in biological research and treatment would have provided a more informed perspective . . . .The report makes clear that there have been important advances in the pharmacological treatment of different clinical disorders. Nevertheless, the review of this literature is incomplete at best. The references are largely dated and current work by major investigators in this field are conspicuously absent . . . .The report underscores the educational problem of finding instructors to provide the necessary training. It does not provide much guidance about how this problem is to be solved . . . .Whereas the Report does provide some caution about the APA promoting Level 3 training [without supervision], it falls far short of recognizing the many problems inherent in psychologists conducting physical exams and the like (p. 321, 322).

These reactions are in strong contrast to claims by advocates that the process was scholarly and "apolitical" (Fox, 1994).

Is This What the Public Wants from Psychology?

Before psychologists expend so much efforts in getting prescription privileges, the wishes and needs of the general consumer should be examined. While the powerful groups supporting prescription privileges have often stated that medication is needed to meet public needs, they have not shown specific data to support this claim.

It is interesting that APA itself has examined public opinion in this area and has found only lukewarm support (Survey of General, 1992). Only 52% of college-educated persons favor "allowing psychologists to prescribe medication after completing additional training." 39% oppose it even though the phrase "after completing additional training" is a powerful element for a positive response. Perhaps more importantly, in response to the question "What is the most important action to take in overcoming a mental problem?," 68% believe that the action to be taken "is helping the person understand the personal or social situations that led to the problem." Only 12% believed that medication is the most important action to take in overcoming a mental health problem and 16% think that "most serious mental health problems are the result of a physical problem such as 'chemical imbalance.'"

The Resistance

The forces aligned against prescription privileges are modest, especially as compared to the enormous war chest retained by drug companies and pro-prescription privilege advocates. However, an organized opposition has finally arisen within psychology, as indicated by the present volume and the conference that led to it. This presents some hope, since legislators in the USA are clearly reluctant to pass bills where there is no consensus in the profession. The medical profession, and its powerful lobby, is rising to the challenge.

Whether this will be enough to stop the prescription privilege movement is unclear. If prescription privileges do come, however, it seems clear that training requirements will be high. It seems unlikely that practicing psychologists will be willing or able to go through the years of additional training that will be needed. The story presented in this chapter is one of a largely disinterested rank and file group being used by political leaders in a powerful association to support a position that is extremely unlikely to benefit either that same rank and file group or the public at large, who neither wants nor needs prescribing psychologists. All of this is lubricated by a continuing flow of drug company money. Meanwhile, the very real intellectual issues involved in this change are being ignored or covered over. It is not a sight that reflects well on organized psychology.

References

Adams, D. (1986). A prescription for psychologists. *Georgia Psychologist, 34*, 13 -15.

American Psychiatric Association details drug industry support for consumers' group. *Psychiatric News, 30*, 1,12, 1995.

American Psychological Association. (August 1995). *Council of Representative Agenda. Prescription privileges for psychologists* (pp. 245-248).

American Psychological Association. (August 1993). *Council of Representatives Agenda. Task Force on Psychopharmacology Report Recommendations* (pp. 301-348).

American Psychological Association. (1993). *The biological revolution: Its significance for psychological research and practice. 101st Annual Convention Program* (p. XXVI). Washington, DC: Author.

Burns, S. M., DeLeon, P. H., Chemtob, C. M., Welch, B. L. & Samuels, R. M. (1988). Psychotropic medication: A new technique for psychology? *Psychotherapy: Theory, Research, Practice, and Training, 25,* 508-515.

Cantor, D. W. (1992). The prescription privilege debate: Not now, may be later. *The Independent Practitioner, 12,* 13-14.

Disclosure (1995). *Program of the College of Physicians and Surgeons of Columbia University. Schizophrenia Conference.*

DeLeon, P. H. (1991). Prescription privileges - Steady progress. *The Independent Practitioner, 11,* 37-38.

DeLeon, P. H. (1991). Legislative Issues. Prescription privileges – Continuing progress. *The Independent Practitioner, 11,* 26-27.

DeLeon, P. H. (1991). On the top of the Hill – The Department of Defense prescription project - Doing fine. *National Register, 17,* 12 -14.

DeLeon, P. H. (1992). Prescription privileges – Significant progress. *The Independent Practitioner, 12,* 70-72.

DeLeon, P. H. (1992). Prescription privileges –An evolving consensus. *The Independent Practitioner, 12,* 169-171.

DeLeon, P. H. (1992). On the top of the Hill – National Health Insurance - Alive and doing well - Prescription Privileges Increasing interest at the State level. *National Register,* 4-6.

DeLeon, P. H. (1993). On the top of the Hill – A nice success story. *National Register, 19,* 17-19.

DeLeon, P. H., Folen, R. A., Jennings, F. L., Wilkis, D. J & Wright, R. H. (1991). The case for prescription privileges: A logical evolution of professional practice. *Journal of Clinical Child Psychology, 20,* 254-267.

DeLeon, P. H., Sammons, M. T. & Sexton, J. (1995). Focusing on society's real needs: Responsibility and prescription privileges. *American Psychologist, 50,* 1022-1032.

DeLeon, P. H. & Wiggins, J. G. (1996). Prescription privileges for psychologists. *American Psychologist, 51,* 225-229.

Egli, D. (Summer 1993) . Psychopharmacology in Independent Practice. *The Independent Practitioner, 13,* 152-153.

Egli, D. (Winter 1994). Psychopharmacology in Independent Practice (PIIP) Report. *The Independent Practitioner, 14,* 18.

Egli, D. (Spring 1994) . Psychopharmacology in Independent Practice (PIIP) Report. *The Independent Practitioner, 14,* 59-60.

Egli, D. (Fall, 1994). Psychopharmacology in Independent Practice: Prescription Privileges. *The Independent Practitioner, 14,* 218-219.

Fact Sheet: Psychopharmacology Demonstration Project (PDP). 13 February 1996.

Fowler, R. D. (1995). Should psychologist prescribe medicine ? *The APA Monitor, 26,* 3.

Fox, R. E. (1988). Prescription privileges: Their implications for the practice of psychology. *Psychotherapy, 37,* 501-507.

Fox, R. E. (1994). The prescription issue at APA. *Psychologist/Psychoanalysis, 14,* 13-18.

Greenberg, R. P. & Fisher, S. (1990). To prescribe or not to prescribe? *National Register, 5*, 10-11.

Kilbey, M. (1995) Letter from the Board of Educational Affairs to State Psychological Association, August, 24, 1995.

Kohout, J., Wicherski, M. & Grocer, S. (1996). *Results on 1995 APA telephone survey of members. Report to the American Psychological Association*, Washington D.C

Mora, M. (1993). Payment calculations under health care reform indicated need for diverse practices. *Psychiatric News, 6*, 4.

Pies, R. W. (1990). Letter to the Editor. *National Register, 5*, 24-26.

Pietrowski, C. (1989). Prescription privileges. A time for some serious thought. *The Psychology Bulletin, 24*, 16-18.

Prescription privileges for psychologists (March, 1996). *Annotated bibliography by the AAAPP Committee concerned about the medicalization of psychology.*

Resnick, R. J. (1995). How come outcome? *The APA Monitor, 26*, 2.

Roan, S. (1993). Tug of war over prescription powers. *Los Angeles Times*, August 7, E6.

Saeman, H. (1995). APA Council ponders prescription privileges then endorses issue with one-sided vote. *The National Psychologist, Sept./Oct, 1*, 7.

Saeman, H. (1996). California prescription bill is dead for 1996. Support "soft" for prescription rights. *The National Psychologist.*

Sanua, V. (1994). *A critical appraisal of DeLeon's columns on prescription privileges which appeared in The National Register and The Independent Practitioner, written from the bottom of the Hill.* Unpublished manuscript.

Sanua, V. (1996) Perceptions of psychologists and psychiatrists. Psychologists do better. *Psychotherapy Patient, 9*, 59-75.

Sanua, V. (1996a). The fallacy of the medical model and the dangers of psychotropic drugs as a mode of treatment for mental disorders. *The Journal of Primary Prevention, 12*, 149173.

Sanua, V. (1996b). The myth of the organicity of mental disorders. *The Humanistic Psychologist, 24*, 1-24.

Sharif, Z. A. & Rao, P. A. (1995, April). Psychopharmacological treatment of schizophrenia. Schizophrenia Research. The last 10 years: What we have learned ? The next ten years: What we can accomplish? *10th Annual Schizophrenia Conference.* Columbia Presbyterian Medical Center New York.

Sleek, S. (1996). Shifting the paradigm for prescribing drugs. *The APA Monitor, 26*, 5, 1, 29.

Survey of general population in the USA on prescription privileges (1992). Washington D.C. Prepared for APA by Frederick/Schneiders.

Wiggins, J. G. (1994). Would you want your child to be a psychologist ? *American Psychologist, 49*, 485-492.

Wright, R. H. (1995). Letter to the Editor. *The APA Monitor, 25*, 4.

Discussion of Sanua

Psychology at a Crossroads

Lois J. Parker, Ph.D.

University of Nevada

By definition, a crossroads is a choice point. A traveler who arrives at such a point (in this case the profession of psychology having arrived at the issue of prescription privileges) has already traversed a road that now intersects with that point. One way to describe that road is in terms of its history, and that is precisely what Dr. Sanua accomplishes in his paper "The Political History of the Prescription Privilege Movement Within the American Psychological Association."

Sanua's method is a multifaceted one, exactly what one would expect in a postmodern world where *narrative*–in this case, historical narrative–tends to take unique forms, or is said to be "over before it begins" (Roemer, 1995, p. 3). No longer tidily arranged by sequential events, this narrative nevertheless is the story of how the profession of psychology has now come to a significant choice point. As presented by Dr. Sanua, the story is comprised not only of chronological events, but of parallel developments within the American Psychological Association (APA), developments that now characterize changes at APA's annual conventions. To highlight these changes, Dr. Sanua provides quick snapshots of the personalities and forces, both within and without the profession, that not only introduced this issue in the first place, but are now seemingly propelling the whole profession of psychology toward its acceptance, which is to say the acceptance of an incorporation of prescription privileges as one part of the health care package that psychologists offer clients.

Because there is much to be gleaned from Dr. Sanua's narrative, a brief review of his major facets may be helpful:

Chronological events are, indeed, present: These may be roughly broken into two segments–those prior to the last ten years, and those of the last ten years. Those prior include, (1) an allusion to a report written as early as 1917 by a psychiatrist objecting to "psychologists diagnosing mental retardation," a report that eventually came to the attention of some of the present promoters of the present issue within the APA; (2) a shift in the 1950s within APA when the research/academic membership "dwindled" from 100% to 50%; and, finally, (3) the establishment, in 1979, of the Psychologists' Use of Physical Interventions (PUPI) committee by APA's Board of Professional Affairs, the first report of this committee being prepared in 1981.

A revision of that report in 1986 seems to have begun a flurry of activities within APA, all aimed at promoting the matter of psychologists gaining the right to prescribe medications. These now constitute the second segment of chronological events leading up to the present. In 1986, this revised report was "adopted by the Board of Directors of the Division of Clinical Psychology (12)," and efforts were begun to incorporate its findings into APA's general policy. In 1987, the issue became a part of this country's main political scene when a suggestion was made by Senator Inouye to the effect that "the Department of Defense sponsor a demonstration project for training psychologists in prescribing medications." In 1988, a rationale aimed at introducing prescription privileges into the profession of psychology was publicized by Patrick DeLeon and others. Then, in 1994, APA's "Expanded Psychological Practice Committee" (EPPC) was renamed the "Psychopharmacology in Independent Practice" (PIP) committee, to more correctly reflect its "historical focus." Following that change, events began to move rapidly. In 1995, Senate Bill #777 supporting prescription privileges for psychologists was introduced in the state of California, following which a motion was presented to APA's Council of Representatives in support of this bill. That same year, a national video conference on psychopharmacology and depression was arranged by APA, but was subsequently cancelled for lack of interest, while a survey focusing on this issue of APA's membership in the same year presented mixed results. And, finally, on February 10, 1996, President Clinton signed the Defense Authorization Act that effectively ended, in 1997, the demonstration project sponsored by the Department of Defense.

Certain parallel changes within the American Psychological Association are next cited by Dr. Sanua, changes that are not only apparent at APA's annual conventions, but apparent also within its sponsored publications. Three of these are noted: one, the steadily increasing number of presentations on programs at annual conventions related to this issue; two, the increasing number of articles appearing in APA sponsored publications that present a pro-prescription privileges stance; and three, the inroads that drug companies have themselves made into the APA conventions, as well as into the sponsorship of psychological research.

And, finally, Dr. Sanua surveys the personalities and forces that are behind this movement. The personalities are, significantly, politically powerful within the American Psychological Association, and are also in positions of control relative to psychological publications. Patrick DeLeon, "an assistant to Senator Inouye, member of the APA Board of Directors, and recording Secretary, Section Editor of the *American Psychologist*," is a key figure, as are a number of recently past APA presidents: Stanley Graham, Jack Wiggins, Raymond Fowler, R. E. Fox, and Robert Resnick.

The forces behind this movement, as seen by Dr. Sanua, are primarily economic. On the one hand, practicing psychologists supporting prescription privileges cite the impact of managed health care and its presumed reduction of available opportunities that psychologists currently have for participating in the mental health market. They suggest that by expanding one's practice to include the right to prescribe medications this threat of a reduction will be alleviated, at least in part. On the other hand, the growing presence of large drug companies at APA conventions and their sponsorship of psychological research suggest the establishment of a working alliance between the profession of psychology and the drug market. In either case, that of the sole practioner or of the profession at large, a critical change is anticipated.

Critical Changes

Critical changes are, of course, the essence of any good story, historical or otherwise. But, as every good therapist knows, stories themselves have a way of changing, depending on who is telling them. Thus, as H. E. L. Mellersh (1970/1993) reminded us over two decades ago, "interpretation is always a dangerous as well as a fascinating business" (p. 58).

What makes the interpretation of this story so dangerous is the simple fact that the future of modern-day psychology hangs in the balances. What makes it so fascinating is that the profession of psychology itself has now come to a significant choice point.

As Dr. Sanua (1995) makes clear elsewhere, the future of psychology, traditionally, has invested itself as a science and a practice, both of which have been ideally anchored in a humanistic approach to human behavior, including its mental operations or private events. To abandon this approach for a more biological one would be to abandon also psychology's traditional investment, as well as the ideology that supports it. That ideology, dating back to Classical Greece and the meaning of the term *psychology*, etymologically speaking, has a long history. And, as Mellersh (1970/1993) also noted, "it is all too easy, in examining the evidence for historical facts . . . to let the dry detail stultify one's imagination" (174).

That imagination is critical to psychology, both as a science and a practice, and I, for one, would not want to see it medicated. It will, in fact, shortly bring us back to that most famous crossroads of all. But first, leaving the matter of science to Dr. Sanua and others, I have a few things to say about psychology as a practice. One hears that *data* must substantiate what we do; indeed, the question arises as to what data can be found to support the practice of psychotherapy. This question was asked in response to Dr. Sanua's presentation of his paper at the conference held on prescription privileges in Reno, Nevada.

If one can rid oneself of a stereotypical view of what constitutes *data*, if one can open oneself to the original meaning of the term *empirical*, namely, the Greek *empeiria*, meaning "trial, attempt, experiment" (Ahsen, 1987, p. 3), then perhaps the *trials and attempts* made in psychotherapy and the storied *data* that result from them can be more clearly validated. That validation constitutes a major part of this story, a part that is now seemingly overlooked by those practicing psychologists who advocate prescription privileges. Yet, when all is said and done, one forgets one's history at a cost.

That cost is clearly visible at the crossroads where our profession has now arrived. Analogously, this arrival evokes in one's imagination that most famous crossroads of all, that one that, traditionally, has had meaning for all psychologists. Simply put, two questions remain: Will the profession of psychology, after killing off its father, which is to say, its tradition of science and psychotherapy, like Oedipus, proceed on down that much traveled road to Thebes? Or will it, unlike Oedipus, take that far less traveled (and, presumably, less economically kingly) road to Daulis (see Eisner, 1987)? The answer to these questions, if favorable to psychology and its tradition, lies ultimately with Dr. Sanua and others who continue to tell the story.

References

Ahsen, A. (1987). Image psychology and the empirical method. *Journal of Mental Imagery, 11*(3&4), 1-38.

APA Board funds advocacy on prescription privileges, changes balloting timelines. *APA Monitor, 27*(8), 22.

Eisner, R. (1987). *The road to Daulis: Psychoanalysis, psychology, and classical mythology.* Syracuse, New York: Syracuse University Press.

Mellersh, H. E. L. (1993). *The destruction of Knossos: The rise and fall of Minoan Crete.* New York: Barnes & Noble.

Roemer, M. (1995). *Telling stories: Postmodernism and the invalidation of traditional narrative.* Lanham, Maryland: Rowman & Littlefield Publishers, Inc.

Sanua, V. D. (1995). "Prescription privileges" vs. psychologists' authority: Psychologists do better without drugs. *The Humanistic Psychologist, 23*(2), 187-212.

Chapter 4

Implications of Prescription Privileges for Psychological Research and Training

Richard M. McFall, Ph.D.
Indiana University–Bloomington

There is a beautiful lake outside Minneapolis where families have vacationed in rustic cabins for generations. But as Minneapolis expanded toward the lake, year-round homes started springing up along the shoreline at an alarming rate, threatening to destroy the very beauty that had attracted everyone to the lake in the first place. To preserve and protect the lake, new zoning ordinances were passed.

The planners who drafted the new regulations included a "grandfather" clause exempting existing properties from the standards for minimum lot size and maximum housing density. Unfortunately, some developers exploited the loophole provided by this clause, cramming oversized homes onto the undersized lakefront lots of existing cabins under the guise of "remodeling." They would tear down all but one tiny part of an old building, and erect a totally new structure around it. Or they would build a totally new structure in two stages, first building a major new addition to an existing structure and then, once the addition was "established," tearing down the original structure entirely.

Zoning authorities wanted to prevent this kind of subterfuge, but were caught in a classic dilemma: On the one hand, they wanted to prevent new construction that might destroy the lake. But on the other hand, they did not want to do anything that might obstruct genuine improvements to existing properties. The crux of this Minnesota dilemma can be summed up in two questions: (1) What defines the boundary separating legitimate positive change from detrimental change? And (2) how much can an existing structure be changed before it becomes something else?

I was reminded of this Minnesota dilemma as I reflected on the implications of granting prescription privileges to psychologists. As you know, the American Psychological Association and others are advocating that qualified psychologists—those with the "requisite" training and credentials—become eligible to prescribe pharmacological treatments for patients with psychological disorders. A bill proposed in the 1996 Missouri legislature—but not passed—is typical of the laws under consideration across the country. It would have granted prescription privileges to Missouri psychologists who met the following conditions:

A licensed psychologist must provide evidence of completion of a pharmacology course, with at least 100 hours of approved clinical training and at least 200 hours of independent course study in the assessment of the need for and the prescription of drugs in the treatment of persons with psychological problems and emotional and mental disorders and illnesses.

Notice that this proposal deals exclusively with training issues. It provides no rationale for the legislation; does not describe the problem that the legislation was supposed to fix; offers no data to document the need for new legislation; and did not explain how the specific proposal was an appropriate solution to any problem or need. Nevertheless, the proposal raised two questions reminiscent of the questions faced by the Minnesota planners: (1) What defines the boundary separating legitimate positive changes in psychological training and practice from detrimental changes? And (2) how much can the training and practice of psychologists be changed before it becomes something else? Like the Minnesota planners, psychologists are caught in a dilemma: On the one hand, we don't want changes that might threaten the integrity of our science and profession. But on the other hand, we don't want to do anything that might obstruct legitimate, evolutionary advancement.

The more I considered the parallels between the battle over environmental protection in Minnesota and the battle over prescription privileges for psychologists, the more fitting and illuminating the analogy seemed. Of course, reasoning by analogy can be risky if the analogy is taken too literally. No two situations are exactly alike, so analogies always must be treated figuratively. But Polya (1957) has argued that analogies can be useful heuristic tools. Like the scaffolding used to erect buildings, analogies serve as conceptual scaffolding, enabling us to step outside of our problem; to reach previously inaccessible parts of a problem; and to gain fresh perspectives on refractory issues. In this spirit, then, I invite you to join me in viewing the issue of prescription privileges for psychologists as though it were an issue of environmental protection. I will argue that the proposed prescription privileges should be resisted because they will contribute significantly to a societal form of toxic pollution.

The Polluting Effects of High Density

The environmental threat of most immediate concern to the Minnesota planners was the likely toxic effect of high-density development along the shoreline. The lake's fragile ecosystem simply could not survive the impact of cramming too many people and structures into too little space, along with all of the secondary consequences. There is a saturation point on the density curve beyond which the environment no longer can absorb the load imposed on it by human use and abuse. The inevitable damage may not be apparent immediately, but once the dynamic process has been set into motion, it can be extremely difficult to halt or reverse.

Legislation granting prescription privileges to psychologists may pose an analogous threat to our social environment, triggering a dynamic process that would be extraordinarily difficult to halt or reverse. The most direct toxic effect would be the increased density of professionals empowered to dispense psychoactive drugs. It is not clear that society could absorb the secondary consequences of this increased density. Currently, public consumption of psychoactive drugs is at an unprecedented high—perhaps approaching a saturation point. Prozac, for instance, is one of the most widely prescribed drugs in the world. Undoubtedly, one main effect of granting prescription privileges to psychologists would be to increase further this high level of drug consumption. What would be the likely impact on society?

I am unaware of anything comparable to an "environmental impact study" of the potential ramifications of granting prescription privileges to psychologists, but clearly such an analysis should be conducted before any such legislation is enacted. We worry about the impact on spotted owls of cutting down trees. Shouldn't we worry at least as much about the potential impact on human beings—on society— of passing legislation that seems likely to increase dramatically the consumption of psychoactive drugs?

I have no doubt that psychologists *with proper training* could perform prescription tasks as well as psychiatrists or physicians. Ph.D. psychologists, as a group, are just as smart, capable, and ethical as M.D.s. My concern simply is with the potential impact of adding tens of thousands of psychologists to the huge army of professionals who already have prescription privileges.

How can I say that there is a "huge army" of prescription-writing professionals when one of the main arguments advanced in favor of allowing psychologists to write prescriptions is that there are not enough psychiatrists to do the job? Well, most of the prescriptions for psychoactive drugs currently are not written by psychiatrists, but by primary-care physicians, with little or no formal training in psychiatry or psychology. These physicians apparently feel competent to treat their patients' psychological problems as well as their physical problems, and are reluctant to refer patients to mental-health specialists for assessment and treatment. This pattern is not likely to change if psychologists suddenly were empowered to write prescriptions. Would physicians who currently don't refer their patients to psychiatrists be any more willing to refer their patients to *psychologists* for pharmacological treatment? Almost certainly, *psychiatrists* would be even less likely than internists and general practitioners to refer patients to psychologists for pharmacological treatment. Thus, the prescriptions that psychologists would write for their patients would represent new, additional prescriptions, thereby increasing the total volume of drug consumption. This increase, in turn, may have a detrimental impact on our social environment.

Whose Interests Would Be Served?

Proponents of prescription privileges for psychologists claim that the legislation would serve the public interest. But, like the "remodeling" claims of the Minnesota builders, this claim has the ring of a subterfuge. The possibility that psychologists' push for prescription privileges may be self-serving arises, in part, from the fact that, under our current health-care system, the professionals who prescribe drugs also gain financially by doing so. In the ideal world, there would be no direct connection between treatment decisions and the compensation derived from providing those treatments. As things stand now, however, there is good reason to wonder whose interests would be served by the proposed legislation, and whose interests would be threatened.

Again, I am not suggesting that psychologists are any more—or any less—likely than other mental health providers to be corrupted by potential conflicts of interest. We know that physicians have a poor record on this score. They have over-prescribed antibiotics to such an extent, for example, that it has led to the evolution of new, drug-resistant strains of bacteria. Tuberculosis, once assumed to be virtually eradicated by the miracle drugs, is staging a comeback as a public health threat. Although some of this excess may be due simply to physicians' ignorance, much of it may be traced to self-serving actions.

Physicians apparently have over-prescribed antibiotics, in part, because they felt compelled to "do something" for patients, even when the "something" clearly was not appropriate, or even was detrimental in the long run. We hear excuses: If the physicians had not written such prescriptions, their patients would have gone to other doctors to get the prescriptions. If the patients were not given a diagnosis and treatment, the doctors would not have been able to collect fees from health insurance companies. If no treatment had been administered and the patients' condition had deteriorated, the doctors might have been sued for malpractice. These excuses suggest that physicians have protected *themselves* from such threats by prescribing something "just to be on the safe side." Whatever the reasons, physicians' prescription pads clearly have been overused—for all drugs, including the psychoactive variety. Almost certainly, this problem of over-prescribing drugs would be magnified if psychologists were given access to prescription pads.

Psychologists with prescription privileges would face strong economic incentives to shift their current treatment patterns from psychological therapies to pharmacological therapies. Psychotherapy—even when it is highly structured—demands more time and patience from the provider than does pharmacological therapy. Reaching for a prescription pad is simply quicker, easier, and more lucrative. Because psychologists could treat more patients in the same amount of time with less effort, while earning more money by writing prescriptions, it seems inevitable that these economic forces would reshape psychologists' treatment patterns.

I am not arguing against *all* uses of drugs. Pharmacological treatments sometimes are the most effective choice for certain conditions, but they are not *always* the safest and most effective treatments. The point is that the choice of treatments for a particular disorder should be based on the empirical evidence concerning the relative costs, benefits, and risks of the available options. Unfortunately, real-world treatment decisions too often are determined primarily by self-serving economic considerations.

If psychologists were given prescription privileges, many eventually would abandon their traditional treatment models in favor of the pharmacological model—regardless of what the scientific evidence might say about treatment efficacy. Am I overstating the case? Let's consider a real-life case example: namely, the current patterns of treatment for panic disorders. Controlled studies have shown that as few as 15 sessions of a specific manualized regimen of psychological treatment—Cognitive Behavior Therapy (CBT)—is effective for 80% to 85% of the patients suffering from panic disorder (Brown & Barlow, 1995; Telch, Lucas, Schmidt, Hanna, Jaimez, & Lucas, 1993). Anxiolytic medications sometimes yield end-of-treatment results nearly this good, but 2-year follow-up data suggest that the gains achieved by CBT are more durable than those achieved by medications.

Ironically, although the comparative outcome data favor CBT over medications, most panic patients do not receive CBT (Barlow, 1994). Perhaps it is understandable that psychiatrists and physicians—who are authorized to prescribe medications—continue to rely almost exclusively on pharmacological treatments. But psychologists—whose inability to prescribe medications limits them to psychological interventions—also are unlikely to employ CBT. When treating patients with panic disorder, most practicing psychologists simply ignore the research evidence and rely instead on outmoded treatments of undocumented or dubious efficacy. Rather than proposing legislation to give psychologists prescription privileges, perhaps psychologists who genuinely wish to serve the public interest ought to propose legislation that would require *all* mental health providers to employ only those treatments that have been shown by controlled empirical research to be the most cost-effective approaches for each disorder (McFall, 1991, 1996).

If psychologists "with additional training" were allowed to apply for a special license to prescribe medications, I foresee a chain of negative consequences: First, within a short time the majority of practicing psychologists would be compelled by market forces to apply for these prescription privileges. Once the prescription option became available, any practicing psychologist who did not pursue the option would be at a competitive disadvantage. Moreover, as typically happens, over time the requirements for acquiring prescription privileges inevitably would become increasingly stringent. Thus, all practicing psychologists would have every incentive to seek the privileges as quickly as possible, rather than delaying. In effect, psychologists soon would be divided into two classes—those with privileges and those without—and this distinction would carry increased weight over time, affecting income, prestige, and professional identity.

Second, psychologists who acquired prescription privileges almost certainly would modify their practice patterns, replacing time-consuming and tedious psychological treatments with simpler and more lucrative pharmacological treatments. Thus, the differences that currently distinguish psychologists from psychiatrists would disappear. Consequently, the availability of effective psychological treatments—although limited now—would all but disappear.

Third, I have noted with disappointment that the majority of practicing psychologists currently are not employing some of the most effective psychological treatments (e.g., Cognitive Behavior Therapy for panic disorders). These same psychologists are among those most likely to seek prescription privileges, once available. In other words, some of the least responsible and conscientious psychologists would be among those prescribing medications in the future. The prospect of

empowering these individuals to dole out potent and potentially dangerous pharmacological treatments is sobering.

I hasten to add that some advocates of prescription privileges legislation are
sincere and responsible, and would do an excellent job if allowed to make selective
use of pharmacological treatments. If we could be highly selective in deciding
which psychologists could prescribe medications, and could limit the scope of the
change, then I would be more sanguine. But we must evaluate the proposed
legislation in terms of the reality, not the ideal. On those grounds, I regard the
proposal with alarm.

Realistically, the people most likely to benefit from psychologists gaining
prescription privileges would be the psychologists. The people most likely to suffer,
in the long run, would be the patients. Access to effective psychological treatments
would diminish while the risks associated with inefficient, inappropriate, or even
dangerous pharmacological treatments for psychological problems would increase.

Why Change the Rules?

Why are some psychologists so interested in acquiring prescription privileges?
The primary motivation for many, I believe, is not altruism, but professional self-
preservation and enhancement. The changing face of the health-care system is a
direct threat to psychological practice. Third-party payers and managed health-care
organizations have begun to look skeptically—often with good reason—at many of
the traditional treatment models for mental health problems. Many psychologists
suddenly are finding that their livelihood is in jeopardy. As a result, they are
scrambling for higher ground—looking for ways to change their professional practice,
to make it more viable, and to survive. Some may see the proposed legislation for
prescription privileges not only as a professional lifeboat, but also as a golden
opportunity to "trade up" in the process—that is, to enter the "psychiatry" profession
through the back door.

As I noted when describing the legislation proposed in Missouri, there has been
little discussion of the rationale behind the move to give psychologists prescription
privileges. The most commonly cited problem that the legislation might address
is the purported difficulty that "under-served populations"—persons living in isolated rural areas or living in poverty—have had getting access to psychopharmacological treatments for their mental or emotional problems. I believe that this
justification is specious. On the one hand, the extent of this problem is not clear.
Access to psychiatric medications is not dictated by the geographical distribution
of psychiatrists because physicians—not psychiatrists—currently write the bulk of the
prescriptions for such medications. On the other hand, it also is not clear that the
best solution to the problem, to the extent that it exists, is to grant prescription
privileges to *psychologists*, who are as likely as psychiatrists to be unavailable to the
rural and poor. Psychologists currently are maldistributed, and are not serving the
"under-served" adequately with psychological treatments. Why would they do a
better job with pharmacological treatments?

But assuming, for the sake of argument, that there were a genuine need to increase the availability of pharmacological treatments among the poor and rural, why fill the void by empowering psychologists to write prescriptions? The doctoral training of psychologists is devoted to the assessment, classification, psychological treatment, experimental study, and prevention of mental and emotional disorders; this training provides relatively little coverage of anatomy, biology, neurochemistry, or pharmacology. In contrast, other professional groups—nurse practitioners and pharmacists, for example—already receive extensive training in these critical areas. Thus, the simplest, most expedient solution to the problem of providing pharmacological treatments to under-served populations would be to capitalize on the training and experience of existing professions; simply empower nurse practitioners and/or pharmacists to handle exceptional psycho-pharmacological needs. There is no justification for creating a whole new system of training and licensing.

In sum, prescription privileges may meet the needs of psychologists, who find their traditional patterns of professional practice under assault; but it is not clear that the proposed legislation is the best way to serve the needs of the public. There are less drastic, more expedient, and safer ways of dealing with pockets of pharmacological need among poor and rural populations. There is no point in creating new systems of training and licensing when existing systems are adequate to deal with special problems. Meanwhile, psychologists who wish to acquire prescription privileges already are capable of doing so within the existing system: they can do it the "old fashioned" way, earning the credentials of a physician or nurse-practitioner.

Increased Risks Associated with a Monoculture

Let's return for a moment to the Minnesota lake where we began. An insidious environmental threat associated with urban development is the drift toward an ecological "monoculture." That is, development promotes an increased homogeneity, or decreased diversity, in flora and fauna. For example, the natural range of grasses is reduced to a few hybrid varieties of beautiful, easy-care lawn grasses. The natural range of trees is narrowed to a few species selected for their decorative and shade properties. And the natural range of animal species is winnowed to a few safe, clean, and unobtrusive types, such as squirrels and robins.

Monocultures are risky. Their lack of diversity makes them vulnerable to collapse. They simply are less adaptive and resilient in the face of unforeseen challenges. Think of all the American towns whose boulevards once were lined with the American Elm tree, but now are denuded. Diversity is critical to the environment's capacity to survive challenge and change. We may be putting society's mental-health environment at risk if we take action that promotes homogeneity, or a monoculture, in the theories and techniques of our mental health-care system. Granting prescription privileges to psychologists would foster just such a pharmacological monoculture.

Ironically, psychiatrists, psychologists, social workers, nurses, and other professional groups for years have championed the merits of the "interdisciplinary team" approach to mental health-care delivery. One of the touted advantages of this approach is its "synergistic diversity," in which the different perspectives of the various disciplines form a unified whole that is greater than the sum of its parts. This synergism would be diminished significantly if the psychological perspective were replaced by a pharmacological perspective redundant to the psychiatric perspective. Thus, granting prescription privileges to psychologists would undermine the vitality of the "interdisciplinary team."

If research had shown that the psychological perspective is invalid, or if psychopharmacological advances had rendered it irrelevant, then there would be little reason to mourn its imminent demise. But the psychological perspective may be more valid, relevant, and valuable than ever. In the long run—if allowed to survive—it may prove to be the *most* important perspective of all. Thus, we should look with dismay upon the prospect of a pharmacological monoculture in mental health. Not only would this diminish patients' access to the valuable psychological perspective, but it also would put the entire mental health field at increased risk by decreasing its diversity and vitality.

Impact on Scientific Research and Training in Clinical Psychology

Although I have outlined a number of good reasons to resist the idea of granting prescription privileges to psychologists, I have waited until last to discuss my most central concern—namely, the probable impact it would have on scientific research and training in clinical psychology. I consider this to be the most insidious of all the threats posed by the legislation to the long-term health and well-being of our society. To explain, I return once again to the environmental analogy.

Of all the threats posed by construction around the Minnesota lake, soil erosion arguably is the most insidious. Wherever there is new construction, the earth's stability and equilibrium are disturbed. Top-soil is moved. The earth's topography is reconfigured. Vegetation that once held the earth in place is stripped away, allowing wind and water to carry away the rich top-soil and to carve new channels that further accelerate the run-off. Streams and lakes then become choked with silt, hastening their death. The remaining land becomes less fertile, fostering an increased reliance on chemical fertilizers, which then are carried away by erosion, too, compounding the problem. Ironically, while the fertility of the land is being diminished, the increasing concentration of nutrients in the streams and lakes makes them *too fertile*, promoting undesirable growth there. In short, erosion destabilizes the ecosystem, undermines healthy growth, promotes negative growth, and strangles the environment.

Prescription privileges for psychologists, in my view, pose an analogous threat to the stability and health of scientific research and training in clinical psychology: With the advent of prescription privileges, the rich environment so essential to nurturing scientific research and training in clinical psychology would be reconfigured, destabilized, and eroded. Critical resources would be diverted to other, less vital purposes. Enterprises antagonistic to scientific research and training would be nurtured. The future of clinical psychology as a science would be diminished. And our society would be deprived of benefits that they otherwise might have enjoyed.

Special Qualities of Scientific Environments

Environments that nurture science and scientific training truly are rare and fragile places. Unlike commercial environments, they do not insist on immediate results or short-term returns on investments, but allow ideas to be pursued for their own sake—for the intrinsic value of the knowledge, without regard for their immediate payoff or application. Unlike political environments, they are not egalitarian, democratic, or authoritarian, but are much more like the natural evolutionary environment, in which the fittest survive (see Rauch, 1993). The "rules" that govern this natural selection process in science are insensitive, for instance, to whether the distribution of "winners" and "losers" seems fair or equitable. The value of competing ideas is not judged on the basis of their relative popularity; "truth" is not decided by a majority vote. The rules also are indifferent to the origins or social status of the people who propose competing ideas; political power and authority are irrelevant to the scientific "truth value" of ideas. In principle, ideas are judged entirely on the basis of their scientific merit. The main criteria for "merit" are theoretical integrity, empirical evidence, predictive power, and resilience in the face of efforts at falsification (e.g., Popper, 1962).

Although science can thrive in a variety of settings, the premier environment for nurturing the growth of scientific knowledge traditionally has been the university. The university also has served as the primary nursery for future generations of scientists. Our leading public and private universities have been remarkably successful over the years at cultivating and nourishing the symbiotic relationship between scientific research and scientific training. The special qualities responsible for this success, however, are extremely fragile and vulnerable to erosion. It is not easy to create a fertile research and training environment in the first place, as evidenced by the fact that not all major universities have achieved success as scientific institutions, despite their best efforts to do so. Nor is the research and training environment easy to sustain, once created, as evidenced by the faded glories of some once-illustrious institutions. This means that our premier research and training institutions cannot be taken for granted, but must be preserved and protected as national treasures.

Threats to Scientific Research and Training

How might the passage of legislation granting prescription privileges to psychologists erode scientific research and training? To begin with, it would reshape the landscape of psychology by creating a new psychological specialty—*psycho-pharmaco-therapy*—and this, in turn, would require the establishment of a new training industry. Pressed by economic hardship, many academic institutions would find the promise of a financial windfall seductive, and be tempted to develop applied training programs for psycho-pharmaco-therapists. Inevitably, however, these new programs would compete with scientific research and training for scarce institutional resources.

Our major research and training institutions would be faced with a stark choice: either take the lead in offering the new training, or allow other institutions to provide the training, thereby relinquishing effective control over the training of clinical psychologists. It would be a difficult and unhappy choice. Universities that decided not to participate would be marginalized; that is, the emerging new specialty would revolutionize the profession of clinical psychology, leaving these institutions behind. But universities that decided to participate would lose in other ways.

First, the new training would require a major commitment in faculty, students, curriculum, and facilities. Regardless of whether the training was offered at the predoctoral or postdoctoral level, either it would extend significantly the minimum training period required of students, or it would displace important content from the current curriculum. To provide expanded training, current teaching resources either would have to be expanded or they would have to be spread more thinly. And to extend the length of training means either that the costs per student would increase, or the total number of students would decrease.

Second, the new training also would invite additional layers of regulation and control over predoctoral and/or postdoctoral training by the external agencies responsible for accreditation and licensing. Thus, a decision to join the new enterprise inevitably would undermine the university's autonomy, would increase the intrusive influences of applied interests, and would erode the traditional academic missions of basic research and scientific training.

Learning from Experience

The detrimental effects of prescription privilege legislation on research institutions would parallel the effects experienced following WWII, when research-training programs, eager to cash in on the new "market demand" for psychotherapeutic training in clinical psychology, adopted the Boulder Model of "scientist-practitioner" training. Initially, there was a vigorous debate—remarkably similar to the current debate—about the wisdom of the proposed changes in psychology, but eventually most major psychology departments across the United States embraced the model. In the years that followed, psychology departments have prospered, but at a very high price to the scientific environment.

Specifically, psychology departments that developed Boulder-Model clinical programs received unprecedented numbers of admission applications from extraordinarily bright students, but most of these applicants were attracted to the field of psychology by the prospects of a career in private practice, as opposed to a career in science. Departments also enjoyed new levels of financial support, thanks to federal training grants to clinical programs, but these funds had strings attached, such as the expectation that the curriculum should emphasize applied and professional content. The special funding of clinical training, in addition, created new tensions within psychology departments—between the "clinical" and "experimental" wings. Students supported by training grants sometimes were obligated to a postdoctoral period of clinical service as repayment for their traineeships; this obligation was yet another obstacle to careers in clinical research. Thanks to the Veterans Administration, clinical students were given access to paid clinical internships; but these internships tended to interfere with students' scholarly and research activities. Psychology departments enjoyed the prestige that came with their clinical training programs being accredited by the American Psychological Association, but formal accreditation opened the door to ever-escalating levels of external regulation and interference. Once accreditation became essential, fear of losing APA accreditation tended to inhibit innovation and foster homogeneity in training programs.

By the 1970s, the professional guild of clinical psychology had grown so large and influential that it was able to persuade individual states to enact licensing laws regulating the practice of psychology. Whether these laws ever achieved their ostensible purpose of protecting the public is debatable, but they clearly have exerted an unwelcome influence on psychology departments. For example, curriculum decisions increasingly are driven by the need to ensure that students are eligible for licensure. At the extreme, recent changes in some states' licensing regulations have raised the requirements for supervised clinical experience to such a level that new Ph.D.s are forced to choose between joining an academic faculty *or* getting the practical experience necessary for a license. Ironically, this means that individuals who choose an academic career may train future clinical psychologists, but may not claim to be one; may construct and validate new psychological tests, but may not administer them to clinical populations; may investigate the origins and indices of psychopathology, but may not engage in diagnosis; and may develop and validate new therapies, but may not administer treatment.

At a Turning Point

After nearly half a century, the Boulder Model's grip on clinical psychology finally has begun to weaken. For example, by the end of the 1980s, professional interests had become so dominant within the American Psychological Association that many research-oriented psychologists concluded that the best hope for preserving scientific psychology was to form a new organization—the American Psychological Society. More recently, changes in the mental health-care system have undermined the market demand for psychotherapy training, thereby encouraging major universities to rededicate their resources to the traditional missions of scientific research and training. In 1994, a coalition of research-oriented clinical training programs formed a new organization—the Academy of Psychological Clinical Science—dedicated to the advancement of *scientific* training in clinical psychology.

In hindsight, many psychologists now regard the postwar professionalization of clinical psychology as a costly mistake (Sechrest, 1992). The commitment to professional clinical training gradually has eroded both the rate of scientific advancement and the quality and quantity of scientific training in psychology. Thus, it would be tragic indeed, if scientific psychology failed to heed the lessons of history. To grant psychologists prescription privileges is to repeat a fundamental mistake: emphasizing professional issues over scientific and training concerns. Once again, the discipline of psychology would be guilty of failing to preserve and protect the very environment that nourishes and sustains it.

So What?

At this point, one might ask, "But why *should* research and training institutions be preserved and protected? *So what* if they were to change? Aren't my arguments, as an academic, merely self-serving? How are they any different, in principle, than the arguments of those who see prescription privileges as essential to the preservation and protection of professional practice in clinical psychology?" These are legitimate questions. Just as environmentalists should be expected to explain convincingly why the protection of flora, fauna, air, and water should be given priority over competing economic interests, defenders of scientific interests should be expected to state their case explicitly and compellingly.

Elsewhere (McFall, 1991, 1995, 1996), I have discussed at length why basic research and scientific training are crucial to the future viability of clinical psychology. Here I only will be able to recap the key points: Clinical psychologists, like all health-care professionals, deal with the problems of some of society's most vulnerable members. Therefore, to guard against potential exploitation, deception, and harm, society increasingly is holding psychologists and other health-care professionals to high standards of "truth in advertising" and accountability for actions. Health-care professions are being required to document empirically that their implicit and explicit claims are valid, and that their interventions are cost-effective and safe. This is as it should be. To meet these rigorous standards, however, the specialty of clinical psychology must rely on its basic research institutions to supply the essential scientific evidence concerning the origins, conceptualization, assessment, prevention, and cost-effective amelioration of psychological problems. Moreover, to continue meeting these standards into the future, clinical psychology must rely upon its training institutions for a continuing supply of clinical scientists capable of advancing our knowledge and technology. Thus, all of society has a stake in preserving and protecting these research and training institutions because the products of these institutions are important to the current and future well being of us all. As a result, society should look very skeptically at any proposal that threatens to undermine these institutions. Advocates should bear the burden of proof concerning the possibility that their proposed changes might have an adverse impact.

Remodeling or Replacement?

This favorable view of research and training institutions is not shared by everyone. A growing chorus of psychologists has been critical of traditional academic institutions, arguing that the research produced by them has failed to provide useful solutions to the problems that practicing psychologists face in the "real world." These critics also have complained that the psychological training provided by traditional academic institutions is not relevant to professional practice in the "real world" (e.g., see the exchange between Peterson, 1996, and McFall, 1996). Finally, they have argued that traditional scientific training may be irrelevant, if not antithetical, to clinical practice.

Such critics have become increasingly bold in challenging what they regard as the hegemony of traditional research and training institutions. For example, they have built their own competing training institutions—mostly free-standing professional schools awarding "doctor of psychology" degrees (Psy.D.), as well as Ph.D. degrees. Many of these new institutions have promulgated an anti-science epistemology, in which the traditional system of controlled, empirical hypothesis testing is replaced with intuitive idiographic analysis grounded in personal experience (see Peterson, 1996). Over the past two decades, the number of students trained at alternative institutions offering alternative epistemologies has increased dramatically, especially relative to the number of students trained in a scientific epistemology by traditional programs. This numerical disparity has contributed to the growing schism within psychology that spawned the American Psychological Society.

These critics probably would not agree with my assertion that our premier research and training institutions are fragile national treasures that must be preserved and protected. Nor would they be dissuaded from seeking prescription privileges simply because it might threaten the essential scientific foundations of the discipline, or undermine our leading academic institutions. I do not believe that these critics—who are among the most vocal proponents of prescription privileges for psychologists—are trying to make only a minor modification in the current professional structure. Like the Minnesota builders, they are in the process of gradually replacing the entire structure under the guise of remodeling. They have already made considerable progress in transforming the long-standing science-based institutions of psychology. Thus, I do not expect my arguments against prescription privileges to change the minds of these critics. I do hope, however, that my arguments might serve as an alarm to those who cherish psychological science, and who wish to preserve and protect the environment that nourishes and sustains that science. Essentially, I have argued (a) that legislation giving prescription privileges to psychologists will have detrimental effects that exceed the bounds of legitimate positive change; and (b) that the legislation is radical in that it would transform clinical psychology into something else entirely. In particular, I have argued that the proposed legislation poses an unacceptable threat to the future well-being of society by undermining the vital research and training institutions of psychological science.

References

Barlow, D. H. (1994). Psychological intervention in the era of managed competition. *Clinical Psychology: Science and Practice, 1,* 109-122.

Brown, T. A., & Barlow, D. H. (1995). Long-term outcome in cognitive-behavioral treatment of panic disorder: Clinical predictors and alternative strategies for assessment. *Journal of Consulting and Clinical Psychology, 63,* 754-765.

McFall, R. M. (1991). Manifesto for a science of clinical psychology. *The Clinical Psychologist, 44,* 75-88.

McFall, R. M. (1995). Models of training and standards of care. In S. C. Hayes, V. F. Follette, R. M. Dawes, & K. E. Grady (Eds.). *Scientific standards of psychological practice: Issues and recommendations (pp. 125-139)*. Reno, NV: Context Press.

McFall, R. M. (1996). Making psychology incorruptible. *Applied and Preventive Psychology, 5*, 9-15.

Peterson, D. (1996). Making psychology indispensable. *Applied and Preventive Psychology, 5*, 1-8.

Polya, G. (1957). *How to solve it: A new aspect of mathematical method (2nd Ed.)*. Princeton: Princeton University Press.

Popper, K. R. (1962). *Conjectures & refutations*. New York: Basic Books.

Rauch, J. (1993). *Kindly inquisitors: The new attacks on free thought*. Chicago: The University of Chicago Press.

Sechrest, L. (1992). The past future of clinical psychology: A reflection on Woodworth (1937). *Journal of Consulting and Clinical Psychology, 60*, 18-23.

Telch, M. J., Lucas, J. A., Schmidt, N. B., Hanna, H. H., Jaimez, T. L., & Lucas, R. A. (1993). Group cognitive-behavioral treatment of panic disorder. *Behaviour Research and Therapy, 31*, 279-287.

Discussion of McFall

Prescription Reforms as Experiments

William O'Donohue, Ph.D.
University of Nevada

Throughout his distinguished career Richard McFall has been one of the strongest and most compelling advocates for a thoroughgoing scientific approach to clinical psychology. Many have used the banner of "science" for its considerable rhetorical value—wrapping something in the aura of science but including little or none of its substance, has been, unfortunately, too often persuasive to various constituencies. McFall, however, has a clear understanding and appreciation of the epistemic value of science. His "Manifesto for a Science of Clinical Psychology" (McFall, 1991) is one of the most lucid statements of how the epistemic duties of the clinical psychologist can only be met by a serious commitment to scientific evaluation.

In the present chapter, McFall considers two questions, "What defines the boundary separating legitimate positive changes in psychological training and practice from detrimental changes? And, how much can the training and practice of psychologists be changed before it becomes something else?" (pg. 101). These are important questions, and McFall presents a series of arguments all pointing to prohibiting prescription privileges for psychologists.

His arguments are varied but rely on some key empirical claims. A partial listing of these claims is included below.

Empirical Claims Contained in McFall's Arguments:

Granting prescription privileges to psychologists will result in an increase in the total volume of drug consumption.

The problem of overprescription would increase if psychologists could prescribe.

If allowed to prescribe, psychologists would do less psychological therapies and shift treatment practices toward pharmacological treatments.

Related to the preceding claim, the availability of effective psychological treatments would "all but disappear."

Requirements for obtaining prescription privileges would over time become increasingly stringent.

Those most likely to gain prescription privileges are the "least responsible and conscientious" (pg. 105) psychologists.

Inefficient, inappropriate, or even dangerous pharmacological treatments for psychological problems would increase (p. 106).

Granting prescription privileges to psychologists will do little or nothing for the problem of providing services to "underserved populations."

Granting prescription priveleges to psychologists will produce a more homogenous "monoculture" in mental health. This decrease in diversity places the field's survival at increased risk.

Granting prescription privileges to psychologists would enhance enterprises antagonistic to scientific research and training.

The new specialty of psycho-pharmaco-therapy would be attractive to academic institutions for financial reasons, and these new programs would compete with scientific research and training for scarce institutional resources.

Prescription privileges would dilute the training of clinical psychologists or increase the expense of such training.

Prescription privileges would result in an increase in oversight by external agencies thus reducing the university's autonomy in training.

Granting prescription privileges to psychologists would harm the movement to make clinical psychology a science–it would "threaten the essential scientific foundations of the discipline" (p. 113).

The reader is asked to note the following five points: 1) McFall has done an excellent job of delineating many different possible situations that may be affected by granting prescription privileges. 2) These are empirical claims. McFall makes claims about (potentially) observable states of the world. They state empirical possibilities, but their contradictions also describe possible states of affairs. That is, it is possible to deny McFall's claims without confronting a logical impossibility. 3) In McFall's analysis these propositions are often involved in causal claims. That is, often these empirical states of affairs are the (presumed) effects of granting prescription priveleges to psychologists, or are the empirical causes of other empirical states of affairs. 4) However, these empirical-causal claims are not particular cases of well-corroborated, general empirical laws. That is, McFall does not (and cannot argue) that there is a, for example, "Gresham's Law of Therapy" that states, "Bad therapy drives out good therapy." Thus, to deny McFall's empirical claims one also does not face physical impossibilities. 5) McFall cites no actual data to show that these empirical states of affairs or these causal relationships actually obtain. Rather, he relies on what may be called plausibility considerations, to suggest that it is plausible to believe that these relations hold or would hold.

Of course, a problem with the epistemic status of McFall's case is that one can plausibly deny the truth of his empirical claims. The critic is faced with no logical impossibility, physical impossibility, or data that such a denial is problematic. McFall in the face of this would have little compelling recourse. This is a serious problem for two reasons: 1) It is the predictable course to be taken by those on the other side of the issue, and thus little movement is made in resolving the questions. The debate is then characterized by statements and denials regarding each side's empirical predictions, with little or no compelling reason to believe either side. 2) It is inconsistent with taking a thoroughgoing scientific approach to this question.

Admittedly, at the current juncture there is little other recourse. There is simply not sufficient data concerning whether these empirical claims of McFall's (or for those on the other side) are true or false. It seems that little can be learned from the Department of Defense initiative, partly because it is such as special case, and partly because it was not designed as a social experiment. Thus, this debate often has the character of one side predicting one state of affairs given prescription priveleges, and the other side claiming this prediction is false, and another prediction to be true.

How is this debate to be advanced? I would suggest the following: Both sides clearly explicate the conditions in which they would regard their position as falsified. What results, if observed, would compel them to admit that they were in error and would cause them to revise their position to that of the other side?

I believe this is a reasonable request. The philosopher of science Karl Popper, whom I know McFall greatly respects, has suggested that error in one's web of belief is most efficiently eliminated if one explicates what observable state of affairs are inconsistent with one's beliefs (i.e., potential falsifiers), and then designs research to see if these observable states of affairs actually obtain. I am suggesting that both sides engage in this process; that is, make this a scientific question, in which the methodology of science can expose error.

Although it would be possible for both sides to conduct this research independently, it would be particularly worthwhile if the project could be conducted conjointly with clear falsifiability criteria agreed upon antecedently for both sides. No ad hoc strategies allowed. This creates the possibility to move this debate by scientific criteria, with all the attendant advantages.

However, how is this to be done? I would suggest that another scholar who I deeply admire, Donald Campbell, has provided an outline of the solution in his classic, "Reforms as Experiments." I propose that both sides agree on a social experiment or a series of social experiments to test their empirical claims. Training programs, state licensing laws, etc., can be randomly assigned and measures developed to see what empirical results obtain.

There are, of course, three major problems to my proposal: 1) The logistical problems and expense of gaining cooperation from diverse entities; 2) McFall could reasonably argue that certain problems will only emerge when prescription privileges are granted on a large scale; and 3) McFall could also reasonably argue that problems will emerge only after the test is concluded and normal "entropy-like" sloppiness comes into play. These are serious concerns, but I do not see any epistemically sound alternative to attempting to include these as best as possible in a scientific trial. Our most important principle should be a commitment to addressing problems through the use of the epistemology of science. We as scientific psychologists need to model this commitment when we address our own policy questions. Campbell argues that we need to be committed to experimentation, not to a particular position or policy. It is unfortunate that the American Psychological Association's establishment insists upon this sort of piecemeal experimental approach before considering enacting such reforms. To the extent that it has, McFall

and others can reasonably be concerned about the epistemic values of the proponents of such reforms.

McFall has an understanding and respect for a scientific approach to clinical
psychology that is admirable. These values appear to be associated with his caution
and concern regarding granting prescription privileges to psychologists. I, too, share
this concern. I have found that a line from a play is often apt—No matter how cynical
one gets, one just can't keep up. However being committed to a fallibilistic
epistemology—we may be wrong—and therefore we must rigorously test our empirical claims. I would strongly recommend that the American Psychological Association become an exemplar of this epistemically sophisticated approach toward
evaluating reforms.

References

Campbell, D.T. (1969). Reforms as experiments. *American Psychologist, 24*, 409-429.
McFall, R. M. (1991). Manifesto for a science of clinical psychology. *The Clinical
Psychologist, 44*, 75-88.

Chapter 5

Medical Training Needed to Prescribe and Monitor Psychoactive Drugs: A Paradigm for the Evaluation, Formulation, and Treatment of Psychiatric Disorders

Michael R. Clark, M.D.
The Johns Hopkins Medical Institutions

The practice of delivering health care encompasses the primary activities of curing the sick and helping the troubled with both often occurring in concert. Patients come to the health care system in distress. Health care professionals must first evaluate the patient in order to make a determination as to the cause of the distress. Only after this process has occurred can treatment be initiated regardless of what type of treatment is being offered. Psychiatry can cite many bad examples of prescribing a treatment without first formulating the individual patient's problem. As a consequence, many patients have received the risks of treatment instead of the benefits. This was largely a result of not thinking carefully about how to define a psychiatrist.

The definition of a psychiatrist has three components: 1) an expert examiner of mental life and behavior; 2) a keeper of a specialized fund of knowledge; and 3) an advocate for the mentally ill. These individual aspects of the definition supply the answers to the questions, "Who are we and what do we do?" The definition provides a framework for how psychiatrists think about examining mental life and behavior, adding to and using the fund of knowledge in research and treatment, and ensuring that patients are not mistreated either in the course of treatment or by society at large. As a result, the mission of psychiatry is born from its identity.

Psychologists are facing a difficult dilemma. Their profession is confronted with the question of whether to prescribe medications. The goals of psychologists are not in debate. They include providing comprehensive care to patients, expanding the profession, and addressing the inadequacies of the current health care delivery system. Yet, this question raises many important issues, such as the training required to prescribe medications, the liability of prescribing medications, and the potential increases in demand for practitioners able to perform pharmacotherapy in addition to psychotherapy. These issues are summarized in two basic questions: "Do psychologists *need* to prescribe medications?" and "do psychologists *have* to prescribe medications?"

Although these questions are important and arise from current external developments in health care, a more crucial question should not be lost. "Do psychologists really *want* to prescribe medications?" The answer to this question lies not in the debate over prescribing privileges, but at the core of the field of psychology. Psychologists must define their profession and then they will be able to decide how to contribute to the delivery of health care. The medical discipline of psychiatry can offer some guidance from the lessons it learned by having made the mistake of not clearly defining psychiatry and its approach to patients before attempting to take care of them (McHugh & Slavney, 1986; Slavney & McHugh, 1987).

The Trap

Within the practice of psychiatry, the ability to provide a treatment such as medication comes with certain risks as well as benefits. The example of a patient complaining of depression demonstrates a common trap for psychiatrists. The trap is an error arising from an excessive reliance on the American Psychiatric Association's Diagnostic and Statistical Manual (DSM) criteria (American Psychiatric Association, 1994). The patient presents with the chief complaint of feeling depressed. The other DSM criteria for a Major Depression are endorsed and the clinician then draws the conclusion that an antidepressant medication is indicated since there is research showing antidepressants are effective in the treatment of Major Depression. Although the reasoning appears sound, it is flawed.

The error comes from an ignorance of basic logical reasoning. Given the premise, "If A is true, then B is true"; then the statement, "If *not* B is true, then *not* A is true," is a logical truth. The converse of the original premise, "If B is true, then A is true" cannot always be concluded. In the example above, 'A' is that group of patients who the experts agreed had Major Depression, and 'B' is then a compilation of the symptoms they report. These symptoms form the DSM criteria for the operationally defined syndrome Major Depression. Therefore, to conclude that an individual who merely reports the criteria for Major Depression ("If B is true,") must actually have a Major Depression ("then A is true.") is an error in reasoning. The only logical conclusion that can be drawn from the DSM is as follows: if an individual does *not* report the criteria of a Major Depression, then that individual does *not* have a Major Depression.

It would now seem impossible ever to make a diagnosis with confidence in an individual patient. Clearly, if only the DSM criteria were available to the clinician, a valid diagnosis would not be possible. However, the cautionary statement at the beginning of the DSM provides the answer (American Psychiatric Association, 1994).

The specified diagnostic criteria for each mental disorder are offered as guidelines for making diagnoses, because it has been demonstrated that the use of such criteria enhances agreement among clinicians and investigators. The proper use of these criteria requires specialized clinical training that provides both a body of knowledge and clinical skills. (p. xxvii)

The DSM acknowledges these are *reliable* criteria for diagnoses and not necessarily *valid* criteria. The validity of any diagnosis is the context in which the patient and their symptoms exist. The biopsychosocial approach was an attempt to define this context (Engel, 1977, 1979, 1980). Unfortunately, it defined only the elements of the context and not the formula by which to produce a diagnosis. Again, the clinician must return to the appropriate training that provides both a fund of knowledge and clinical skills for the examination and diagnosis of the patient.

Psychiatrists possess a fund of knowledge about the body as a whole. Medical school includes courses on anatomy, biochemistry, pathology, physiology, and neuroscience to give some examples. These parts combine to produce an integrated comprehension of the body as a whole that is greater than just the sum of these disciplines. Similarly, medical students also take pharmacology to gain a more specific fund of knowledge about drug actions, interactions, side effects, and toxicity. The clinical experience of internship and residency provides the training within a given specialty of medicine, and then builds upon this foundation.

These experiences over many years result in the development of clinical skills. Not only does the physician become adept at the physical examination but, more importantly, develops the ability to formulate the individual patient's case from which he constructs a valid diagnosis. The formulation of what is wrong with a patient includes the patient's core symptoms, associated symptoms, course, duration, precipitating factors, predisposing factors, and signs from the physical examination as well as results from objective testing including laboratory and imaging studies. This composite of many facts about the patient's illness initially leads to the production of a differential diagnosis of the patient's condition. The differential diagnosis is a priority list of all the possible conditions that could be causing the patient's illness. For example, depression could result from a medical disorder such as stroke, hypothyroidism, or pancreatic cancer. Ultimately, the final diagnosis is made and only then is rational treatment initiated.

The Conflict

The primary conflict for any profession attempting to take care of patients with disorders of mental life and behavior is between mind and brain (Slavney, 1993). This dualism can finally be resolved by recognizing that both entities exist, problems can arise from both realms, and although they are linked, the connections are still unclear. Mind and brain remain distinct and cannot be merged to form a unifying theory of mental life. The conflict arises from the concepts of explanation and understanding (Peirce, 1957). Explanation describes the linear reasoning of cause and effect (see figure to the left). An event 'A' results in an outcome 'B'. Many complex phenom-

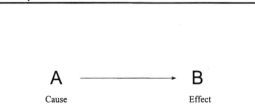

Explanation

A ⟶ B

Cause   Effect

ena in the environment can be broken down into a series of these two component steps or dyads. In contrast, understanding involves the process by which an aspect of the *environment* becomes meaningful in a person's *world*.

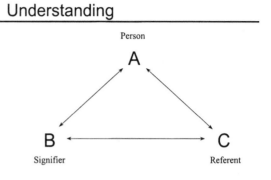

Understanding

Understanding requires the person to interact with some event, and then assign a symbol to it that embodies the unique and personal qualities of the event (see figure to the right). All three components of this triad are essential to a meaningful understanding. The triad cannot be reduced to a dyad.

In medicine, the dyad is present within a series of cause and effect relationships that describe an altered circumstance in the body and produce disease pathology (see figure below). In the end, the collected signs and symptoms of the pathology are recognized as a clinical syndrome. A significant portion of the practice of medicine involves working backward through these steps. For example, a patient presents with shortness of breath and lower extremity edema. After an examination, he is formulated as having the syndrome of congestive heart failure (CHF). Further examination attempts to determine what pathology is present. The patient may have an arrhythmia, mitral stenosis, or constrictive pericarditis. Each of these pathologies, for example an arrhythmia, has an associated list of potential etiologies such as being on the medication nortriptyline, having developed coronary artery disease, or having contracted bacterial endocarditis. This process is often referred to as the medical model and will be discussed later as the Disease perspective.

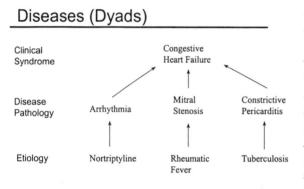

Diseases (Dyads)

In contrast, the triad is constructed out of the interaction of the patient with a situation, and their unique interpretation of that particular situation. When another person, such as a therapist, is introduced to the triad, several different triads are now formed (see figure top of facing page). However, one of the more important is the new triad of the second person's interaction with the first and subsequent reinterpretation of the original situation. In this circumstance, a new meaning emerges out of the interaction between the two people. Although this process

Life Events (Triads)

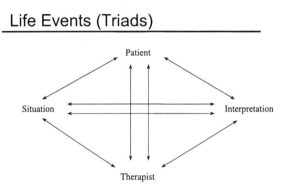

occurs in every aspect of daily life, psychiatrists and psychotherapists practice psychotherapy as triads. A problem is presented, and through a meaningful interaction some solution is derived.

In returning to the example of a patient presenting with the complaint of depression, the "gap" between dyads and triads becomes more obvious. If the patient's depression is the result of a disease such as a deficiency of norepinephrine in the brain, then the required treatment will be the prescription of a medication that provides an increase in norepinephrine by inhibiting its metabolism (see figure to the right). If, however, the depression is due to the patient having just been fired from his job and fearing financial disaster, the therapist will need to provide an understanding of this problem. He will help the patient to re-interpret

Diseases

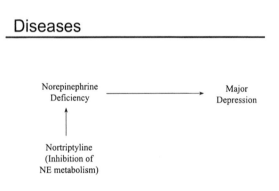

the situation as not disastrous and having the potential for developing greater rewards than those of the previous job (see figure below).

In comparing dyads and triads, there is no way to close the gap between them. They are unable to be combined; however, both may be present in a given patient. Dyads are open to external forces such as bacteria or drugs that alter normal physiology in a series of events. Triads are closed systems, with their meaning being the product only of the principal components. Hence, the triad is based on the relationships of the components, while the dyad is based on a cause and its linked effect. Psychiatrists deal with both situations. They bridge this gap by virtue of their training as both doctors and psychotherapists.

Life Events

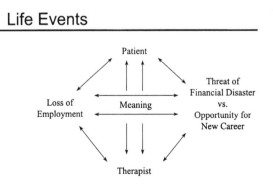

Causality and meaning are still inadequate in the description of human consciousness and behavior. Even though individuals can be affected by the external world and form an interpretation of that world, they still have internal characteristics and actions that can shape the distress they experience. The psychiatrist's initial role in the evaluation of a patient in distress is to produce a differential diagnosis attempting to sort out whether the patient is sick with a disease, in trouble from an inappropriate compelling behavior, frustrated by their own psychological vulnerabilities, or demoralized by a particular stressor. Clearly, a different paradigm is needed for the evaluation of patients if such a comprehensive, integrated, differential diagnosis is to become possible.

The Paradigm

The goal of any evaluation of a patient's complaints is to recognize the contribution of several types of processes involved in the generation of distress (McHugh, 1987, 1987a, 1992). McHugh and Slavney described four perspectives applicable to the evaluation and treatment of psychiatric disorders (McHugh & Slavney, 1986). The four perspectives are Diseases, Life Stories, Dimensions, and Behaviors (Table 1).

Diseases

The disease perspective utilizes the logic of cause and effect as described above. It is a linear approach most often described as the medical model. The objective lies in using the patient's symptoms and signs to make a categorical and, therefore, mutually exclusive diagnosis. The patient either has a particular disease or he does not. One diagnosis is ruled in, and all other diagnoses are ruled out.

The disease perspective assumes an abnormality in the structure or function of a bodily part as described above in the example of CHF. This is an example of the power of Nature to "break" individuals. The broken part transforms physiology into pathophysiology and health into sickness. As a consequence, signs and symptoms of the disease emerge and cluster together as a recognizable syndrome. Treatment is then designed to prevent or repair the broken part and restore function to premorbid levels. Definitive cures can be developed to combat specific etiologies when they are discovered to produce the abnormality. Unfortunately, the etiology of many conditions is elusive and treatments can only be approximations at cure. In addition, every treatment has the potential for causing even more damage and making the patient worse.

The disease perspective's limitations are its rigid linear view of mutually exclusive conditions and presumption that all mental distress emerges from broken parts. Psychiatric disorders are often the responses of perfectly intact individuals facing life's difficulties. Other perspectives than disease are required to comprehend these conditions and expand the process of evaluation, formulation and treatment.

Table 1: Summary of the Perspectives of Psychiatry

	Diseases	Life Stories	Behaviors	Dimensions
Logic	causal relationships define categories	accumulated events produce a unique narrative	acts have design and purpose	personal features are described along spectrums of measurement
Essence	abnormal structure or function of a bodily part	meaningful connections between past events and present circumstances	altered drives and goals can produce problem behaviors	the relative amount of a trait predisposes to inherent strengths and vulnerabilities
Goal	prevent or correct the abnormality to restore function	understand patterns and re-interpret meaning to restore mastery	stop behavior to restore drives/goals and prevent relapse	guide toward strengths and avoid provocation of vulnerabilities to restore balance
Risk	all treatments can cause more damage	all interpretations are hostile	all demands to stop behavior are stigmatizing	all advice is paternalistic

Life Stories

The life story perspective relies on the narrative of an individual's unique sequence of events to generate meaning. Life events are those specific items of a person's story that have been encountered. Each person has a *unique* life story or series of events. The person's life produces new experiences demonstrating patterns based on an understanding of how and why those particular events occurred. Meaningful connections are made between past events and present circumstances. These connections generate a sense of how a life is unfolding.

A person may become distressed when he experiences the unintended consequences of past intentional interactions, their sequence, or the setting in which they occurred. This distress is the result of a perceived loss of mastery over one's life, and becomes the logical outcome of past events. This loss is the result not of Nature's power but of individual motives becoming entangled with events. Treatment in this instance is designed to increase understanding by re-writing the story in such a way that the person can now appreciate the patterns and outcomes of his intentions. This new understanding leads to making better choices for the future. Unfortunately, there is never one "true" story about the patient's life but an infinite number. In the successful therapy, the patient accepts the interpretation because he sees it as useful in his approach to life.

The patient who develops lung cancer can be shown that even though he has a terminal illness, he can contribute to the future and maintain a sense of control. This contribution may not have been previously considered, such as supporting smoking cessation programs. Similarly, a patient who presents to a psychiatrist feeling overwhelmed by his third divorce would benefit from discussing each marriage to understand recurrent mistakes. Recognizing this pattern would allow for changes to avoid future mistakes of the same kind, and restore the individual's desire for companionship.

Dimensions

The dimensional perspective is based on the logic of a continuous distribution. Individual variation exists for many characteristics and bodily processes occurring along a continuum or normal distribution. Traits are aspects of who people are. Most individuals possess an average amount of a particular trait, however, a few individuals will exist at both extremes. These differences define individual variation. The trait itself conveys certain strengths and weaknesses upon the individual that vary depending on the quantity of the trait. At times, these people will be vulnerable to distress by virtue of their unusual "dose" of a characteristic. The qualities inherent to the trait itself determine the type of susceptibility. Different aspects of life could then potentially provoke difficulty.

For example, the person with low levels of aldehyde dehydrogenase is usually unaware of his position along the continuum. However, consuming a significant quantity of alcohol will overwhelm the capacity to metabolize this substance and result in poisoning. The individual with a low IQ may function without substantial difficulty in a highly structured environment. When the structure is disrupted, this person will display their limitations in abstract reasoning and problem-solving. They will become distressed. The solution is often found in restoring structure or providing the person with new skills to solve specific problems.

Another example of the dimensional perspective lies in affective temperament. Personality traits vary along spectrums of particular characteristics such as extroversion/introversion. The person who is extremely introverted will be vulnerable to different problems than the one who is very extroverted. Treatments within the dimensional perspective focus on illuminating the strengths and weaknesses that are the manifestations of particular characteristics such as being anxious in unfamiliar situations. With guidance, these vulnerabilities can be avoided; however, the advice can be excessively paternalistic if simply prescribed. Specific methods should be devised to compensate for vulnerabilities. Psychiatrists not only help patients with their weaknesses, but also recognize their strengths so potential can be fulfilled. The major weakness of the dimensional perspective is the arbitrary definition of the difference between "normal" and "abnormal."

Behaviors

The behavioral perspective rests on the logic of design and purpose. People have reasons for what they do, and often have trouble recognizing the factors influencing their behavior. Behavior is typically described with respect to time. The behavior itself is preceded by antecedents forming the foundation for the emergence of a specific behavior. Consequences then develop as an outcome of that behavior, and may increase or decrease the potential for the behavior to occur in the future. These principles have been refined in both the fields of classical and operant conditioning. Many techniques have been developed to shape, generalize, and extinguish different types of behavior. These methods focus primarily on the innate drives of behavior and its reinforcements. This view limits the potential for altering a problematic behavior that is producing distress by ignoring the accompanying ideas or self-imposed goals of the individual.

Behavior can also be discussed in terms of a repeating cycle with several important components. These include the appetites or drives to engage in the behavior and the satiety or satisfaction occurring when the goals of the behavior have been accomplished. This conception of behavior recognizes that treatment of behavioral disorders must first stop the behavior. The potential for preventing its recurrence is increased if the specific motivations and goals of these purposeful acts are discovered. The individual components precipitate, sustain, and reinforce the behavior. Both the consequences of behavior and the drives motivating the behavior must be appreciated. For example, a drive may need to be reduced or a goal changed in order to break the vicious cycle of repetitive problematic behaviors.

The patient with chronic renal failure requiring hemodialysis who is repeatedly admitted to the hospital with CHF secondary to fluid overload is often discovered to be drinking too much water. Attempts to discourage him from this dangerous behavior will be unsuccessful unless it is recognized that his thirst is high and the

goal of the behavior is to satisfy this intense craving. Substance abuse can be
formulated in a similar fashion. The drives, behaviors, and goals of using excessive
medications or illicit drugs must each be determined. This allows treatment to
move beyond stopping the act to altering the associated drives and goals. Demanding a behavior be stopped without appreciating these other features will only
stigmatize the behavior creating arguments about rights and freedoms, instead of
responsibilities and consequences.

Summary

Together, these four perspectives provide a comprehensive yet flexible approach to the evaluation of a patient in distress. Each individual patient will have
a different combination of the four perspectives (Clark, 1994, 1996; Slavney, 1990).
The patient does not have to fit into one theoretical approach in order to receive
treatment. Treatment is now designed out of the formulation and diagnosis.

If a patient's distress continues, the physician must consider other factors that
may have been overlooked before abandoning or adjusting a treatment plan. Usually
these factors are within one of the perspectives initially thought to be less important.
A new combination of approaches is then required to treat the patient successfully.

The perspectives of psychiatry identify the patient as a person who is a composite of vulnerabilities and strengths but afflicted with diseases, struggling through
life events, and motivated for various reasons. Each individual perspective has its
own logical process for evaluation and subsequently directed treatment. Although
the perspectives are complimentary, they each remain distinct and essential.

The "Prescription"

Psychiatrists have struggled to define themselves in order to avoid the pitfalls
in taking care of patients. Psychologists must do the same. Not because it is "wrong"
to prescribe medications but because the question of whether psychologists *want*
to prescribe medication has not been answered.

Before the answer can be found, psychologists must continue to examine
patients using the methods they know best, apply their fund of knowledge with
ingenuity and energy, and advocate for patients with problems in mental life and
behavior. Then they will discover who they are, and what it is they do.

Undoubtedly the future will bring change, but psychologists will survive. All
health care providers must work together to design actively the integrated and,
therefore, more comprehensive health care delivery systems. In this way, each
profession will control its own destiny rather than simply be told what to do by
others who really do not understand them.

References

American Psychiatric Association. (1994). *Diagnostic and statistical manual of mental
disorders* (4th ed.). Washington, DC: American Psychiatric Association.
Clark, M. R. (1994). Chronic dizziness: An integrated approach. *Hospital Practice,
29*, 57-64.

Clark, M. R. (1996). The role of psychiatry in the treatment of chronic pain. In j. Campbell & M. Cohen (Eds.), *Pain treatmant centers at a crossroads: A practical and conceptual reappraisal* (pp. 59-68). Seattle, WA: IASP Press.

Engel, G. L. (1977). The need for a new medical model. *Science, 196*, 129-36.

Engel, G. L. (1979). The biopsychosocial model and the education of health professionals. *General Hospital Psychiatry, 1*, 156-65.

Engel, G. L. (1980). The clinical application of the biospychosocial model. *American Journal of Psychiatry, 137*, 535-44.

McHugh, P. R. (1987). William Osler and the new psychiatry. *Annals of Internal Msedicine, 107*, 914-8.

McHugh, P. R. (1987a). Psychiatry and its scientific relatives: "A little more than kin and less than kind." *Journal of Nervous and Mental Disorders, 175*, 597-83.

McHugh, P. R. (1992). A structure for psychiatry at the century's turn—the view from Johns Hopkins. *Journal of the Royal Society of Medicine, 85*, 483-7.

McHugh, P. R. & Slavney, P. R. (1982). Methods of reasoning in psychopathology: Conflict and resolution. *Comprehensive Psychiatry, 23*, 197-215.

McHugh, P. R. & Slavney, P. R. (1986). *The perspectives of psychiatry.* Baltimore, MD: Johns Hopkins University Press.

Peirce, C. S. & Thomas, V. (1957). *Essays in the philosophy of science.* New York, NY: Liberal Arts Press.

Slavney, P. R. (1993). The mind-brain problem, epistemology, and psychiatyric education. *Academic psychiatry, 17*, 59-66.

Slavney, P. R. & McHugh, P. R. (1987). *Psychiatric polarities: Methodology and practice.* Baltimore, MD: Johns Hopkins University Press.

Discussion of Clark

A New Era or Pandora's Box?

Gregory J. Hayes, M.D., M.P.H.
University of Nevada School of Medicine

As one of the few physicians participating in this conference, I must state clearly my personal stance on the granting of prescription privileges to psychologists: it will produce more harm than good. I must also immediately say that I feel strangely schizophrenic in making such a statement.

As a physician I have long supported the sharing of prescription privileges with other members of the health care team. For example, over the last six years I have repeatedly testified in favor of a bill before the Nevada state legislature which would grant limited prescription privileges to optometrists; in our most recent legislative session we were, in fact, successful in this effort. My support for granting these privileges to optometrists, allowing them to be "general practitioners" of the eye, stemmed from repeated personal experiences. Many times during my years in general practice, I turned to my optometric colleagues for help in handling an eye problem at the primary care level. What I learned was that optometrists often knew a good deal more than I did; their training had exceeded my own. Given that reality, I felt it was a waste of time, energy, and money to insist that an optometrist refer non-surgical eye problems to primary care physicians only to have these same physicians call the referring optometrist many times for advise on how to handle the problem. Optometrists, given their training and with some additional pharmacology training, are well placed to simplify this sequence of events and handle many of the problems they discover themselves.

Yet in the case of psychologists, I find myself siding, although probably for different reasons, with the more conservative members of my profession. I find myself frightened by the potentially detrimental effects of such a change. The obvious question is: Why the difference?

There is no doubt that well-trained psychologists could do a very professional job with the prescribing of medications. It is not a matter of mental acumen certainly—at least among psychologists who are products of top-quality programs. In fact, because psychologists are so much better skilled in psychotherapy than their psychiatric counterparts, it could also be argued that psychologists, given adequate training, could do a better job than psychiatrists of deciding when and if the prescribing of a psychoactive drug were appropriate.

But there is an important difference between psychologists and other members of the health care team—optometrists, nurse practitioners, podiatrists, physician assistants, etc.—when it comes to prescribing drugs. All these other disciplines are oriented to the medical model of health care; psychologists are not. All these other disciplines receive a great deal of training and undergraduate and graduate course work relevant to the use of drugs; psychologists do not. So in contrast to other health professions, we are speaking of an overwhelmingly radical change in the focus of psychology should the ability to prescribe be granted.

As Dr. Clark has pointed out, the interaction of diseases, life events, behaviors, and traits which allow us to describe and understand mental illness are so complex that, even after the training of medical school, without additional specialization physicians are ill-equipped to diagnose properly and treat such problems. In fact, in my view, because non-psychiatrists are disproportionately responsible for the gross overuse and misuse of psychoactive drugs we observe today, they should be denied the ability to prescribe them without obtaining adequate specialty training. But could not psychologists be among those with such "adequate specialty training"? As I have noted, of course they could. But there would be a big price to pay.

First would be the added years of training. To be adequately trained, an array of undergraduate courses in biology, chemistry, anatomy, and physiology would be a must. And then something on the order of the first two years of medical school would seem essential as well. All that, coupled with the psychologist's superior training in psychotherapy, would theoretically produce a specialist with a more balanced view of psychotherapy and psychopharmacology than that observed among psychiatrists.

But for those willing put forth the effort to extend their graduate training so substantially, there would be other dangers. Most important of all would be the temptation to decrease the use of psychotherapy and to rely more and more heavily on medications to treat mental health problems. In the interest of keeping the time commitment for graduate training under control, there would a push to limit the amount of training in psychotherapy as well. That is precisely what occurred in psychiatry with the discovery of the benzodiazapines and the subsequent litany of ever more potent anti-psychotics, anti-depressants, and the like: Psychotherapeutic skills among psychiatrists atrophied from disuse.

Would that happen to most psychologists? I believe it would. All of us would like to feel we are immune to the problems which others may experience. But if the profession of psychology moves into the world of the prescribing of drugs, they should do so with clear understanding that a very powerful force will be unleashed. In our culture there is a strong demand on the part of the consumer for access to all available treatments. To date, with only a few experimental exceptions, persons seeking help from psychologists did not have the expectation of receiving medications. In fact, some portion of these clients probably chose psychology expressly because they were not going to be "forced" to include a drug in their treatment plan. If prescription privileges become the norm, however, the demand on the part of the client for the use of these seemingly "magical" pills will unrelentingly increase. The amount of time a psychologist will be required to dedicate to considering, prescribing, evaluating, and studying psychoactive drugs will grow substantially. And the amount of time available for psychotherapy will decrease substantially at the same time. It will be unavoidable. If most psychologists are ultimately able to prescribe, the very skills which today make psychology so viable will steadily disappear.

There are other dangers as well. If, in the final analysis, only a few hundred hours of psychopharmacology are required to be allowed to prescribe as a psychologist, Pandora's box will open wide. Psychologists prescribing in this manner will be in over their heads (I am especially fearful of psychologists from programs of dubious quality), even more so than non-psychiatrist physicians, and will undoubtedly overuse such medications, including inappropriate treatment of cases in which serious and even life-threatening iatrogenic harm will result. As Dr. Piasecki will later describe, the potential problems with drug interactions and drug side effects is very serious business indeed. A few hundred hours of additional training would be so inadequate to the task as to be patently unethical.

The more prudent alternative would pattern the substantial additional training along the lines of that received by Morgan Sammons, a thoughtful and important contributor to this important conference. Creating such a large hurdle would mean that relatively few psychologists would ever be given prescription privileges, and the more widespread potential for negative consequences on the professions would be averted. But even here there is a potential danger. Psychologists seem exceedingly unaware of just how seductive drugs can be. Our society, our culture, thrives on them. Once a few psychologists are allowed to obtain the training, the demand will be for more and more psychologists to be allowed to do the same. At one level there is nothing wrong with that. As I have noted, I believe someone like Morgan Sammons could do a demonstrably better job than most psychiatrists and would be, at least at the outset, less likely to overuse medications. But once the genie is out of the lamp there is no sure way to contain it. Given our cultural enthusiasm for access to all available therapies, the risk is very real that demand for drugs and all the time commitment that that implies will lead to ever-shrinking psychotherapeutic skills. And that would be sad indeed. A profession focusing on effective, non-medical interventions in mental illness is an important counterbalance to psychiatry's strongly drug-oriented model. Although I welcome the granting of prescription privileges to many health-related disciplines, for psychology I feel it is a terrible mistake.

Chapter 6

The Implications of Basic Research in Behavioral Pharmacology for Prescription Privileges for Psychologists

Alan Poling, Ph.D., LeeAnn Christian, Ph.D.,
and Kristal Ehrhardt, Ph.D.
Western Michigan University

Over the last decade, there has been much controversy within the professional psychology community regarding prescription privileges for psychologists. In response to the growing interest in the acquisition of prescription privileges for psychologists, an ad hoc task force on psychopharmacology was established during the 1990 APA convention in Boston. The goals of the task force were to examine issues relating to the "desirability and feasibility" of the use of psychopharmacological agents by psychologists, and to determine training and competence criteria (see Smyer et al., 1993 for a summary of the task force's recommendations).

Some psychologists view the obtainment of prescription privilege as a logical next step in the evolution of a maturing profession (e.g., Brentar & McNamara, 1991; DeLeon, Fox & Graham, 1991). Others envision it leading to the demise of a profession that already struggles to define itself (e.g., DeNelsky, 1991). Arguments for and against prescription privileges for psychologists have appeared in many venues (e.g., DeLeon & Wiggins, 1996; DeLeon, Folen, Jennings, Willis, & Wright, 1991; DeNelsky, 1991, 1996; Fox, 1988a, b; Hayes & Heiby, 1996; Kingsbury, 1992; Klein, 1996; Kubiszyn, 1994); they will not be repeated here.

Conspicuous by their absence in the debate concerning prescription privileges are psychologists who conduct basic research with psychoactive substances, including psychotropic medications. The purpose of the present chapter is to describe the kinds of basic research characteristically conducted by behavioral pharmacologists, and to consider the relevance of such research for prescription privileges for psychologists.

Overview of Behavioral Pharmacology

There is no clear and absolute distinction between psychopharmacology and behavioral pharmacology. The former term was coined years ago to describe an emerging science dealing with the behavioral effects of drugs (Macht & Mora, 1921). In an influential textbook that helped to popularize the term, "behavioral pharmacology," Thompson and Schuster (1968) defined it as "a branch of biological science that uses the tools and concepts of experimental psychology and pharmacology to explore the behavioral actions of drugs" (p.1). Behavioral pharmacologists often, but not always, use concepts and procedure characteristic of the experimental analysis of behavior to explain the drug effects. The experimental analysis of behavior is a unique approach to the study of behavior popularized by the late B.F. Skinner, although many other people contributed to its development (see Michael, 1980; O'Donnell, 1985; Zuriff, 1985). Table 1 contrasts the research strategies characteristic of the experimental analysis of behavior with those characteristic of traditional experimental psychology. Behavioral pharmacologists often favor the former strategies, but this is not always the case.

A crucial step in the development of behavioral pharmacology was the demonstration that behavior is lawfully related to measurable changes in the environment, and can be explained without recourse to unobserved, hypothetical entities. Ivan Pavlov's studies of classical conditioning were among the first experiments to demonstrate the orderliness of overt behavior and its susceptibility to scientific analysis. One of Pavlov's students, Igor Zavadskii, conducted a study that is thought to be the first in the tradition of behavioral pharmacology. In this study, Zavadskii measured the effects of caffeine, cocaine, ethanol, and morphine on the classically conditioned salivation of dogs (Laties, 1979). Zavadskii's procedures share much with those used by behavioral pharmacologists today: A wide range of doses was studied, within-subject controls were employed, and effects were measured under a range of conditions. This line of research apparently held little appeal for the Soviets, however, and the emergence of behavioral pharmacology as an organized discipline awaited the birth of behavioral psychology in America.

As an infant science, behavioral psychology attempted to discover general principles of behavior by studying seemingly simple organisms (rats, pigeons, non-human primates) under controlled laboratory conditions. As early as 1920, researchers at Johns Hopkins University examined how drugs influences maze learning by rats (Macht & Mora, 1921). However, systematic examinations of the behavioral actions of drugs occurred only sporadically from the turn of the century until its midpoint. In the 1950s, interest in the area skyrocketed; Pickens (1977) reported that between 1917 and 1954 only 28 studies examining drug effects on learned behavior were published in English-language journals, whereas 274 such studies appeared from 1955 to 1963. The factors responsible for this remarkable increase are complex (see Pickens, 1977), but certain momentous happenings bear note.

By 1955, behavioral pharmacology had matured into an accepted, if controversial, discipline. In two major books, Skinner (1938,1953) espoused the theme that behavior is orderly, therefore subject to scientific analysis, and described a technology for this analysis. In 1956, the potential value of this technology for studying drug effects was emphasized at a conference called Techniques for the Study of the Behavioral Effects of Drugs, sponsored by the New York Academy of Sciences and chaired by Skinner and Dews (Annals, 1956). Researchers studying drug-behavior interactions were quick to adopt Skinner's operant conditioning methodology,

Table 1: *Characteristics of the Experimental Analysis of Behavior and Traditional Experimental Psychology*

Dimension	Experimental Analysis of Behavior	Traditional Experimental Psychology
Number of subjects	Few	Many
Research design	Within-subject	Between-subjects
Importance of behavior	Significant in its own right	Significant as an indication of events at *another level* of analysis
Data collection	Direct, repeated measures of behavior	Various methods used, often indirect and non-repeated measures of behavior
Data analysis	Graphical	Statistical
Approach to variable data	Consider the variability as imposed; isolate and control the responsible extraneous variables	Consider the variability as intrinsic; use statistics to detect effects of the independent variable despite the variability

especially in the areas of drug self-administration and drug effects on the performance of learned behaviors.

Studies of Behavioral Loci of Drug Action

The striking clinical effectiveness of chlorpromazine raised questions concerning the precise behavioral actions of the drug, and researchers attempted to detail the drug's actions in laboratory studies. The term, behavioral loci of drug action, is often used to refer to the specific changes in behavior produced by a drug (Thompson, 1981), and studies of behavioral loci of drug action have always been a major part of behavioral pharmacology.

As indicated in several reviews (e.g., Baldessarini, 1990; Fielding & Lal, 1978; Jannsen & Van Bever, 1978; Seiden & Dykstra, 1977), laboratory studies with nonhumans have revealed that chlorpromazine and related neuroleptics generally produce dose-dependent decreases in the rate of occurrence of positively-reinforced operants. They reduce spontaneous motor activity and exploratory behavior, while increasing the latency to respond to (but not necessarily the ability to discriminate) various stimuli. At high doses, they produce catalepsy.

The effects of neuroleptics on learning are complex and difficult to summarize. A study by Poling, Cleary, Berens, and Thompson (1990) provides an example of a study designed to examine how four neuroleptics influence learning, specifically, pigeons' behavior under a repeated acquisition procedure. The rationale for this study was described by Poling et al. (1990) as follows:

> Learning impairment is [a] serious side effect associated with these [neuroleptic] drugs (Aman, 1984; Lipman, DiMascio, Reatig, & Kirson, 1978). Like other behavioral side effects of neuroleptics, learning impairment has been little studied in humans. Clinical investigations have not revealed whether various neuroleptics differ with respect to likelihood and severity of learning impairment.
>
> Laboratory studies of the effects of neuroleptics on learning also are few (e.g., Picker, Cleary, Berens, Oliveto, & Dykstra, 1989; Thompson, 1974), and no direct comparisons of the effects of different neuroleptic drugs have appeared. It is, however, apparent that there are substantial differences in the behavioral effects of various neuroleptics. For example, studies using the delayed-matching-to-sample procedure [an index of short-term memory] and other assays of discrimination suggest that, although the effects of specific agents from the same chemical class may differ substantially, phenothiazines, thioxanthenes, dibenzodiazepines, dihytroindolines and tricyclic dibenzoxazepines typically disrupt accuracy to a greater extent than butyrophenones and benzamines (Laties, 1972; Newland & Marr, 1985; Nielson & Appel, 1983; Picker & Massie, 1988; Poling, Picker, & Thompson, 1984). The purpose of the present study was to compare systematically the effects of four neuroleptic drugs—haloperidol, molindone, mesoridazine and thioridazine—on the behavior of pigeons under a re-

peated acquisition procedure. This procedure requires subjects to learn a spatially defined sequence of responses that changes from session to session (Thompson, 1978).

Haloperidol is a butyrophenone; mesoridazine and thioridazine are phenothiazines; and molindone is a dihydroindoline. Results obtained with the delayed-matching-to-sample procedure suggest that haloperidol might well disrupt learning to a lesser extent than the other three drugs. Determining whether this is so requires more than a comparison of simple dose-response relations for the four drugs, for they differ appreciably in potency. In view of this, dose-response relations in the present study are expressed both in terms of the actual amount of drug given and in terms of chlorpromazine-equivalent dose. (p. 1240)

The repeated acquisition schedule was arranged in three-key operant conditioning chambers. It comprised a four-link response chain. A different key color was correlated with each link and key position defined which response was correct during each link. Correct positions for each link changed on a daily basis, and completion of the chain of four correct responses resulted in food delivery. For example, on Monday food might be delivered dependent on completing the sequence peck left, peck center, peck right, peck center, whereas the sequence center, right, left, center might be required for food delivery on Tuesday.

Under this procedure, most errors were made relatively early in the session in the absence of drugs, and stable error rates appeared with extended training. When this occurred, several doses of each of the four drugs were administered. At sufficiently high doses, each drug increased errors and reduced response rates relative to control values. Doses at which these effects occurred differed substantially across drugs, however. For example, haloperidol disrupted learning (increased errors) and reduced rates of responding at substantially lower doses than any of the three other drugs, a finding consistent with other laboratory reports (e.g., Picker, 1987, 1989). But, as Poling et al. (1990) indicated:

It is erroneous to assume on this basis that in clinical applications haloperidol would be more likely than molindone, mesoridazine, or thioridazine to interfere with learning. The four drugs differ dramatically in therapeutic potency and, when they are compared in terms of chlorpromazine-equivalent doses, haloperidol appears to be considerably less disruptive than mesoridazine or thioridazine, and somewhat less disruptive than molindone. (p. 1243)

The study by Poling et al. (1990) was discussed at some length because it is an example of basic research intended to explore an issue of obvious clinical importance, specifically, neuroleptic-induced learning impairment. Despite this focus, obvious care is needed in making extrapolations to humans treated with neuroleptics. As Poling et al. Pointed out,

Correction for human therapeutic potency [i.e., comparing chlorpromazine-equivalent doses] does not address the pharmacological relevance of these findings. The issue is whether any of the drugs tested in the present study interfered with learning or performance at doses relevant to those used with humans. Unlike drugs such as opioid analgesics, in which behavior in the presence of pain allows an independent reference point from which interspecies drug effects may be compared, neuroleptics have no obvious objective measures which will correlate the dose range in laboratory animals with the therapeutically relevant human range. Difference in route of administration, metabolism, receptor distribution, and chronicity of exposure, etc. make it impossible to extrapolate doses directly from clinical practice to laboratory investigation. Behavioral changes in learning or performance under the drug may be the best objective measure available to relate human and nonhuman drug effects. Once this relative does range is established the benefits of the animal model may be fully utilized. Unfortunately, much of the necessary human behavioral pharmacology has not yet been done. (p. 1244)

Studies such as this suggest probable adverse effects of psychotropic drugs when used with human patients, and also suggest topics for investigation by clinical psychopharmacologists. They do not, however, provide information of direct value to practitioners. It would, for example, be naive and misguided to favor haloperidol over mesaridizine in clinical practice on the basis of the data reported by Poling et al. (1990).

Studies of Psychotropic Screening Procedures

Because the widespread adoption of chlorpromazine led to substantial profits for its manufacturer, researchers also attempted to develop procedures useful for detecting other drugs with clinical actions similar to those of chlorpromazine. Procedures used to screen drugs for potential psychotropic (or other useful) properties are termed "models" or "tests." Although the terms sometimes are used interchangeably, Porsolt, McArthur, and Lenegre (1993) differentiate them as follows:

The word 'model' implies an attempt by the experimenter to imitate the pathology for which the drug is destined. The word 'test' is applied more generally to any procedure used to characterize a psychotropic agent. Models in psychopharmacology are usually based on behavioral changes induced in animals by manipulation of their internal or external environment. The underlying assumption is that the environmental manipulations are analogous to those inducing the pathology in man. For example, anxious-like behavior can be induced in animals by placing them in unknown environments or in environments in which they have been punished (p. 24)

The pole-jump escape/avoidance procedure was one of the first assays demonstrated to be selectively affected by chlorpromazine and other neuroleptics (Cook & Weidley, 1957). In this assay, rats can avoid a forthcoming electric shock by climbing a pole during the presence of a tone, or escape the shock by climbing after the tone ends and shock begins. In the absence of drugs, subjects learn the signaled avoidance task rapidly and well, and receive very few shocks. Neuroleptic drugs, but not most other substances, interfere with avoidance behavior at doses that leave escape behavior intact. Recognizing this allowed researchers working at various drug houses to screen potential neuroleptics quickly and accurately.

Over the years, other tests for neuroleptics were developed. Tests for additional classes of psychotropic medication, including antidepressants and anxiolytics, also are available (see Porsolt et al., 1993). Using extant tests to screen novel tests, developing new tests (in particular, those based on biological models of mental illness and drug action), and evaluating the adequacy of particular tests as practical screens and animal models continues to be of interest to basic researchers.

Animal models are of partial benefit for isolating useful new psychotropic medication. They may also be beneficial for detecting deleterious side effects, and for revealing the neuropharmacological mechanisms through which psychotropic drugs produce their effects. For example, the capacity of neuroleptic drugs to induce catalepsy in laboratory animals appears to correlate highly with their ability to produce extrapyramidal side effects, and all the older neuroleptics act as antagonists at dopamine receptor sites (Porsolt et al., 1993).

The latter observation gave rise to the dopamine hypothesis of schizophrenia (Carlsson, 1988), and the two observations together led to the popularity of neuro-leptic screens that compare drug doses that induce catalepsy with those that block hyperactivity (or stereotypy) induced by dopamine agonists, such as d-amphetamine or apomorphine (e.g., Heffner, Downs, Meltzer, Wiley, & Williams, 1989; Moyer, Abou-Gharbia, & Muth, 1998). Drugs for which the ratio is high (i.e., much larger doses are necessary to produce catalepsy than to block the effects of dopamine agonists) are apt to produce clinically beneficial effects without excessive risk of extrapyramidal side effects. The discovery that some neuroleptics, such as clozapine, are not potent dopamine antagonists has, however, called the dopamine model of schizophrenia into question and led to the development of screens that do not index dopaminergic activity (Porsolt et al., 1993).

Like procedures used to examine behavioral loci of drug action, procedures used to screen psychotropic drugs do not yield information that can be directly or simply applied to issues of everyday clinical practice. Understanding psychotropic screen-ing procedures and the information they yield makes a practitioner better informed about the substances she or he administers, but does not appear to affect his or her ability to prescribe those drugs in appropriate fashion.

Studies of Mechanisms of Drug Action

After researchers isolate the behavioral effects of a drug (i.e., determine its behavioral loci of action), they often attempt to determine the mechanism through which these effects are produced. "Mechanism of action" refers to a general drug effect at one level of analysis that produces (or at least, covaries with) another, usually more specific, effect at another level of analysis. In lay terms, a drug's mechanism of action refers to how the drug "causes" or "works to produce," whatever effects are of interest. For example, chlorpromazine generally is effective in reducing what are referred to as the "positive" symptoms of schizophrenia (hallucinations, thought disorders, bizarre behavior), which is one of the drug's most noteworthy effects (e.g., Baldessarini, 1990). The drug also produces extrapyramidal side effects (rigidity, tremor, slowed movement, restlessness). These effects, which can be directly observed, appear to covary with events at another level of analysis, specifically, antagonism of the neurotransmitter actions of dopamine by competitively blocking dopamine$_2$ receptors (Julien, 1995). Thus, it has been proposed that blockade of dopamine receptors is the mechanism of action responsible for the beneficial effects of chlorpromazine in people with schizophrenia, and for the extrapyramidal side effects of the drug.

Much of the interest in mechanisms of drug action has focused on the relation between neuropharmacological and behavioral events, and receptor models of drug action have proven invaluable in predicting and explaining drug effects. Moreover, research dealing with the neuropharmacological mechanisms of action of psychotropic drugs have led to influential biological models of mental illness, such as the dopamine theory of schizophrenia, which posits that the disorder arises from excessive dopaminergic activity in certain areas of the brain (Sedvall, 1990). Although support for the dopamine theory of schizophrenia is only correlational and its validity has recently been called into question (e.g., Julien, 1995; Sedvall, 1990), the model has played an important role in organizing research and theorizing. It appears that any person who prescribes psychotropic drugs should be abreast of current notions concerning neuropharmacological mechanisms of drug action, and associated biochemical models of mental illness, if only to be able to explain to patients how their medications "work."

Gaining this level of knowledge does not, however, require familiarity with specific studies. Moreover, much of the evidence on which neurochemical models of drug action rest resulted from clinical, not basic, research. And, with some notable exceptions, the basic research that has been conducted has been done by neurscientists other than behavioral pharmacologists.

Although behavioral pharmacologists appear to be attending with increasing regularity to relations between neurochemical and behavioral events, they historically have emphasized behavioral, not neuropharmacological, mechanisms of drug action. "behavioral mechanisms of drug action" involve the stimulus properties of a drug and the manner in which the drug modulates the actions of nondrug stimuli (Thompson & Schuster, 1968, Thompson, 1981). More specifically:

> By behavioral mechanism of drug action, we refer to a description of a drug's effect on a given behavioral system (locus) in terms of some more general set of environmental principles regulating behavior. Specifying the behavioral mechanism(s) responsible for an observed effect involves: a) identifying the environmental variables which typically regulate the behavior in question, and b) characterizing the manner in which the influence of these variables is altered by the drug. In some instances, the drug

assumes the status of a behavioral variable, per se, rather than modulating an existing environmental variable. (p.3)

One of a drug's potential mechanisms of action involves its own stimulus properties. Other important behavioral mechanisms of action can be discerned by examining how the drug influences the behavioral control exercised by antecedent and consequence variables. A major contribution of behavioral pharmacologists to understanding drug effects is the demonstration that drugs have, or can acquire, unconditional, conditional, discriminative, reinforcing, and punishing stimulus properties (Thompson & Pickins, 1971). Much of the early research involving stimulus properties of drugs examined the capacity of abused substances to serve as positive reinforcers in laboratory animals.

Over 50 years ago, Spragg (1940) observed that chimpanzees made physically dependent on morphine would learn to select one of two boxes if the experimenter then injected the animal with morphine contained in a syringe hidden under the box, and Headlee, Coppeck, and Nichols (1955) demonstrated that intraperitoneal injections of morphine served as a reinforcer for physically dependent rats. Since these studies appeared, hundreds of investigations have examined the reinforcing effects of various substances, including a variety of psychotropic medications (see Griffiths, Bigelow, & Henningfield, 1980; Henningfield, Lukas, & Bigelow, 1986; Young & Herling, 1986). In general, anxiolytics and stimulants serve as positive reinforcers, whereas neuroleptics and antidepressants do not.

Discriminative stimulus functions of drugs have also generated great research interest, and studies in this area have yielded valuable information concerning the sensory consequences of drugs and the biochemical mechanisms that mediate these consequences (e.g., Copaert & Balster, 1988; Stolerman, 1993). Basic research exploring stimulus properties of drugs makes it abundantly clear that the effects of many substances, including psychotropic medications, often depend upon a complicated interplay of environmental and pharmacological variables. Contextual analysis is a necessary part of behavioral pharmacology.

Of course, behavioral mechanisms of action involve more than a drug's stimulus properties. Other important behavioral mechanisms involve the capacity of drugs to modulate in a general way the effects of other stimuli that control behavior in the context of operant or respondent conditioning. For example, sedative-hypnotic drugs, including clinically-effective anxiolytics (e.g., chlordiazepoxide), appear to have antipunishment effects (e.g., Commissaris, 1993; Geller & Seifter, 1960; Graeff, 1987). That is, behavior that historically has been suppressed by punishment increases when such drugs are administered, but similar behavior not suppressed by punishment does not increase. On the whole, it appears to be more difficult to determine how a drug modulates the behavioral control effected by nondrug variables than to examine the drug's stimulus properties, and most studies of behavioral mechanisms of drug action have been in the latter area.

Studies of behavioral mechanisms of drug action show that drugs may possess stimulus effects acquired through conditioning, as well as the ability to affect behavior in the absence of conditioning (i.e., act as unconditional stimuli). More-over, drugs may modulate the effects of nondrug variables in the context of operant and respondent conditioning. Knowing this has two important implications for understanding drug effects in humans. The first is that the behavioral actions of a given drug may differ dramatically across individuals. One person may dance while intoxicated at a party because that response was richly reinforced in similar circum-stances in the past, another may sing for the same reason. In both cases, ethanol would be affecting behavior as a discriminative, as well as an unconditional, stimu-lus (i.e., these stimulus functions would constitute the drug's behavioral mecha-nisms of action).

The second implication is that a drug's behavioral actions within an individual may vary over time. Ethanol, for instance, possesses aversive taste properties and typically does not serve as a positive reinforcer upon initial exposure. With repeated exposure to the drug's pharmacological properties, however, it frequently comes to serve as a powerful positive reinforcer. If nothing else, studies of behavioral loci and mechanisms of drug action have made it abundantly clear that psychoactive drugs, including psychotropic medications, are not magic bullets that selectively and inevitably change behavior in specifiable ways. They are, rather, stimuli and as such produce effects that may differ as a function of the conditions under which they are, and have been, administered. Anyone who prescribes drugs should know this, but mastery of the extensive basic research literature relating to mechanisms of drug action is not necessary to prescribe psychotropic medications wisely.

Studies of Variables that Modulate Drug Effects

Basic research studies have revealed that a wide range of variables influence the behavioral effects of drugs (see Poling, 1986; van Haaren, 1993). Included among these variables are some, such as dose, time of administration, drug history, geno-type, health, and age, that are recognized to be important in all areas of pharmacol-ogy. Other, less obvious variables that may modulate drug effects include 1) the response rate in the absence of the drug (e.g., Thompson, Dews, & McKim, 1981); 2) the consequences that maintain (or suppress) behavior (e.g., Barrett, 1981); 3) the degree to which responding is stimulus-controlled (e.g., Laties, 1975); 4) the topog-raphy of behavior in question (e.g., Fowler, 1987); 5) the behavioral history of the individual (e.g., Barret & Witkin, 1986); and 6) the presence of rule-governed behavior relevant to the drug (e.g., Poling & LeSage, 1992).

The extent to which nondrug variables can modulate drug effects is clearly evident in a study by Siegel, Hison, Krank, and McCully (1093), who examined the lethality of a large does (15 mg/kg) of heroin in three groups of rats. During the first part of the study, all rats in the two experimental groups received 15 injections of heroin over a 30-day period. Heroin was injected every other day, and the dose was gradually increased from 1 to 8 mg/kg. On days when heroin was not given, rats received an injection of dextrose. Heroin injections and dextrose injections were given in markedly different environments, specifically the animals' colony area or another room where loud noise was present. Half of the rats received heroin in the colony area; the remainder were given drug in the room with white noise present. On the final day of the study; rats in one of the experimental groups (Same) received 15 mg/kg heroin in the environment where they historically had received smaller doses, and rats in the other experimental group (Different) received 15 mg/kg heroin in the environment where dextrose had been given in the past. Control rats, which had not previously received only dextrose, also received 15 mg/kg heroin. Half of these rats were given the drug in the colony room, whereas the remaining rats received heroin in the room with the white noise.

The lethality of heroin differed widely in the three groups of subjects. Although exposure to heroin alone produced some tolerance to the drug, as evidenced by the lower lethality (64% deaths) in the Different group than in the Control group (96% deaths), the environment in which the drug was administered strongly affected the degree of tolerance observed. In fact, mortality was twice as great in the group (Different) that received heroin in a novel environment (64%) as in the group (Same) that received the drug in the usual environment (32%).

Such findings cannot be explained in terms of heroin's pharmacological properties alone, but Siegel (e.g., 1989) has developed a classical conditioning model that accounts for them nicely. He proposes that stimuli reliably correlated with drug administration are established as conditional stimuli that come to evoke conditional responses that are opposite in direction to the unconditional responses elicited by the drug, which is an unconditional stimulus. These conditional responses compensate for (i.e., counteract) the unconditional responses elicited by the drug and, as the conditional responses increase in magnitude as a result of repeated conditional stimulus-unconditional stimulus pairings, reduce the magnitude of the observed response to the drug, for example, morphine-induced analgesia. Diminution of the observed response with repeated administrations of a drug is by definition tolerance.

Siegel's studies of drug tolerance provide especially compelling evidence of the potential importance of nonpharmacological variables in modulating drug effects. Similarly compelling evidence is available in other contexts, and for psychotropic drugs as well as substances of abuse. Because drug effects are influenced by a wide range of factors, both currently operative and historical, it stands to reason that a given drug can produce dramatically different behavioral actions in different people, or in the same individual at different times and places. Consider two adolescents with autistic impairments who engage in self-injurious biting, for which each is treated with the same dose of a neuroleptic drug. Self-injury allows adolescent one to terminate aversive encounters with staff, but enables adolescent two to prevent such encounters. Here, biting would be maintained as an escape response for adolescent one and as an avoidance response for adolescent two. It would not be surprising if the drug's effects on self-biting differed in these individuals for neuroleptics often interfere with avoidance responding at doses that have no effect on escape responding. If this held true in the present example, adolescent one's self-biting would be unaffected by doses of neuroleptic that suppressed the response in adolescent two. This is perfectly lawful and comprehensible if the role of behavioral and environmental variables in determining drug effects is acknowledged, but a mystery if they are ignored. A drug's behavioral effects are rarely simple, but they are always lawful. Making this point clear and isolating the factors that contribute to a drug's behavioral actions are two major contributions to the understanding of drug effects in humans that have arisen from the efforts of behavioral pharmacologists.

Recent Research in Behavioral Pharmacology

We have introduced the general approaches to research characteristic of behavioral pharmacology and provided examples of basic research findings over the past 20 years. These examples and our summaries of findings in various research areas are intended to introduce nonspecialists to the kinds of studies characteristic of basic research in behavioral pharmacology. To provide a more detailed picture of contemporary basic-science research in the area, Table 2 summarizes every research article published in *Behavioral Pharmacology* in 1995. This journal, although established relatively recently (in 1989), is one of the major outlets for studies in behavioral pharmacology, and its contents should reveal the research topics that are currently popular in the discipline.

The table lists each research article according to the surname of the first author, in the order that the articles appeared. For each article, information is provided concerning the species studied, whether or not a psychotropic drug was used, the experimental question, whether or not physiological measures were reported, and whether or not implications for clinical practice were noted.

Drugs were considered to be psychotropic if they have a recognized use in dealing with behavioral disorders (or mental illness), even if they are used infrequently. For example, amphetamines were considered as psychotropic drugs because they are sometimes used to treat attention deficit disorder (hyperactivity), although methylphenidate is the drug of choice for this purpose (Poling, Gadow, & Cleary, 1991). Experimental questions were phrased (in most cases by us, not by the original authors) to capture the essence of the studies. They do not necessarily describe every purpose of particular investigations.

Four noteworthy patterns are evident in the data. First, psychotropic drugs were evaluated in nearly 40% of the articles, with amphetamines being the compounds studied most often. Second, although many different kinds of experimental questions were addressed, the majority of investigations were in one way or another concerned with relations between behavioral and neurochemical events. Third, as expected given the pattern just described, most studies reported both behavioral and physiological outcome measures. Fourth, very few articles discussed the implications of findings for practitioners.

If the 77 studies described in Table 2 are taken to be representative of contemporary behavioral pharmacology, the discipline appears to be heavily oriented towards neuropharmacological analyses of drug action. Developing models that

Table 2. Characteristics of 1995 Behavioral Pharmacology Articles

First Author	Species	Psychotropic Drug(s) Used	Experimental Question Asked	Physiological Outcomes Measured	Implications for Practitioners Noted
Essman	rats	no	Does genotype affect the behavior and neurochemical responses of mice to a dopamine agonist?	yes	no
Flores	rats	yes (*d*-amphetamine)	Are the affects of *d*-amphetamine on schedule-induced drinking (of water) rate dependent?	no	no
Gyertyan	mice	yes (chlorpromazine, chlordiazepoxide)	Do marbles evoke digging and/or burying by mice and how do anxiolytic drugs affect these behaviors?	no	no
Chiamulera	rats	no	Does ethanol re-exposure reinstate enthanol-seeking behavior in rats with a history of ethanol self-administration?	no	no
Ferger	rats	no	Are different kinds of sensory stimuli (auditory, olfactory, tactile) similarly effective in producing conditioned drug (apomorphine) effects?	no	no
Weiner	rats	no	How does the experimental drug BMXY-1482 affect latent inhibition in rats?	no	no
Sams-Dodd	rats	yes (*d*-amphetamine)	What are the effects of *d*-amphetamine and phencyclidine on the social behavior, locomotor activity and stereotyped responses of rats?	no	no

First Author	Species	Psychotropic Drug(s) Used	Experimental Question Asked	Physiological Outcomes Measured	Implications for Practitioners Noted
Gambarana	rats	yes (imipramine)	How does long term exposure to imipramine or fluoxetine affect escape deficits produced by unavoidable shocks?	yes	yes
Heinrichs	rats	no	Does suppressing corticotropin-releasing factor in the amygdela attenuate the aversive consequences of morphine withdrawal as indexed in a place conditioning procedure?	yes	no
Weddell	humans	no	What are the effects of bromocriptine on psychomotor function, cognition, and mood in *de novo* patients with Parkinson's disease?	no	no
Shippenberg	rats	yes (desipramine)	How is the mesolimbic dompamine system involved in mediating the aversive effects of opiold antagonists as indexed by conditioned place preference?	yes	no
Kling-Petersen	rats	yes (d-amphetamine)	What are the effects of the dopamine D3-and autoreceptor-preferring antagonist (-)-DS121 on locomotor activity, conditioned place preference and intracranial self-stimulation?	yes	no
Sanger	rats	yes (several anxiolytics)	How do benzodiazepine ω receptor agonists and partial agonists affect punished and unpunished operant responding and the capacity of pentylenetetra-zole to act as a discriminative stimulus?	no	no

Cheeta	rats	no	How do reinforcer sweetness and raclopride affect progressive-ratio operant performance?	no	no
Ohmori	rats	yes (methamphetamine)	Does the training environment modify the expression of behavioral sensitization produced by methamphetamine?	no	no
Katz	squirrel monkeys	yes (amphetamine)	What are the effects of D 1 dopamine antagonists on schedule-controlled behavior?	no	no
Jarbe	rats	yes (lithium chloride)	Are discriminated taste aversion procedures viable for studying the contextual control of drugs as discriminative stimuli?	no	no
Pakarinen	squirrel monkeys	yes (d-amphetamine)	What are the effects of $GABA_A$ antagonists on repeated acquisition (learning)?	no	no
Maurice	mice	no	What are the effects of nimodipine (a calcium channel antagonist) on learning?	no	no
Evans	humans	yes (alprazolam)	What are the behavioral and subjective effects on DN-2327 (pazinaclone) and alprazolam in normal volunteers?	no	yes
Kamien	humans	yes (triazolam)	Do placebo effects influence the acquisition of drug discrimination?	no	no
Commissaris	rats	no	How do selective and non-selective monoamine oxidase inhibitors affect performance in a conditioned suppression assay?	no	no
Johnson	mice	no	Does nicotine treatment affect ethanol-induced locomotor stimulation and dopamine turnover?	yes	no

First Author	Species	Psychotropic Drug(s) Used	Experimental Question Asked	Physiological Outcomes Measured	Implications for Practitioners Noted
Broqua	rats	no	What are the behavioral effects of neuropeptide Y receptor agonists in the elevated plus-maze and fear potentiated startle procedures?	no	no
French	rats	no	Does the reinforcing efficacy of PCP, TCP, BTCP, and cocaine differ when indexed with a progressive ratio schedule?	no	no
Ambosio	rats	no	How does genotype influence locomotor activity and morphine self-administration?	no	no
Herremans	rats	yes (midazolam)	What are the effects of benzodiazepine receptor ligands in a delayed conditional discrimination task?	no	yes
Witkin	mice	no	What are the effects of ifenprodil on the stimulatory, discriminative stimulus, and convulsant effects of cocaine?	no	no
Wolgin	rats	yes (amphetamine)	Can rats learn to inhibit amphetamine-induced stereotypy?	no	yes
Baker	rats	yes (d-amphetamine)	How do the discriminative stimulus effects of the optical isomers of MDMA compare?	no	no
Arnone	rats	no	What are the effects of SR 59026A on male sexual activity?	no	no

Name	Species	Drug	Question		
Rodgers	mice	no	What are the effects of scopolamine and its quaternary analogue in the murine elevated plus-maze test?	no	no
Didriksen	rats	yes (risperidone)	What are the effects of resperidone on schedule-induced polydipsia?	no	no
Wenger	pigeons	yes (d-amphetamine)	How do drugs of abuse affect temporal discrimination?	no	no
Ciano	rats	yes (d-amphetamine)	Are extracellular dopamine receptors in the nucleus accumbens different during the intravenous self-administration of cocaine and d-amphetamine?	yes	no
Auta	monkeys	yes (triazolam)	What are the effects of full and partial allosteric modulators of $GABA_A$ receptors on complex behavioral processes as indexed by repeated acquisition procedures?	no	yes
Caine	rats	no	What are the effects of the dopamine agonist 7-OH-DPAT on cocaine self-administration?	no	no
Sobel	rats	yes (diazepam)	Does within session averaging of data produce graded dose response functions in drug discrimination learning?	no	no
Mitchell	humans	no	How does ethanol consumption affect cigarette smoking?	no	no
Bell	rats	no	Does cocaine serve as an orally self-administered reinforcer?	no	no
Shoaib	rats	no	Is intracerebral administration of nicotine effective in producing conditioned taste aversions?	yes	no
Doty	humans	no	Does naltrexone influence the subjective and performance effects of ethanol in social drinkers?	no	no

First Author	Species	Psychotropic Drug(s) Used	Experimental Question Asked	Physiological Outcomes Measured	Implications for Practitioners Noted
Broersen	rats	no	How do pharmacological manipulations of prefrontal dopamine affect punished and unpunished behavior?	yes	no
Cherek	humans	no	Does provocation frequency influence the effects of smoked marijuana on aggressive responding?	no	no
Melo	rats	no	How do drugs that affect 5-HT_{1A} and 5-HT_2 receptors in the inferior colliculus influence elevated plus-maze performance?	yes	no
Mitchell	marmosets	no	How do drugs that influence excitatory amino acid and dopamine transmission affect parkinsonian symptoms induced by 6-OHDA?	no	no
Amalric	rats	no	Does the blockade of excitatory amino acid transmission in the basal ganglia reverse reaction time deficits induced by dopamine inactivation?	yes	no
Sanger	rats	yes (d-amphetamine)	Does eliprodil block spermine-induced hyperactivity?	no	no
Maldonado-Irizarry	rats	no	How do excitatory amino acid antagonists affect performance in a food searching assay of spatial learning?	yes	no
Murray	rats	no	What are the effects of dizocilpine on spatial and visual discrimination in a Y-maze task?	no	no

Misztal	rats	no	How do various glutamate antagonists affect dark avoidance?	no	no
DeMontis	rats	yes (imipramine, fluoxetine)	What are the effects on learned behaviors of drugs that affect NMDA receptors?	no	no
Shoaib	rats	no	What are the effects of the glycine partial agonist (+)-HA966 on cocaine-induced locomotor activity and self administration?	no	no
Balster	rats, monkeys	no	What are the effects of two novel substituted quinoxaline-dione glutamate antagonists in a complex behavioral test battery?	no	no
Koek	rats	yes (d-amphetamine, chlordiazepoxide)	What are the effects of the NMDA antagonist, dizocilpine, in subjects trained to discriminate various drugs from saline?	no	no
Gatto	rats	no	Can a three-choice ethanol- dizocilpine -water discrimination be established?	no	no
Vanecek	pigeons	no	Is a procedure with two doses of morphine and saline as discriminative stimuli useful for the pharmacological characterization of opioids?	no	no
Moreau	rats	no	How does electroshock treatment affect intracranial self-stimulation in subjects that are and are not stressed?	yes	no
Cesana	mice	yes (buspirone, desipramine, fluoxetine)	What are the effects of BIMT 17, a new potential antidepressant, in a forced swimming test?	yes	no

First Author	Species	Psychotropic Drug(s) Used	Experimental Question Asked	Physiological Outcomes Measured	Implications for Practitioners Noted
Drinkenburg	rats	no	What are the effects on visual discrimination of drugs that antagonize or deplete acetylcholine?	no	no
Smith	rats	no	How do training dose and intrinsic efficacy influence the actions of kappa opioid agonists and antagonists in a drug discrimination procedure?	no	no
Gingras	rats	no	Does ethanol self-administration differ in high and low responders to novelty?	no	no
Li	pigeons, rats	no	Does food deprivation and satiation influence sensitivity to the discriminative-stimulus effects of pentobarbitol and morphine?	no	no
Griebel	mice	yes (chlordiazepoxide)	How do benzodiazepine receptor ligands with different intrinsic activities affect defensive (antipredator) behavior?	no	no
Wolgin	rats	no	What are the effects of acute and chronic cocaine on milk intake, body weight, and activity in bottle- and cannula-fed subjects?	no	no
VanEtten	humans	no	What are the effects of response cost and unit dose on alcohol self-administration in moderate drinkers?	no	no
Negus	monkeys	no	Are there diurnal patterns of cocaine and heroin self-administration?	no	no
Hughes	monkeys	no	Does tolerance and cross-tolerance occur to the response rate decreasing effects of μ opioids in morphine maintained subjects?	no	no

Beninger	rats	no	What are the effects of dopamine D1-like receptor agonists on behavior maintained by conditioned reinforcement?	no	no
Elmer	mice	no	Does genotype influence the rate depressant effects of ethanol on schedule-controlled behavior?	no	no
Bakshi	rats	yes (amphetamine)	What are the effects of amphetamine, strychnine, and caffeine on prepulse inhibition and latent inhibition of a startle response?	no	no
Poulous	rats	no	Does impulsivity predict individual susceptibility to high levels of alcohol self-administration?	no	no
Jewett	pigeons	no	What are the effects of nor-binaltorphimine and related substances on food reinforced responding?	no	no
Rowlett	rats	no	How do cocaine, heroin, and naltrexone, alone and in combination, affect milk drinking?	no	no
Bruhwyler	rats, mice	yes (clozapine, haloperidol, diazepam, imipramine, chlorpromazine)	What are the effects of new benzodiazepine derivatives with disinhibitory and/or antidepressant potential on neurochemistry and behavior in open-field and forced-swimming tests?	no	no
Sipes	rats	no	Is DOI disruption of prepulse inhibition of startle mediated by 5-HT_{2A} or 5-HT_{2C}?	no	yes
Garrett	rats	yes (d-amphetamine)	What are the effects of dopamine agonists on rotational behavior in nontolerant and caffeine tolerant rats?	no	no

may be of value in understanding the clinical actions of psychotropic drugs and the biochemical basis of behavioral disorders (mental illness) is of interest to many researchers, but studies in this area are not of direct relevance to prescribing practices. A few studies that essentially address the behavioral side effects of psychotropic medications appear but, as discussed previously with respect to the study of neuroleptic-induced learning impairment conducted by Poling et al. (1990), data from such studies are more useful to clinical researchers than to practitioners.

Basic Research and Sound Clinical Practice

Basic research in behavioral pharmacology has yielded a great deal of information concerning the behavioral effects of drugs (including psychotropes), the behavioral and neuropharmacological mechanisms responsible for those effects, and the variables that modulate loci and mechanisms of drug action. Moreover, the within-subject experimental designs and sensitive measures of behavior favored by behavioral pharmacologists are most appropriate for clinical drug evaluations (e.g., Poling & Cleary, 1986a, b; Singh & Beale, 1986). Some of the assays might also be useful for everyday drug evaluation. For instance, the repeated acquisition procedure might provide a sensitive assay of drug-induced learning impairment, and the delayed-matching-to-sample procedure might pick up short-term memory deficits caused by medications.

In our opinion, a solid background in behavioral pharmacology will prove useful in helping practitioners to understand the importance of environmental variables in modulating drug effects, the relationship between behavioral and neuropharmacological events, and the value of animal models. Such a background may also prove helpful for developing sensitive everyday drug evaluation procedures, especially when the people who receive medication are not highly verbal. Training in behavioral pharmacology (or, for the terms are approximately synonymous, preclinical psychopharmacology) should be required for anyone who prescribes psychotrpic medications. Several curricula have been proposed for training psychologists to prescribe drugs (see Chafetz & Buelow, 1994; Fox, Schwelitz, & Barclay, 1992; Sammons, Sexton, & Meredith, 1996; Smyer et al., 1993), and all of them appear to allow for (although not necessarily ensure) adequate training in the basic research aspects of behavioral pharmacology.

We have considered elsewhere what constitutes appropriate use of psychotropic medications in general (e.g., Poling & Bradshaw, 1993; Poling et al., 1991), and when such drugs are prescribed for people with mental retardation (e.g., Gadow & Poling, 1988; Poling, 1994). Adequate training in behavioral pharmacology may be a necessary prerequisite if psychologists are to use drugs appropriately, but it surely is not sufficient to allow them to do so. Behavioral pharmacologists recognize this; at least, none have claimed to merit prescription privileges. Of course, with sufficient training, people with basic research backgrounds can certainly acquire the skills necessary to become competent in the clinical use of psychotropic medication. Whether they, or other psychologists, are well advised to do so is a topic for

others to debate. As they say in Appalachia, "We don't have a dog in that fight."
The pack's big enough already.

References

Aman, M. G. (1984). Drugs and learning in mentally retarded people. In C. D.
 Burrows & J. S. Were (Eds.) *Advances in human psychopharmacology* (Vol. 3, pp.
 121-163). Greenwhich, CT: JAI Press.

Aman, M. G. (1990). Drugs and the treatment of psychiatric disorders. In A. G.
 Gilman, T. W. Rall, A. S. Nies, & P. Taylor (Eds.). *The pharmacological basis of
 therapeutics* (pp. 383-405). New York: Pergamon Press.

Barrett, J. E. (1981). Differential drug effects as a function of the controlling
 consequences. In T. Thompson & C. Johanson (Eds.). *Behavioral pharmacology
 of human drug dependence* (pp. 159-81). Washington, D.C.: U. S. Government
 Printing Office.

Barrett, J. E. & Witkin, J. M. (1986). The role of behavioral and pharmacological
 history in determining the effect of abused drugs. In S. R. Goldberg & I .P.
 Stolerman (Eds.). *Behavior analysis of drug dependence.* New York: Academic Press.

Brentar, J. & Mcnamara, J. R. (1991). Prescription privileges for psychology: The
 next step in its evolution as a profession. *Professional Psychology: Research and
 Practice, 22* (3), 194-95.

Carlsson, A. (1988). The current status of the dopamine hypothesis of schizophrenia. *Neuropsychopharmacology, 1,* 179-86.

Chaftez, M. D. & Beulow, G. (1994). A training model for psychologists with
 prescription privileges: Clinical pharmacopsychologists. *Professional Psychology:
 Research and Practice, 25,* 149-153.

Colpeart, F. C., & Balster, R. L. (1988). *Transduction mechanisms of drug stimuli.* Berlin:
 Springer.

Commissaris, R. L. (1993). Conflict behaviors as animal models for the study of
 anxiety. In F. van Haaren (Ed.). *Methods in behavioral pharmacology* (pp. 443-474).
 New York: Elsevier.

Cook, L., & Wedley, E. (1957). Behavioral effects of some psychopharmacological
 agents. *Annals of the New York Academy of Sciences, 66,* 740-762. New York:
 Elsevier.

De Leon, P. H., Folen, R. E., and Graham, S .R. (1991). The case for prescription
 privileges: Psychology's new frontier? *American Psychologist, 46,* 384-393.

DeLeon, P. H. & Wiggens, J. G. (1996). Prescription priveleges for psychologists.
 American psychologist, 51, 207-212.

DeNelsky, G. Y. (1991). Prescription privileges for psychologists: The case against.
 Professional Psychology: Research and Practice, 22, 188-193.

DeNelsky, G. Y. (1996). The case against prescription privileges for psychologists.
 American psychologist, 51, 207-212.

Fielding, S., & Lal, H. (1978) Behavioral action of neuroleptics. In L. L. Ivers, S.
 D. Iverson, & S. H. Snyder (Eds.). *Handbook of psychopharmacology* (Vol. 10, pp.
 91-128). New York: Pergamon Press.

Fowler, S. C. (1987). Force and duration of operant responses as dependent variables in behavioral pharmacology. In T. Thomson, P. B. Dews, & J. E. Barrett (Eds.). *Neurobehavioral pharmacology* (pp. 83-127). Hillsdale, NJ: Erlbaum.

Fox, R. E. (1988a). Prescription privileges: Their implications for the practice of psychology. *Psychotherapy, 25*, 501-507.

Fox, R. E. (1988b). Some practical and legal objections to prescription privileges for psychologists. *Psychotherapy in Private Practice, 6*, 23-30.

Fox, R. E., Schwelitz, F. D. & Barclay, A. G. (1992). A proposed curriculum for psychopharmacology training for professional psychologists. *Professional Psychology: Research and Practice, 23*, 216-219.

Gadow, K., & Poling, A. (1988). *Pharmacotherapy in mental retardation.* San Diego: College-Hill Press.

Geller, I., & Seifter, J. (1960). The effects of meprobamate, barbituates, *d*-amphetamine and promazine on experimenatally-induced conflict in the rat. *Psychopharmacology, 3*, 374-385.

Graeff, F. G. (1987). The antiaversive action of drugs. In T. Thompson, P. B. Dews, & J. E. Barrett (Eds.). *Neurobehavioral pharmacology* (pp.129-156.) Hillsdale, NJ: Earlbaum.

Griffiths, R. R., Bigelow, G. E., & Henningfield, J. E. (1980). Similarities in animal and human drug-taking behavior. In N. K. Mello (Ed.). *Advances in substance abuse: Behavioral and biological research* (pp. 1-90). Greenwich, CT: JAI Press.

Hayes, S.C., & Heiby, E. (1996). Psychology's drug problem: Do we need a fix or should we just say no? *American Psychologist, 51*, 198-206.

Headlee, C. P., Coppock, H. W., & Nichols, J. R. (1995). Apparatus and technique involved in a labaoratory method of detecting addictiveness of drugs. *Journal of the American Pharmacological Association, 44*, 229-231.

Heffner, T. G. , Downs, D. A., Meltzer, L. T., Wiley, J. N., & Williams, A. E. (1989). CI-943: A potential antipsychotic agent: Preclinical behavioral effects. *Journal of Pharmacology and Experimental Therapeutics, 251*, 105-112.

Henningfield, J. E., Lukas, S. E., & Bigelow, G. E. (1986). Human studies of drugs as reinforcers. In S. R. Goldberg & I. B. Stolerman (Eds.) *Behavioral analysis of drug dependence* (pp. 69-122). New York: Academic Press.

Jannsen, P. A., & Van Bever, W. F. (1978). Preclinical psychopharmacology of neuroleptics. In W. G. Clark, & J. del Guidice (Eds.). *Principles of psychopharmacology* (pp. 279-295). New York: Academic Press.

Julien, R. M. (1995). *A primer of drug action.* New York: Freeman.

Kingsbury, S. J. (1992). Some effects of prescribing privileges. *Professional Psychology: Research and Practice, 23*, 3-5.

Klein, R. G. (1996). Comments on expanding the role of clinical psychologists. *American Psychologist, 51*, 216-218.

Kubiszyn, T. (1994). Pediatric psychopharmacology and prescription privileges: Implications and opportunities for school psychology. *School Psychology Quarterly, 9*, 26-40.

Laties, V. G. (1972). The modifications of drug effects on behavior by external discriminative stimuli. *Journal of Pharmacology and Experimental Therapeutics, 183,* 1-13.

Laties, V. G. (1975). The role of discriminative stimuli in modulating drug effects. *Federation Proceedings, 34,* 1880-1888.

Laties, V. G. (1979). I. V. Zavadkii and the beginnings of behavioral pharmacology: An historical note and translation. *Journal of the Experimental Analysis of Behavior, 32,* 463-472.

Lipman, R. S., DiMascio, A., Reating, N., & Kirson, T. (1978). Psychotropic drugs and mentally retarded children. In M.A. Lipton, A. DiMascio, & K. F. Killam (Eds.). *Psychopharmacology: A generation of progress* (pp. 1437-1449). New York: Raven Press.

Macht, D. L., & Mora, C. F. (1921). Effects of opim alkaloids on the behavior of rats on the circular maze. *Journal of Pharmacology and Experimental Therapeutics, 16,* 219-235.

Michael, J. (1980). Flight from behavior analysis. *The Behavior Analyst, 3,* 1-24.

Moyer, J. A., Abou-Chariba, M., & Muth, E. A. (1988). Behavioral pharmacology of the gamma carboline WT 47384: A potential antipsychotic agent. *Drug Development Research, 13,* 11-28.

Newland, M. C., & Marr, M. A. (1985). The effect of chlorpromazine and imipramine on rate and stimulus control of matching-to-sample. *Journal of the Experimental Analysis of Behavior, 44,* 49-68.

Neilson, E. B.,& Appel, J. B. (1983). The effect of drugs on the discrimination of color following a variable delay period: A signal detection analysis. *Psychopharmacology, 80,* 24-28.

O'Donnell, J. M. (1985). *The origins of behaviorism: American psychology 1920-1970.* New York: New York University Press.

Pickens, R. (1977). Behavioral pharmacology: A brief history. In T. Thompson & P. B. Dews (Eds.). *Advances in behavioral pharmacology* (Vol. 1, pp. 230-261). New York: Academic Press.

Picker, M. (1987). Effects of clozapine on fixed-consecutive-number responding in rats: A comparison to other neuroleptic drugs. *Pharmacology Biochemistry and Behavior, 30,* 603-612.

Picker, M. (1989). Neuroleptics and conditional discrimination tasks: Cholinergic mediation of the accuracy-and-response-rate-altering effects of chlorpromazine but not haloperidol. *Behavioral Pharmacology, 1,* 141-152.

Picker, M., Cleary, J., Berens, K., Oliveto, A., & Dykstra, L. A. (1989). Molidone: Effects in pigeons responding under conditional discrimination tasks. *Pharmacology Biochemistry and Behavior, 32,* 439-445.

Picker, M., & Massie, C. A. (1988). Differential effects of neuroleptic drugs on the delayed matching-to-sample performances of pigeons. *Pharmacology Biochemistry and Behavior, 31,* 952-957.

Poling, A. (1986). *A primer of human behavioral pharmacology*. New York: Plenum Press.

Poling, A. (1994). Pharmacological treatment of behavioral problems in people with mental retardation: Some ethical considerations. In L. J. Hayes, G. J. Hayes, S. C. Moore, & P. M. Ghezzi (Eds.). *Ethical issues in developmental disabilites* (pp. 149-177). Reno, NV: Context Press.

Poling, A., & Bradshaw, A. L. (1993). Psychopharmacology. In A. S. Bellack and M. Hersen (Eds.). *Handbook of behavior therapy in the psychiatric setting* (pp. 113-132). New York: Plenum Press.

Poling, A., and Cleary, J. (1986a). The role of applied behavior analysis in evaluating medication effects. In A. Poling, & R. Fuqua, (Eds.). *Research methods in applied behavior analysis: Issues and advances* (pp. 299-332). New York: Plenum Press.

Poling, A., & Cleary, J. (1986b). Within-subject designs. In K. Gadow and A. Poling (Eds.). *Methodological issues in human psychopharmacology* (pp. 115-136). Greenwich, CT: JAI Press.

Poling, A., Cleary, J., Berens, K., & Thompson, T. (1990). Neuroleptics and learning: Effects of haloperidol, molindone, mesoridazine, and thioridizine on the behavior of pigeons under a repeated acquisition procedure. *Journal of Pharmacology and Experimental Therapeutics, 255*, 1240-1245.

Poling, A., Gadow, K., & Cleary, J. (1991). *Drug therapy for behavior disorders: An Introduction*. New York: Pergamon Press.

Poling, A., & LeSage, M. (1992). Rule-governed behavior and human behavioral pharmacology: A brief commentary on an important topic. *The Analysis of Verbal Behavior, 10*, 37-44.

Poling, A., Picker, M., & Thompson, J. (1984). Effects of chlorprothixene, haloperidol, trifluoperazine on the delayed matching-to-sample performance of pigeons. *Pharmacology Biochemistry and Behavior, 21*, 721-726.

Porsolt, R.D., McArthur, R. A., & Lenegre, A. (1993). Psychotropic drug screening procedures. In F. van Haaren (Ed.). *Methods in behavioral pharmacology* (pp. 23-51). New York: Elsevier.

Sammons, M. T., Sexton, J. L., & Meredith, J. M. (1996). Basic science training in psychopharmacology: How much is enough? *American Psychologist, 51*, 230-234

Sedvall, G. (1990). Monoamines and schizophrenia. *Acta Psychiatrica Scandavica, 82* (Suppl. 358), 7-13.

Seiden, L. S., & Dykstra, L.A. (1977). *Psychopharmacology: A biochemical and behavioral approach*. New York: Van Nostrand Reinhold.

Siegel, S. (1989). Pharmacological conditioning and drug effects. In A. J. Goudie & M. W. Emmet-Oglesby (Eds.) *Psychoactive drugs: Tolerance and sensitization* (pp. 115-180). Clifton, NJ: Humana Press.

Seigel, S., Hinson, R. E., Krank, M. D., & McCully, J. (1982). Heroin "overdose" death: Contribution of drug-associated environmental cues. *Science, 216*, 436-437.

Singh, N. N., & Beale, I. L. (1986). Behavioral assessment of pharmacotherapy. In S. R. Schroeder (Ed.). *Ecobehavioral analysis and developmental disabilities* (pp. 82-100). New York: Springer-Verlag.

Skinner, B. F. (1938). *The behavior of organisms.* New York: Appleton-Century-Crofts.

Skinner, B. F. (1953). *Science and human behavior.* New York: Macmillan.

Smyer, M. A., Balster, R. L., Egli, D., Johnson, D. L., Kilbey, M. M., Leith, N. J., & Puente, A. J. (1993). Summary of the ad hoc task force on psychopharmacology of the American Psychological Association. *Professional Psychology: Research and Practice, 24,* 394-403.

Spragg, S. R. S. (1940). Morphine addiction in chimpanzees. *Comparative Psychology Monograph, 15,* 7.

Stolerman, I. P. (1993). Drug discrimination. In F. van Haaren (Ed.). *Methods in behavioral pharmacology* (pp. 159-208). New York: Plenum Press.

Thompson, D. M. (1974). Repeated acquisition of response sequences: Effects of *d*-amphetimine and chlorpromazine. *Pharmacology Biochemistry and Behavior, 2,* 741-746.

Thompson, D. M. (1978). Stimulus control and drug effects. In D. E. Blackman & D. J. Sanger (Eds.), *Contemporary research in behavioral pharmacology* (pp. 159-208). New York: Plenum Press.

Thompson, T. (1981). Behavioral mechanisms and loci of drug action: An overview. In T. Thompson & C. Johanson (Eds.), *Behavioral Pharmacology of human drug dependence* (pp. 1-10). Washington, DC: U.S. Government Printing Office.

Thompson, T., Dews, P. B., & McKim, W. M. (1981). *Advances in behavioral pharmacology* (Vol. 3). New York: Academic Press.

Thompson, T., & Pickens, R. (1971). *Stimulus properties of drugs.* New York: Appleton-Century-Crofts.

Thompson, T., & Schuster, C. R. (1968). *Behavioral pharmacology.* Englewood Cliffs, NJ: Prentice-Hall.

van Haaren, F. (1993). *Methods in behavioral pharmacology.* New York: Elsevier.

Young, A. M., & Herling, S. (1986). Drugs as reinforcers: Studies in laboratory animals. In S. R. Goldberg & I. P. Stolerman (Eds.) *Behavioral analysis of drug dependence* (pp. 9-67). New York: Academic Press.

Zuriff, G. E. (1985). *Behaviorism: A conceptual reconstruction.* New York: Columbia University Press.

Discussion of Poling, Christian, and Ehrhardt

Clinical Decision Making Practices

W. Larry Williams, Ph.D.

University of Nevada

The chapter by Poling, Christian, and Ehrhardt provides an elegant and timely overview of the general history and current practices in the field of Behavioral Pharmacology. A major theme of the chapter is that knowledge and training in basic behavioral pharmacology, while certainly beneficial for appropriate clinical application of psychotropic medications, is not sufficient. The authors not only make the observation that those most knowledgeable in basic behavioral pharmacology have not themselves suggested or indicated a desire for prescription privileges, but end their chapter with a clear message that the decision to extend prescription privileges to psychologists, or any other group of clinical practitioners, must be based on other variables. I support this position, and will argue that increasing the numbers of professionals who will prescribe psychotropic medications, without a re-examination of the general clinical decision-making practices in psychology and related helping disciplines, will be disastrous for those professionals and their consumers. Although I feel this will be true for clinical practice with all populations, I will restrict my observations and arguments to the area of developmental and related disabilities.

Poling, Christian and Ehrhardt provide us with several examples of the actions and functions of psychotropic medications that have been demonstrated to date. For example, the fact that neuroleptics produce learning impairment; that drugs have or can acquire unconditional, conditional, discriminative, reinforcing and punishing stimulus properties; that drugs modulate the effects of non drug variables in the context of operant and respondent conditioning, such that behavioral reactions to a drug can differ widely across individuals, and within individuals over time. A particularly useful observation they provide concerns the importance of the knowledge of the differential drug action on avoidance and escape performance. The current development of functional analysis technology in the applied behavior analysis field (e.g., Iwata, 1994), has revealed the precision with which clinical interventions can now be applied when appropriate clinical assessment methods are employed. The combination of information on drug effects with that of the effect of environmental contingencies, provides even greater precision. Unfortunately, many practitioners in the Developmental Disability field will be unaware of these features of the nature of behavior, while others will be aware of them and still choose to ignore them in prescribing treatment. The contribution of behavioral pharmacology to pharmacology in general, and what differentiates behavior analysis from many areas of psychology is a foundation in empirical decision making. That this is not common as a basis for typical clinical decision making, is central, I believe, to several problematic issues in service provision and clinical treatment in Developmental Disabilities.

While multi, trans, and interdisciplinary assessment and treatment methods have long been described for comprehensive services in Developmental Disabilities (e.g., Garner & Orelove 1994), all too often they do not exist. It is becoming apparent that once trained in a particular profession or theoretical orientation within a profession, we find it extremely difficult to cooperate and relinquish control to others in a coordinated treatment effort. Successful interdisciplinary work requires a common set of principles and constant prompting of people to follow them. I would argue that where different orientations collaborate effectively, these principles involve the use of agreed upon measures and descriptions of relevant therapeutic, educational, or other service activities and their effects with patients, students and consumers. Such measures and descriptions will by definition probably be empirical in nature. Basic to this process is the availability of trained professionals and their willing communication. The lack of sufficient personnel or their willingness to function together is the basis of recently discussed problems in the appropriate prescription of psychotropic medications for persons with Developmental Disability.

Fredericks and Hayes (1995) for example, reported on the lack of relationship between medication changes and available behavioral measures in an analysis of the long term treatment of three persons with Developmental Disability in a public interdisciplinary setting. Physician's medication change decisions were not at all based on information from other professional's empirical data on client performance. Thus, lack of communication renders treatment ineffective or even dangerous. Sturmey (1995) has recently reported on the problems involved in the prescription of psychotropic medications for persons with Developmental Disability based on traditional diagnostic parameters. Here, the issues of inferring pathology from behavioral symptoms, when the same behaviors are seen to support the presence of a different underlying pathology, or different behaviors, the same pathology, mitigate against furthering knowledge and practice in the effective use of medications and other treatments. Again, it is a problem of refusal to be guided by agreed upon empirical practices.

I have argued elsewhere (Williams & Murray 1993), that much of the service delivery in the Developmental Disabilities field is the product of "superstitious" decision making by service providers. This is the case if educational, vocational, or clinical activities are not determined by regular review of consumer relevant outcomes from such services. This may be recognized as the behavioral clinical intervention model, where progress toward objectives is constantly monitored in order to adjust or replace treatment procedures, until the objective is met. An analysis of complex decision making by Goltz (1992) demonstrated that larger groups or "chunks" of separate performances, such as those involved in financial investment decisions, can come under schedule control and consequently demonstrate an increased resistance to extinction. Thus, investors continue to invest in loosing situations. Given that assessment and treatment behaviors could easily be under such control, and especially in the case where empirical outcome measures are not involved and procedural reliability is ignored, clinical treatment decisions can be superstitiously maintained.

In conclusion, and returning to the position indicated by Poling, Christian, and Ehrhardt, prescribers of medication require training in appropriate clinical application of medications. This will probably require knowledge of basic behavioral pharmacology. I have argued that it will necessarily involve adoption of empirical decision making methods that are strongly associated with a behavior analysis perspective. The reluctance to find in favor of allowing prescription privileges for psychologists, therefore, follows from problems that current prescribers have not addressed. Specifically in the field of Developmental Disability, where consumers' benefits from medication must be inferred from behavior, there are currently major issues concerning appropriate use of psychotropics. Whether increasing the number of professionals, theoretical orientations, and likely non-empirical practices will benefit consumers is, for me, unlikely . . . but of course an empirical question.

References

Federicks, D., & Hayes, L.J.(1995). Effects of drug changes and physician prescribing practices on the behavior of persons with mental retardation. *Journal of Developmental and Physical Disabilities, 7*, (2), 105-122.

Garner, H.G. & Orelove, F.P.(1994) *Teamwork in Human Services: models and applications accross the lifespan.* Boston: Butterworth-Heinemann.

Goltz, S. M. (1992). A sequential learning analysis of decisions in organizations to escalate investments despite continuing cost or losses. *Journal of Applied Behavior Analysis, 25*, 561-574.

Iwata, B., A., Dorsey, M. F., Slifer, K. J., Bauman, K. E., & Richman, G.S.(1994). Toward a functional analysis of self-injury. *Journal of Applied Behavior Analysis, 28*, 3, 1-34.

Sturmey, P.(1995). Diagnostic-based pharmacological treatment of behavior disorders in persons with Developmental Disabilities: A review and a decision-making typology. *Research in Developmental Disabilities, 16*, 4, 235-252.

Williams, W. L. & Murray, P. (May, 1993). Service Review: A management procedure for establishing decision-making under control of service outcome data. Paper presented at the *19th Annual Association for Behavior Analysis Conference*, Chicago, Il. May 27, 1993.

Chapter 7

Current Status of Combined Treatments: Implications for Prescription Authority

Michael J. Telch, Ph.D., Tracy Sloan, M.A., and
Victoria Beckner
The University of Texas at Austin

In the debate over prescription privileges for psychologists, the argument is often made that psychologists would be able to provide more *effective* treatment if they could prescribe medications in conjunction with psychotherapy. Phrases such as "integrated care" or "treat the whole person" are often used to argue the case for prescription authority.

At the heart of this argument lie several core assumptions:

1. Treatments combining psychotherapy with medication(s) are *generally* more effective than either medication or psychological monotherapies;

2. Psychologists are in a better position to offer truly integrative drug-psychological treatments than other mental health professionals;

3. If granted prescription privileges, prescribing psychologists will continue to provide psychotherapy along with medications.[1]

Whether psychologists are better suited for delivering combined treatments (i.e., Assumption 2) and whether prescribing psychologists will choose to deliver combined treatments (Assumption 3) are addressed elsewhere in this volume. Suffice it to say that while the validity of Assumptions 2 & 3 do not depend on Assumption 1, their importance surely does.

Our remarks will focus primarily on the efficacy of treatments that combine a psychosocial treatment with medication. For efficiency, we refer to these treatments as "combined treatments." We have organized this chapter around the following questions: (a) What is the prevailing attitude about combined treatments and the rationales for using them? (b) What is the current scientific knowledge base on combined treatments? (c) What does this knowledge base tell us about the efficacy of combined treatments relative to single modality treatments? (d) What are the research priorities for advancing our understanding of combined treatments? and (e) What implications do the research findings have for prescription privileges?

The *belief* that combined treatments are generally superior to drug or psychosocial treatments is pervasive and definitely not restricted to only those psychologists in favor of prescription authority. Rather, it is a view held strongly across mental health disciplines. Even the National Institute of Mental Health, in their public education materials for depression and anxiety disorders, indicate that combined approaches may offer the most effective treatment for these problems (NIH, 1993; 1994).

Survey data collected from recipients of outpatient mental health services reveal that most patients receive *both* pharmacotherapy and psychotherapy (Consumer Reports, 1995; Taylor, King, Margraf, Ehlers, Telch, Roth, & Agras, 1989). Although it is not clear that the singular treatments being combined in day-to-day clinical practice are those with established efficacy, there appears to be a pervasive attitude that combined drug-psychological treatments are superior to single modality treatments.

Combined Treatments

The rationale(s) for using a combined drug-psychological approach in treating mental disorders are inextricably linked to how one conceptualizes psychological dysfunction and the presumed efficacy and mechanisms of action of the single modality treatments being combined. In general, evidence from well-controlled clinical trials provide compelling evidence that certain forms of psychotherapy and certain classes of pharmacotherapy each are beneficial in the treatment of many specific mental disorders. It is then *assumed* that the combination of these two treatment modalities will confer some added benefit over either treatment alone. The additivity assumption plays a pivotal role in the debate over prescription authority. As Sammons (this volume) notes, "the additive effects of psych and pharmacotherapy is one supposition (not entirely without empirical support) which undergrids many of my arguments."

It is our contention that the additivity assumption is partly governed by the erroneous assumption that psychotherapy and pharmacotherapy operate via different mechanisms, and thus specifically address different symptoms within a disorder.

Treatment Specificity

Treatment specificity is often given as a reason for favoring combined treatments. The argument hinges on the assumption that medications and psychological treatments exert their primary effect on different loci of a syndrome—presumably the physical and psychological (or cognitive) facets respectively. To the extent that medication and psychological treatments appear to affect different symptom clusters within a syndrome, their combined use offers the advantage of treating multiple loci concurrently and hence may be more effective. For example, in treating panic disorder, Klein (1981) stressed the specific action of certain classes of medication in blocking spontaneous panic. It was *assumed* that psychosocial treatments were *ineffective* for the spontaneous panic feature of the disorder, but quite helpful in treating the psychological complications of spontaneous panic, namely anticipatory anxiety and phobic avoidance. The assumption of treatment specificity for tricyclic antidepressants and the monoamine oxidase (MAO) inhibitors, along with the recognition that panic disorder is a multifaceted syndrome, led to the recommendation of administering panic blocking medication in conjunction with psychological treatment that encouraged patients to confront fear-provoking cues (Klein, 1981). Although widely accepted, tests of the specificity hypothesis in panic disorder have failed to support it. Antidepressants such as imipramine exert their effects across multiple symptom clusters including panic attacks, anticipatory anxiety, and phobic avoidance (Telch & Lucas, 1994). Similarly, graduated exposure and other cognitive-behavioral procedures result in significant improvements across multiple symptom clusters as well.

Data from diverse lines of inquiry suggest that it is time to jettison the mind-body dualism that underlies the specificity assumption. Biological and psychological processes operate via dynamic reciprocal causal linkages, and thus can be seen as different perspectives of the same phenomenon. There is substantial evidence that pharmacologic agents are capable of producing measurable changes in cognition (DeRubeis, Holon, & Garvey, 1990; Holon, DeRubeis, & Evans, 1987). More recent studies have also demonstrated that psychosocial treatments, such as exposure and response prevention for obsessive-compulsive disorder, are capable of producing measurable changes in neurophysiology similar to those produced by selective serotonergic medications (Schwartz, Stoessel, Baxter, Martin, et al., 1996).

We do not mean to say that medication and psychosocial treatments are generally equivalent across the board with respect to either potency or mechanism of action. Rather, our aim is to dispel the myth that combined treatments exert their effects across a broader range of symptom facets compared with single modality treatments alone. Of course, the extent to which a specific pharmacologic, psychosocial, or combined treatment demonstrates generalization of effects across symptom clusters within a given syndrome remains an empirical question.

Facilitation Effects

A commonly voiced rationale for combining medication and psychosocial treatments is facilitation effects (Telch & Lucas, 1994). These refer to conditions where the effects of either medication or psychotherapy is enhanced by the presence of the other treatment modality. We distinguish two major types – (1) Medication-assisted psychotherapy and (2) psychotherapy-assisted pharmacotherapy. At first glance this distinction may appear silly. We provide it simply to highlight that the *primary* treatment may be either psychotherapy or medication, and the decision is made to supplement this primary treatment with the other modality.

Medication-Assisted Psychotherapy

In the case of drug-assisted psychotherapy, the primary treatment is psychotherapy, and medication(s) are used to promote the psychotherapy process. For example, patients displaying marked depression while undergoing psychological treatment for an anxiety disorder may possess insufficient energy or motivation to comply with the within-session or between-session demands of the psychosocial treatment. The suggestion to add an antidepressant may be made in an effort to stabilize mood so as to allow psychotherapy to continue more productively. Similarly, extreme anxiety may serve as an obstacle for patients in psychotherapy, and the administration of an anxiolytic may allow the patient to calm down sufficiently so that psychological treatment may proceed.

Although the examples provided above appear quite reasonable, several cautionary remarks deserve mention. First, the potential facilitative effects of medication on psychotherapy ought to be considered in light of the potential for negative effects. Examples of these are provided later in this chapter. Second, one should consider whether alternatives to pharmacotherapy (e.g., exercise, dietary prescriptions) might also facilitate psychotherapy with less risk potential.

Facilitation of Pharmacotherapy Through Psychological Treatment

A third rationale for combining medication and psychological treatments involves the potential facilitative effects that psychological interventions may have for patients undergoing drug treatments. One such facilitative function may be increased compliance to medication. As noted in previous reviews of pharmacological treatments, many patients display a fear of taking medications (Telch, Tearnan, & Taylor, 1983; Telch, 1988). Although reassurance by the physician may be sufficient for some, psychological treatment specifically targeting medication fears may be needed for the patient displaying severe anxiety surrounding medication use.

Psychological treatments may also serve a facilitative role in assisting patients during medication withdrawal. Patients who are provided education on withdrawal effects and additional strategies aimed at enhancing their sense of mastery and control of withdrawal symptoms may be more likely to withdraw from medications successfully. For instance, it has been recently demonstrated that compared to a drug taper control, drug taper plus CBT was markedly more effective in reducing the rate of relapse among panic patients withdrawing from high potency benzodiazepines (Otto et al., 1993; Spiegel, Bruce, Gregg, & Nuzzarello, 1994).

Possible Outcomes When Combining Psychotherapy and Medication

Although many assume that combined treatments will outperform the individual monotherapies, this does not have to be the case. In turning to the issue of efficacy, we should keep in mind that the combination of pharmacological and psychological treatments may result in one of several possible outcomes. These outcomes are illustrated in Figure 1.

The first two outcomes, additivity and potentiation, are favorable in that the combination treatment outperforms either of the singular treatments. *Additivity* is displayed when the effects of the combined treatment resemble the sum of the effects of each singular treatment. *Potentiation* is demonstrated when the outcome of the combined treatment significantly surpasses the additive effects of the singular treatments.

Unfortunately, combining drug and psychological treatments do not always lead to additive or potentiation effects. Three additional outcomes are possible. *Inhibition* refers to a negative interaction between the treatments resulting in a combined effect that is less than either treatment administered individually. *Reciprocation*

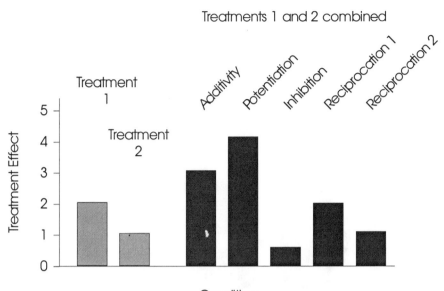

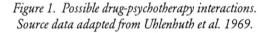

Figure 1. Possible drug-psychotherapy interactions.
Source data adapted from Uhlenhuth et al. 1969.

effects are also possible. These refer to combined treatment effects that are equivalent to one or both of the singular treatments.

Let us illustrate a few of these possible outcomes with real data from the panic disorder/agoraphobia literature. Figure 2 presents behavioral approach data at post-treatment from a combined treatment study of imipramine and exposure (Agras et al., 1990). Notice the additive effects of imipramine and exposure homework on this particular measure.

Figure 3 illustrates the potentiation of imipramine and exposure therapy reported by Telch et al. (1985). Notice how the magnitude of change for the combination treatment exceeds the additive effects of the individual treatments.

We recently observed a significant negative interaction between imipramine and exposure on agoraphobics' panic appraisals. Notice that imipramine appears to be inhibiting the effectiveness of exposure on this measure of panic-related cognitions.

Current Scientific Knowledge Base on Combined Treatments

The present review is limited to those controlled studies that have compared one or more drug-psychotherapy combination treatments to one or more singular treatments (drug or psychotherapy). Comparative studies of two or more singular treatments, whether drug or psychological, have been omitted since they do not directly address combined treatments. Several additional studies were excluded for failure to report the necessary statistics to calculate effect sizes.

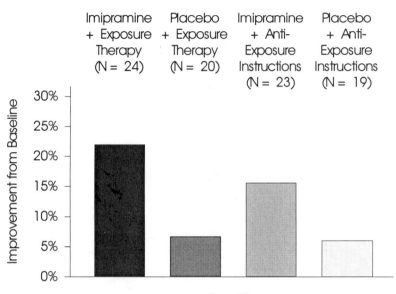

Figure 2. Improvement in Behavioral Approach Test (BAT) scores from pre- to posttreatment. Source data from Agras et al. 1991.

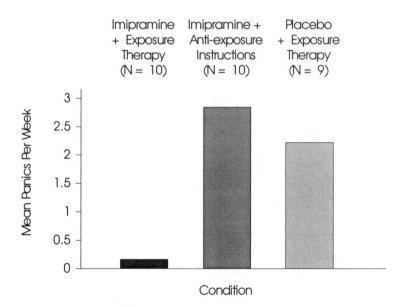

Figure 3. Mean number of panic attacks at 26 weeks posttreatment. Source data from Telch et al. 1985.

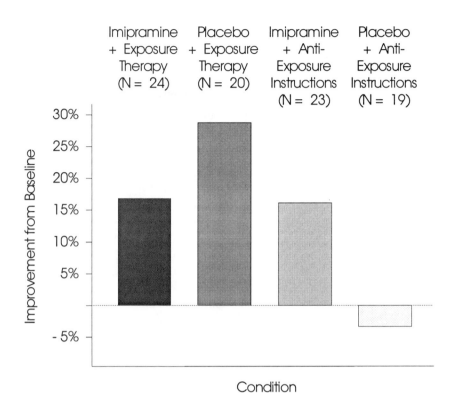

Figure 4. Improvement in panic appraisals from pre- to posttreatment.
Source data from Agras et al. 1991.

In general, the scientific knowledge base on combined treatments is quite poor. Controlled studies have been limited to just a few specific disorders. In addition to the problem of too few studies, limitations in the existing studies further complicate matters. Some of the more notable problems of the studies reviewed were: (a) failure to assess outcome after withdrawal of medication; (b) failure to compare the combined treatment to *both* medication alone and psychotherapy alone; and (c) inadequate statistical power due to small sample size.

What constitutes sufficient evidence for judging a combined treatment superior? At first glance this appears to be a relatively straightforward question. Should we not judge a combined treatment to be superior if it outperforms medication alone? One should exercise caution here. For what appears to be a superior performance for the combined treatment may instead simply reflect a superiority of psychological treatment over medication. Thus, in studies which fail to include a treatment group consisting of psychotherapy with no active drug, one cannot rule out the possibility that the superiority of the combined treatment is due to a reciprocation effect (i.e., combined treatment equaling psychotherapy alone).

What about a study showing combined treatment outperforming psychotherapy alone (or psychotherapy with pill placebo)? One runs into a similar interpretive problem here as well. In the absence of a medication only comparison group, demonstration that a combined treatment outperforms psychotherapy without medication may reflect the mere superiority of medication over psychotherapy.

One solution to this problem is to exclude any combined treatment study that doesn't compare a combined treatment to both psychotherapy alone (or psychotherapy with pill placebo) and medication alone. We rejected this solution on the grounds that the number of controlled outcome studies on combined treatments was already meager and thus further exclusion seemed counterproductive. Rather, we adopted an alternative solution. First, for each study we calculated effect sizes for two major comparisons: (a) combined treatment vs. medication alone, and (b) combined treatment versus psychotherapy alone (or psychotherapy plus pill placebo). Effect sizes across multiple outcome measures within a study were averaged to produce one overall effect size for each comparison. This procedure was repeated for studies that included follow-up outcome data. Next, these effect sizes were averaged across studies for each of the sampled disorders resulting in the following four summary effect sizes for each disorder: (a) combined versus medication at posttreatment; (b) combined versus psychotherapy at posttreatment; (c) combined versus medication at follow-up; and (d) combined versus psychotherapy at follow-up. We considered combining the posttreatment and follow-up effect sizes, but decided against it in order to provide some estimate of both the relative efficacy of combined treatments in the short-term, as well as their relative durability. We adopted the decision rule to classify a combined treatment as superior *only* if it outperforms *both* pharmacotherapy alone and psychotherapy alone.

Combined Treatments for Panic Disorder/Agoraphobia

Scientific Knowledge Base

Studies on the combined treatment of panic disorder/agoraphobia reviewed in the meta-analysis by Telch and Lucas (1994) are presented in Table 1. Despite the respectable number of combined treatment studies in this area, tremendous knowledge gaps exist. Most (8 of 13) of the combined treatment studies employed imipramine as the pharmacologic treatment (Agras, Telch, Taylor, Roth, & Brouillard, 1991; Marks, Grey, Cohen, Hill, Mawson, Ramm & Stern, 1983; Michelson & Mavissakalian, 1985; Sheehan, Ballenger & Jacobsen, 1980; Telch et al., 1985; Zitrin, Klein & Woerner, 1980; Zitrin, Klein, Woerner & Ross, 1983). MAO inhibitors were used in three of the earlier studies (Lipsedge, Hajioff, Napier, Pearce, Pike & Rich, 1973; Sheehan et al., 1980; Solyom, Heseltine, McClure, Solyom, Ledwidge & Steinberg, 1973). A low-potency benzodiazepine was used in one early study (Hafner & Marks, 1976), as was a barbiturate (Chambless et al., 1976). One multi-center study examined the high-potency benzodiazepine alprazolam (Marks & Swinson, 1990). Finally, one study (Sheehan et al., 1980) included two separate

Table 1. Treatment Outcome for Panic Disorder

Study	Treatment	Drug Dosage	N	Assmt. Period (weeks)	Duration of Treatment (weeks)	Short-term Assmt. after Drug Withdrawl	Post-treatment Effect Size	
							Drug vs. Combined	Psychotherapy vs. Combined
Agras et al 1991	IM+EX IM+AX PL+EX PL+AEX	Week 8: 142 mg/day Week 16: 168 mg/day	24 23 20 20	0, 8, 16, 24	Drug: 24 EX: 8	Yes	0.16	-0.08
Hafner & Marks 1976	GE+DZ (waning) GE+DZ (peak) GE+PL IE (high anxiety)+PL IE (low anxiety)+PL	.1 mg/kg	14 13 14 6 6	0, 2	2	No		
Lipsedge et al. 1973	MSD+IZ SD+IZ IZ MSD+PL SD+PL PL	IP: 50 mg/day BR: 1%IV solution	10 13 9 10 8 10	0, 8	8	No		
Marks et al 1983	IM+EX or IM+RT PL+EX or PL+RT	Week 14: 158 mg/day Week 26: 110 mg/day	23 22	0, 14, 28, 35 52, 104	Drug: 24 EX: 12	Yes		0.16

Study	Treatment	Drug Dosage	N	Assmt. Period (weeks)	Duration of Treatment (weeks)	Short-term Assmt. after Drug Withdrawl	Drug vs. Combined	Psychotherapy vs. Combined
Marks & Swinson 1993	AZ+EX AZ+RT PL+EX PL+RT	Week 8: 6 mg/day	34 34 30 31	0, 8, 18, 23, 43	18	Yes		0.31
Mavissakalian et al 1983	IM IM+PR	125 mg/day	7 8	0, 12	12	No	.65	
Mavissakalian & Peral 1985	IM+FL IM+PR	Month 1: 80 mg/day	14 17	0, 4, 8, 12	12	Yes		0.36
Mavissakalian et al 1986a, 1986b	PL+FL PL+PR	Month 2: 125 mg/day Month 3: 123 mg/day	17 14					
Sheehan et al 1980	PH+SG IM+SG PL+SG	PH: 45 mg/day IM: 150 mg/day	17 18 22	0, 6, 12	12	No		1.19 0.91
Solyom et al 1981	PH+EX PH PL+EX PL	PH: 45 mg/day	10 10 10 10	0, 8, 16	8	No		

Study	Groups	Dose	N	Assessment	Follow-up			
Tekh et al 1985	IM+EX IM+AEX PL+EX	Week 8: 190 mg/day Week 26: 179 mg/day	10 10 9	0, 8, 26	Drug: 26 EX: 8	No	0.71	0.48
Zitrin et al 1980	IM+EX PL+EX	200 mg/day	29 24	0, 14, 26	Drug: 26 EX: 10	No		0.65
Zitrin et al 1983	IM+ST PL+SD	204 mg/day	18 24 21	0, 26	26	No		0.51
Pooled Effect Size							0.39	0.45

Note. EX=exposure therapy; AEX=anti-exposure instructions; GE=group exposure; IE=individual exposure; SD=systematic desensitization; RT=relaxation training; PR=programmed practice; FL=flooding; SG=support group; ST=supportive therapy; IM=imipramine; PL=placebo; DZ=diazepam; MSD= methohexitane-assisted systematic desensitization; IZ=iproniazid; AZ=aprazolam; PH=phenelzine combination treatments - imipramine plus supportive psychotherapy, and phenelzine plus supportive psychotherapy.

What are the psychological treatments employed in the combined studies? As was the case with imipramine and pharmacotherapy, exposure-based therapies are overly represented. Eleven of the 13 studies examined a medication combined with an exposure-based treatment; two studies (Sheehan et al., 1980; Zitrin et al., 1983) combined medication with non-behavioral supportive psychotherapy; and one study (Zitrin et al., 1983) included two separate combined treatments - imipramine plus supportive psychotherapy, and imipramine plus imaginal desensitization.

With the exception of the combined treatment of imipramine and exposure, our knowledge base for combined drug-psychological treatments is quite limited. For instance, despite the widespread use of high potency benzodiazepines in the treatment of panic disorder, only one study (Marks et al., 1993) has examined their efficacy in combination with a psychological treatment. Of particular importance is the absence of data on the combined effects of pharmacotherapy and the new genre of cognitive-behavioral treatments for panic, as well as the absence of data on the combined effects of SSRIs and CBT.

A few remarks about the studies deserve highlighting. First, the patient samples are composed of agoraphobics exclusively. Patients with uncomplicated panic disorder or panic disorder with minimal avoidance are not represented. Only three of the studies included an active drug without psychological treatment as a comparison group. Moreover, none of the studies included a psychological treatment without placebo. Five of the 13 studies did not report outcome data for panic attacks.

How effective are combined treatments for panic disorder in the short-term? To address this issue, we examined controlled studies comparing one or more combined treatments with one or more singular treatments. Effect sizes were calculated separately for each of the following five domains: (a) panic, (b) phobic anxiety, (c) phobics avoidance, (d) depression, and (e) global functioning.

Combined Versus Psychological Treatments

Results of the eight studies which directly compared a combined treatment with a psychological treatment are presented in Table 1. Several studies were excluded from the analyses for failing to report group means and standard deviations. Note the double listing of the Sheehan et al. (1980) study. This is not an error. The study has two entries because it contributed two separate combined versus psychological comparisons to the analysis (imipramine plus supportive psychotherapy and phenelzine plus supportive psychotherapy). Note that row summaries represent the pooled effect size across the five assessment domains for each study, whereas column summaries represent the average effect size for a particular assessment domain pooled across studies. Effect sizes with a positive sign signify an advantage for the combined treatment.

Results of these analyses reveal a significant overall short-term advantage of combined treatment for most of the studies. Moreover, inspection of the column summaries indicate that the short-term superiority of the combined treatment was consistent across the five major assessment domains, rather than being limited to one domain such as panic. A modest but significant overall advantage for combined treatments over psychological treatment alone was observed at posttreatment (overall pooled effect size = .45).

These data are at odds with a review by Clum (1989) in which he concluded that combined treatments were less effective than behavior therapies alone. It should be noted that Clum (1989) based his conclusion on comparisons of author-defined success rates for individual studies. Unfortunately, this analytic approach is flawed when one considers that the differences in success rates may simply reflect between-study differences in the criteria used to define successful outcome.

Combined Versus Pharmacological Treatments

A second set of analyses were conducted in order to examine the relative efficacy of combined versus pharmacological treatments. Only three studies included a direct comparison of a combined treatment with pharmacotherapy alone (Agras, Telch et al. 1991; Mavissakalian & Michelson, 1983; Telch et al., 1985). In all three studies the combined treatment was imipramine plus exposure. Although limited by the small number of studies, this set of results reveal a clear short-term advantage of the combined treatment over pharmacological treatment alone. As in the previous comparison, the advantage of the combined treatment over drug alone was present across each of the major assessment domains (overall effect size = .39).

Evaluation of the Long-Term Efficacy of Combined Treatments for Panic

Few studies included an evaluation of the longer term effects of combined treatments. In a follow-up study of the patients originally treated in the Marks et al. (1983) study, Cohen et al. (1984) reported that approximately two-thirds of the patients interviewed (90% of the original cohort) at the two-year follow-up were improved or much improved from their pretreatment level of functioning. No significant advantage of the combined treatment was observed on any of the major clinical outcome measures. Mavissakalian and Michelson (1986) conducted a two-year follow-up of agoraphobics treated in their original study, comparing the singular and combined efficacy of imipramine and therapist-assisted exposure. All subjects received a systematic program of self-directed exposure. Seventy-six percent of the original cohort were interviewed. The overall improvement was maintained throughout follow-up. However, the superiority of the combined treatment over exposure alone, which was present at week 12, was no longer present at follow-up due to higher relapse among the imipramine treated patients and the continued improvement for patients in the self-directed exposure control. Consistent with the follow-up findings from the Marks et al. (1983) study, approximately two-thirds of the patients assessed cross-sectionally at the two-year follow-up were markedly improved.

The London-Toronto multicenter study (Marks et al. 1993) reported 43-week follow-up data on the single and combined effects of alprazolam and exposure therapy. These data are of particular interest since they represent the only available information on the efficacy of a combined alprazolam plus exposure treatment. Our effect size analyses presented earlier suggested a slight advantage of the combined alprazolam- exposure treatment over exposure plus placebo at the posttreatment assessment. In contrast to the short-term results, data on the combined treatment's long-term efficacy after medication withdrawal revealed that patients receiving the combination treatment evidenced a significantly poorer outcome at follow-up, compared to those patients treated with exposure plus placebo. The poorer long-term outcome for the combined alprazolam-exposure group was due to a markedly higher relapse rate among those receiving the combined treatment, rather than further gains made by the placebo plus exposure group. These findings are consistent with early reports suggesting that tranquilizing medication may interfere with the therapeutic effects of exposure (Chambless et al., 1979).

The deleterious long-term effects of adding medication to behavior therapy are not limited to the high potency benzodiazepines. Results from the long-awaited NIMH-funded multi-center panic disorder treatment study are just becoming available (Barlow, Personal Communication; October 1, 1977). This state-of-the-art multi-site clinical trial tested the singular and combined effects of imipramine, pill placebo, and CBT. Five treatment conditions were compared: (a) imipramine alone, (b) pill placebo, (c) CBT, (d) CBT plus pill placebo, and (e) CBT plus imipramine. The study represents a quantum leap in methodological sophistication and sets a new standard for the scientific evaluation of combined treatments. Contrary to expectation, preliminary analysis at follow-up shows the combined treatment performing significantly less well than either CBT alone or CBT plus placebo (Barlow, Personal Communication; October 1, 1977).

Conclusions Regarding the Efficacy of Combined Treatments for Panic

Our analysis suggests that in the short-term, combined treatments provide panic patients with agoraphobia greater benefit than either medication alone or psychosocial treatment alone. However, given the narrow range of treatments studied and the sample characteristics (i.e., all had agoraphobia), we feel that the above conclusion is limited to the combined treatment of imipramine plus exposure. We found no evidence to support the superiority of combined treatment at follow-up. On the contrary, data from two multi-site clinical trials suggest that adding medication (either alprazolam or imipramine) to behavior therapy may worsen patient outcome in the long-run. Consequently, we conclude that at the current time, combined treatments offer no overall advantage over psychosocial treatment alone.

Combined Treatments for Depression

Current Scientific Knowledge Base

Eight studies comparing combined treatment to singular treatment(s) for depression were reviewed. In all of the studies, the combined treatment consisted of a psychosocial treatment plus a tricyclic antidepressant (TCA). One study (Bellack, Hersen, & Himmelhoch, 1981) was excluded from Table 2 because it lacked sufficient information for calculating effect sizes. However, results from this study showed the combined treatment of social skills training (SST) plus a TCA was no more effective than either social skills training alone or medication alone. At posttreatment, Bellack and colleagues found no significant difference between combined treatment (social skills training and a tricyclic antidepressant) and each singular treatment (social skills training plus placebo, and medication alone). These findings were similar to the results of other studies presented in Table 2.

No differences between combined treatment and singular treatments were also found when cognitive therapy (CT) was employed (Murphy, Simons, Wetzel, & Lustman, 1984; Beck, Hollon, Young, Bedrosian, & Budenz, 1985). Murphy and colleagues compared combined treatment to CT, CT plus placebo, and a tricyclic antidepressant alone, while Beck and colleagues compared combined treatment to CT alone. Hersen and colleagues found that social skills training plus a tricyclic antidepressant was as effective as the tricyclic alone, but less effective than SST plus placebo (Hersen, Bellack, Himmelhoch, & Thase, 1984). On the other hand, combined treatment was found to be more effective than CT alone, cognitive behavioral therapy (CBT) alone, and interpersonal psychotherapy alone (Covi & Lipman, 1987; Hollon, DeRubeis, Evans, et al., 1992; Weissman et al., 1979). Combined treatment (CT or CBT plus an antidepressant) was also more effective than psychodynamic therapy alone (Covi & Lipman, 1987) and antidepressant alone (Hollon, DeRubeis, Evans, et al., 1992). All seven studies assessed outcome before drug withdrawal.

The three studies that assessed outcome at follow-up found no differences between combined and singular treatments (Beck, et al., 1985; Hersen, et al., 1984; Murphy, et al., 1984). One study (Hersen et al., 1984) assessed outcome before drug withdrawal, while the other two studies (Murphy et al., 1984; Beck et al., 1985) assessed outcome after drug withdrawal. Treatment integrity was not assessed for two of the studies (Beck et al. 1985; & Hersen et al. 1984). Hollon and colleagues assessed treatment integrity through the use of independent judges who rated the sessions on the quality of execution and adherence to the cognitive model. Murphy and colleagues assessed treatment integrity through the reviewing of audiotapes and weekly supervision.

Overall Findings

Effect sizes for the two comparisons (pharmacotherapy versus combined, psychotherapy versus combined) are presented in Table 2. Two studies (Covi & Lipman, 1987; Murphy, et al., 1984) have two effect sizes listed because they contributed two separate combined versus psychological comparisons to the analysis (CT alone and CT -plus-placebo versus combined CT-plus-medication; and CBT alone and pschodynamic therapy alone versus CBT-plus-medication).

Results revealed mixed findings across studies. At posttreatment, the psychological treatment showed a small advantage over combined treatment (pooled effect size = -.25), whereas at follow-up, the treatments no longer differed (pooled effect size =.08). Comparisons between pharmacotherapy versus combined treatment

Table 2. Treatment Outcome for Depression

Study	Treatment	Drug Dosage	N	Assmt. Periods (weeks)	Duration of Tx (weeks)	Short-term Assmt. after Drug Withdrawl	Long-term Assmt. after Drug Withdrawl	Outcome Measure	Post-Tx Effect Size		Follow-up Effect Size	
									Psycho-therapy vs. Combined	Drug vs. Combined	Psycho-therapy vs. Combined	Drug vs. Combined
Hersen et al 1984	SST+PL SST+AM AM	50-300 mg/day	33 30 26	12, 36	12	No	No	BDI HRSD	-0.55	-0.14	-0.32	-0.07
Murphy et al 1984	CT CT+PL NH CT+NH	50-150 mg/mL	24 24 22	12, 28	12	No	Yes	BDI HRSD	0.02 -0.11	0.03	0.18 0.34	0.16
Beck et al 1985	CT CT+AM	75-200 mg/day	18 15	12, 36, 60	12	No	Yes	BDI HRSD	-0.03		0.47	
Hollon et al 1992	CT IM CT+IM	200-450 mg/day	16 32 16	6, 12	12	No	N/A	BDI HRSD	0.34	0.46		
Weissman et al 1979	P AM IP+AM	100-200 mg/day	25 24 24	1, 4, 8, 12, 16	16	No	N/A	SF	0.29	0.51		

Covi & Lipman 1987	CBT TRAD CBT+IM	100-300 mg/day	27 20 23	14	14	No	N/A	BDI	0.48 1.47			
Pooled Effect Size									-0.25	0.14	0.08	0.06

Note. SST=social support therapy; CT=cognitive therapy; IP=interpersonal psychotherapy; TRAD=traditional group psychotherapy (psychodynamic); SF=symptomatic failure (a Raskin depression score of 9 or more); BDI=Beck Depression Inventory; HRSD=Hamilton Rating Scale for Depression; PL=placebo; NH=nortriptyline hydrochloride; AM=amitriptiline; IM=imipramine.

Positive effect signs denote superiority for combined treatment

Table 3. Treatment Outcome for Obesity

Study	Treatment	Drug Dosage	N	Assmt. Periods (weeks)	Duration of Tx (weeks)	Short-term Assmt. after Drug Withdrawl	Long-term Assmt. after Drug Withdrawl	Outcome Measure	Post-Tx Psychotherapy vs. Combined	Post-Tx Drug vs. Combined	Follow-up Psychotherapy vs. Combined	Follow-up Drug vs. Combined
Craighead et al 1981	BT / BT+FF / FF	120 mg/day max.	32 / 23 / 25	24, 72	24	Yes	Yes	weight change	3.99	0.68	-3.03	-1.08
Marcus et al 1990	BT+PL / BT+FL	60 mg/day	10 / 11	2, 8, 20, 36, 52	52	No	N/A	weight change	1.42			
Brightwell & Naylor 1979	BT+PL / BT+PH/PL / BT+PL/PH / R+PL/PH	30 mg/day	9 / 5 / 12 / 6	8, 16, 24	24	No	N/A	weight change	1.13 / 0.45			
Rodin et al 1988	CBT / CBT+PL / CBT+DH	75 mg/day	17 / 16 / 16	16, 20, 24, 48	20	No	Yes	weight change	0.66 / 0.02		-0.17 / 0.37	
Craighead 1984	BT / BT+FF / FF	60-160 mg/day	16 / 14 / 16	16, 32, 64	16	Yes	Yes	weight change	0.28	0.46	0.10	0.69

Brownell & Stunkard 1981	BT BT+FF	60-160 mg/day	43 69	16, 48	16	No	Yes	weight change	4.03		0.74	
Pooled Effect Size									1.51	0.60	0.01	-0.34

Note. BT=behavior therapy; CBT=cognitive behavior therapy; FF=fenfluramine; FL=fluoxetine; PH=phentermine; PL=placebo; R=relaxation; DH=diethylpropion hydrochloride.

Positive effect signs denote superiority for combined treatment

revealed no significant advantage for combined treatment at either posttreatment (effect size =.14) or follow-up up (effect size = .06).

Based on these analyses, we conclude that combined treatment is no more effective than single modality treatment for depression. This conclusion is similar to that drawn by Manning, Markowitz, and Francis (1992) in their review of combined treatments for depression.

Combined Treatments for Obesity

Current Scientific Knowledge Base

Six studies comparing combined treatment to singular treatment(s) are presented in Table 3. A consistent pattern of findings emerged at posttreatment. Patients treated with pharmacotherapy plus behavior therapy lost significantly more weight than those treated with placebo plus behavior therapy (Marcus, Wing, Ewing, Kern, McDermott, & Gooding, 1990; Brightwell & Naylor, 1979; Rodin, Elias, Silberstein, and Wagner, 1988) or behavior therapy alone (Brownell & Stunkard, 1981; Craighead, 1984; Rodin, Elias, Silberstein, and Wagner, 1988; Craighead, Stunkard, & O'Brien, 1981). Marcus and colleagues used an SSRI for the drug treatment, while the rest used an anorectic.

Only two studies directly compared a combined treatment to pharmacotherapy. Craighead (1984) found that combined treatment (BT plus an anorectic) was more effective than the anorectic alone. However, Craighead, Stunkard, & O'Brien (1981) found no significant difference between BT plus an anorectic and the anorectic alone. Outcome was assessed before drug withdrawal in four of the studies (Marcus et al., 1990; Brightwell & Naylor, 1979; Rodin et al., 1988; Brownell & Stunkard, 1981), and after drug withdrawal in two others (Craighead et al., 1981; Craighead, 1984).

The pattern of results at follow-up reveal a somewhat different picture. Those receiving combined treatment regained more weight than those receiving an anorectic alone (Craighead et al., 1981; Craighead, 1984), or those receiving behavior therapy alone (Craighead et al., 1981; Rodin et al., 1988; Brownell & Stunkard, 1981). All studies assessed outcome after drug withdrawal. Treatment integrity was not assessed in any of the studies.

Overall Findings

Effect sizes for the two comparisons (pharmacotherapy versus combined, psychotherapy versus combined) are presented in Table 3. Two studies (Brightwell & Naylor, 1979; Rodin et al., 1988) have two effect sizes listed because these studies contributed two separate combined versus psychological comparisons to the analysis (BT or CBT alone and plus placebo versus combined treatment).

Combined therapy was markedly more effective than psychotherapy alone at posttreatment (pooled effect size = 1.50). However, at follow-up the differences were negligible (pooled effect size = .01). Similarly, combined therapy was also significantly more effective than medication alone at posttreatment (pooled effect size =

.60). However, an interesting reversal of findings emerged at follow-up. Patients receiving combined treatments displayed less overall weight loss relative to patients receiving medication alone (pooled effect size = -.34).

Our review of the effects of combined treatment for weight loss suggests a definite short-term advantage compared with either behavior therapy or medication alone. However, the greater efficacy of combined treatment over either single modality treatment is not present at follow-up. Indeed, there is some suggestion that combined treatment may have a deleterious effect relative to medication alone in the long run.

Combined Treatments for Bulimia

Current Scientific Knowledge Base

A description of the controlled studies in bulimia that compared a combined treatment to at least one singular treatment are presented in Table 4. One study comparing CBT + TCA (Mitchell, Pyle, Eckert, et al., 1990) was excluded because it failed to provide sufficient information to allow the calculation of effect sizes. Mitchell et al. (1990) found a significant posttreatment advantage for combined treatment over CBT alone on an index of global improvement. However, no significant differences were observed on eating behavior or global severity ratings. Agras and colleagues (Agras, Rossiter, Arnow, et al., 1992) found that a 24-week combined treatment of CBT plus desipramine was superior to a 16-week treatment with desipramine alone in reducing binge eating and purging, and superior to 24 weeks of desipramine alone in reducing purging. Additionally, the combined treatment was superior to CBT alone in reducing dietary preoccupation and disinhibition. In another study (Agras, Telch, Arnow, et al., 1994b), the addition of desipramine to CBT plus a weight loss program resulted in greater weight loss, and greater reductions in disinhibition. Fichter and colleagues (Fichter, Leibl, Reif, Brunner, Schmidt-Auberger, & Engel, 1991) found that the use of fluoxetine in combination with BT resulted in a significantly greater reduction in body weight when compared to BT plus placebo.

Walsh and colleagues (Walsh, Wilson, Loeb, et al., 1997) conducted an ambitious study comparing medication (desipramine + fluoxetine), CBT + medication, CBT + Placebo, Supportive Psychotherapy + Medication, and supportive psychotherapy + placebo. They found the combined treatment of CBT plus medication showed greater reductions in binge eating and dysfunctional eating attitudes than either CBT plus placebo or medication alone. Interestingly, participants receiving medication alone lost significantly more weight relative to the group receiving the combined treatment. Similarly, the combined treatment of supportive psychotherapy plus medication was less effective than medication alone in reducing frequency of binge eating. All outcomes were assessed before drug withdrawal.

The Agras et al. (1994) study was the only one to assess the outcome for medication-free subjects at follow-up. The study found that a 24-week combined treatment (desipramine plus CBT) was more effective in reducing binge eating than a 16-

Table 4. Treatment Outcome for Bulimia

Study	Treatment	Drug Dosage	N	Assmt. Periods (weeks)	Duration of Tx (weeks)	Short-term Assmt. after Drug Withdrawl	Long-term Assmt. after Drug Withdrawl	Outcome Measure	Post-Tx Effect Size		Follow-up Effect Size	
									Psycho-therapy vs. Combined	Drug vs. Combined	Psycho-therapy vs. Combined	Drug vs. Combined
Agras et al 1992	CBT CBT+DP (wk 16) CBT+DP (wk 24) DP (wk 16) DP (wk 24)	130.8 ng/mL	23 12 12 12 12	16, 24, 32	16 or 24	No	Yes	binges/wk purges/wk hunger/dis-inhibition dietary preoccu-pation	0.35	-0.03 0.26		
Agras et al 1994a	CBT CBT+DP (wk 16) CBT+DP (wk 24) DP (wk 16) DP (wk 24)	130.8 ng/mL	22 10 9 11 9	72	16 or 24	N/A	Yes	binges/wk purges/wk hunger/dis-inhibition dietary preoccu-pation restraint depression self-esteem			0.3 -0.14	0.07 0.04
Agras et al 1994b	CBT/WL CBT/WL+DP	285 mg/day	36 36	12, 24, 36	36	No		weight binges/wk disinhibition hunger restraint	0.10			

Study	Treatment	Dose	N			Blind	Measures			
Fichter et al 1991	BT+PL BT+FL	60 mg/day	20 19	1, 2, 3, 4, 5	5	No	EDI urge to binge binges weight (kg) HAMD	0.27		
Walsh et al 1997	CBT+PL SP+PL CBT+DP/FL SP+DP/FL DP/FL	DP: 188 mg/day FL: 55 mg/day	25 22 23 22 28	16	16	No	binges/wk vomiting/wk EAT restraint disinhibition hunger weight	0.54 0.04	0.31 -0.09	
Pooled Effect Size								0.24	0.11	0.08	0.03

Note. BT=behavior therapy; CBT=cognitive behavior therapy; WL=weight loss program; SP=supportive psychotherapy; DP=desopramine; FF=fenfluramine; FL=fluoxetine; PL=placebo; EDI=Eating Disorder Inventory; EAT=Eating Attitude Test; HAMD=Hamilton Depression Rating Scale

Positive effect signs denote superiority for combined treatment

week treatment with desipramine alone. On measures of dietary preoccupation and disinhibition, the 24 week combined treatment was superior to 16 weeks of desipramine treatment alone. Outcome was assessed after drug withdrawal. The one study (Walsh, Wilson, Loeb, et al., 1997) that assessed treatment integrity had an independent rater assess 227 audiotaped therapy sessions.

Overall Findings

Effect sizes for the two major comparisons are presented in Table 4. The study conducted by Agras and colleagues (1992, 1994a) has two effect sizes listed because it contributed two separate combined versus pharmacological comparisons to the analysis (CBT plus desipramine at week 16 and week 24 was compared to desipramine alone at week 16 and 24 respectively). The study conducted by Walsh and colleagues (1997) also has two effect sizes listed because it contributed two separate combined versus psychological comparisons (CBT plus placebo versus CBT plus desipramine; and supportive psychotherapy plus placebo versus supportive psychotherapy plus desipramine).

At post-treatment, combined treatment showed a slight advantage over psychological treatment (pooled effect size = .24), but no real advantage over medication alone (pooled effect size = .11). At follow-up, combined treatments did not outperform psychological treatment alone (pooled effect size = .08) nor pharmacotherapy alone (pooled effect size = .03). Overall, results of these analyses do not meet our criteria for demonstrating superiority of combined treatment.

Combined Treatments for ADHD

Current Scientific Knowledge Base

One between group trial (Hinshaw, Henker, & Whalen, 1984) and two within-group trials (Carlson, Pelham, Milich, & Dixon, 1992; Pelham, Carlson, Sama, Vallano, Dixon, & Hoza, 1993) comparing combined treatment to singular treatment(s) are presented in Table 5. Both Pelham and colleagues (1993), and Carlson and colleagues (1992), found that methylphenidate (MPH) alone yielded improvements on both behavioral and cognitive measures, while behavior therapy (BT) yielded improvements on only behavioral measures. In comparing combined treatment to the two singular treatments, Pelham and colleagues found that BT plus MPH was more effective than BT alone across all outcome measures, but was no more effective than MPH alone. However, when MPH dosages were low, the addition of BT enhanced improvements. Carlson and colleagues' (1992) results were similar. Subjects in the regular classroom condition showed significant improvement for on-task behavior and disruptive behavior on higher doses (.6 mg/kg) of MPH as compared to a lower dosage (.3 mg/kg). However, those in the behavior modification program evidenced similar improvements for on-task and disruptive behavior whether prescribed a high or low dosage of MPH. Thus children's behavior improved with lower dosages of MPH when BT and MPH were combined. Outcome was assessed before drug withdrawal in both studies. Neither assessed treatment integrity.

Table 5. Treatment Outcome for ADHD

Study	Treatment	N	Assmt. Periods (weeks)	Duration of Tx (weeks)	Short-term Assmt. after Drug Withdrawal	Outcome Measure	Short-term Effect Size	
							Psychotherapy vs. Combined	Drug vs. Combined
Pelham et al 1993	BM	31	8	8	No	seatwork completed	0.57[cd]	0.03[cd]
	8.1 mg MPH (low dose)	31				seatwork accuracy	0.64[ce]	0.10[ce]
	16 mg MPH (high dose)	31				time on task	-0.30[bd]	0.05[bd]
	BM+8.1 mg MPH	31				Iowa I/O	-0.40[ba]	-0.05[be]
	BM+16 mg MPH	31				Iowa O/D	0.30[cd]	0.00[cd]
Carlson et al 1992	BM	24	8	8	No	seatwork completed	0.44[ce]	0.30[ce]
	.3 mg/kg MPH (low dose)	24				seatwork accuracy	0.69[bd]	0.31[bd]
	.6 mg/kg MPH (high dose)	24				time on task	0.93[be]	-0.18[be]
	BM+.3 mg/kg MPH	24						
	BM+.6 mg/kg MPH	24						
Hinshaw et al 1984	RSE+placebo	12	5	5	No	neg. social behav.	0.91[a]	
	RA+placebo	12				approp. social behav.		
	RSE+MPH	12				cooperation		
	RA+MPH	12				social/peer interaction	0.91	
Pooled Effect Size						behavioral	-.09[d]	0.10[d]
							-0.12[e]	-0.07[e]
						cognitive	0.45[d]	0.02[d]
							0.55[e]	0.08[e]

Note. BM=behavior modification; MPH=methylphenidate; I/O=inattention/overactivity; O/D=oppositional/defiant; a=social peer interactions; b=behavioral measures; c=cognitive measures; d=low drug dose; e=high drug dose.

Positive effect signs denote superiority for combined treatment

Hinshaw and colleagues (1984) compared the combined effects of MPH and reinforced self-evaluation (RSE) to RSE alone for improving social/peer interactions among ADHD children. The combined MPH plus RSE treatment was more effective in positively changing social behavior than RSE alone. Since the combined treatment was not compared to medication alone, one cannot rule out the possibility that the superiority of the combined treatment was due to the greater effectiveness of methylphenidate over reinforced self-evaluation

Overall Findings

The effect sizes for the ADHD studies are presented in Table 5. In calculating effect sizes, data were separated into behavioral measures and academic performance measures, as the interaction of drugs and BT affect these domains differently. Behavioral measures included time on task, Iowa I/O, and Iowa O/D. The academic performance measures included seatwork completed, and seatwork accuracy. Additionally, since it is known that combined methylphenidate and CBT have differing efficacy depending on the dosage level, the analysis was also split by high and low medication dosage (when reported).

On measures of cognitive performance, combined treatment showed a clear advantage over behavior therapy alone (pooled effect size = .45 low dose; pooled effect size = .55 high dose), but did not show an advantage over medication alone either at the low dose (pooled effect size = .02) or the high dose (pooled effect size = .08). For measures of disruptive behavior, a different pattern of findings emerged. Combined treatments were no more effective than behavior therapy alone (pooled effect size = -.09 - low dose; pooled effect size = -.12 high dose) and no more effective than medication alone (pooled effect size = .10 low dose; pooled effect size = -.07 high dose). Overall, results of these analyses do not meet our criteria for demonstrating superiority of combined treatment.

General Conclusions Regarding
the Efficacy of Combined Treatments

What conclusions can be drawn from our review of combined treatments? Given the pervasive bias that combined treatments are more effective, we were quite surprised by the results of our efficacy analyses. Using a relatively straightforward analytic approach, we found little evidence to support the claim that combined treatments provide greater benefit than single modality treatments. Our specific conclusions are presented below. They differ somewhat depending on the timing of assessment and the specific disorder being treated.

1. In the treatment of panic disorder and obesity, combined treatments clearly outperformed single modality treatments in the *short-term*;

2. In the treatment of bulimia, depression, and ADHD, combined treatments were not significantly more effective in the short-term than single modality treatments;

3. At follow-up, combined treatments were not significantly more effective than single modality treatments for any of the disorders reviewed;

4. Patients receiving combined treatments for panic disorder showed poorer outcome at follow-up relative to patients receiving behavioral or cognitive-behavioral treatment without active medication.

Some might argue that the conclusions above are premature given the existing gaps in our knowledge base. Others might argue that randomized clinical trials are limited in the information they provide with respect to the effectiveness of treatments as they are delivered in the real world (Seligman, 1995). What other source of data might inform us about the effectiveness of combined treatments? In 1995, *Consumer Reports* published the results of a large-scale survey on the effectiveness of psychotherapy. The study has been described as "the most extensive study of psychotherapy effectiveness on record" (Seligman, 1995, p. 969). Among the almost 3000 survey respondents, *there were no differences between psychotherapy alone and psychotherapy plus medication for any disorder.* Too few respondents reported receiving medication alone to allow for a comparison with combined treatment. These results converge with our conclusions from the clinical trial data suggesting that the administration of psychoactive agents in combination with psychotherapy provides no appreciable added benefit relative to psychotherapy alone.

Priorities for Future Research on Combined Treatments

Where do we go from here? The gaps in our current knowledge base and the conceptual and methodological limitations in the research to date suggest a tentative listing of recommendations. The order of listing in no way implies a ranking of importance.

1. Clinical trials are needed to examine the efficacy of new psychoactive agents in combination with new psychological treatments.

Many of the studies on combined treatments involve medications that are no longer widely prescribed in day-to-day clinical practice. For example, TCAs and MAOIs have been the focus of almost all the combined treatment investigations in panic disorder. Yet these drugs are no longer widely prescribed in clinical practice. As new medications and psychosocial treatments become widely used in clinical practice, there exists a corresponding need to evaluate their combined effects.

2. Patient selection criteria should be less stringent in order to enhance the generalization of study findings to clinical practice.

The ecological validity of findings from randomized clinical trials can be significantly enhanced if investigators would adopt less stringent patient exclusion criteria. Inclusion of patients with (a) comorbid Axis I conditions such as substance abuse, (b) personality disorders, and (c) suicidal inclusion can be achieved without sacrificing internal validity. Increasing the heterogeneity of the sample has the added advantage of facilitating the identification of treatment moderators. Funding agencies such as the National Institute of Mental Health should encourage this by being sensitive to the larger sample size requirements brought about by increased sample heterogeneity.

3. Future studies require experimental designs that correct for the (a) confounding of drug effects and psychological treatment effects, and (b) the inappropriate use of placebo + psychotherapy to represent psychotherapy alone.

Few of the studies reviewed included a "pure" psychological treatment without pill placebo. The problems associated with using pill placebo plus psychotherapy to represent psychotherapy alone have been cogently discussed (Hollon & Beck, 1978; Hollon & DeRubeis, 1981). In short, the presence of a placebo may add to the effectiveness of psychotherapy in the short-run (the classic placebo effect), but may also undermine the long-term gains of psychotherapy when patients misattribute improvement to the "drug." For instance, Klerman et al. (1974), found that depressives receiving placebo plus interpersonal psychotherapy had twice the relapse (i.e., 28% vs. 14%) of a similar group receiving interpersonal psychotherapy alone. Designs which rely on placebo-plus-psychotherapy comparisons, although useful in illuminating the mechanisms governing the interaction of medication and psychotherapy, are inadequate for drawing valid inferences about differential outcome. The scant empirical evidence directly comparing placebo plus psychotherapy with psychotherapy alone suggests it is misguided to assume equivalence.

4. Research aimed at identifying optimal sequencing and dosing of combined treatments is needed.

We have yet to even scratch the surface in understanding how best to sequence combination treatments. Systematic examination of sequencing variations is needed to deliver combined treatment in an optimal fashion. In addition to sequencing, the dosing of psychological treatments deserves study. For instance, it is not uncommon for pharmacological studies to continue medication for six months. Yet, the dosing of psychological treatments in the combined treatment studies have been relatively "low."

5. Research is needed which aims to identify patient subtypes for whom combined treatments are indicated, and patient subtypes for whom combined treatments are contraindicated.

Moderator analyses aimed at identifying patient variables that predict response to combined treatment is critical for attaining an effective system of matching treatment modality and patient characteristics. Indices of problem severity, and the presence of comorbid conditions are just a few of the factors that deserve careful study. To assist in meeting the large sample size requirements for moderator analyses, outcome data from several research centers might be pooled and re-analyzed.

6. A broader assessment of treatment utility that integrates information along several evaluative dimensions is necessary.

Outcome evaluation has been too limited in scope. We need to move beyond unitary indices of treatment efficacy to a more multidimensional mapping of treatment utility that integrates information from several evaluative dimensions such as: (a) degree of symptom improvement, (b) clinical significance of improvements, (c) quickness of action, (d) attrition, (e) adverse effects, and (f) treatment durability. The development of evaluative algorithms for integrating information from these various dimensions into a composite index of treatment utility would be a major advance. Preliminary work along these lines has recently appeared (Michelson, 1991).

Implications for Prescription Authority

The argument that psychologists will be more effective in their delivery of clinical services if they are authorized to prescribe medications hinges on the assumption that psychoactive medications given concurrently with a psychosocial treatment enhances patients' clinical status. Based on the available data, this assumption appears false. More importantly, our knowledge base is limited, and additional research is clearly needed. Until we have substantial evidence in hand which demonstrates the superiority of combined treatments, there is no justification for a "full steam ahead" approach in the endorsement of prescription authority.

References

Agras, W.S., Rossiter, E.M., Arnow, B., Schneider, J.A., Telch, C.F., Raeburn, S.D., Bruce, B., Perl, M., Koran, L.M. (1992). Pharmacologic and cognitive-behavioral treatment for bulimia nervosa: A controlled comparison. *American Journal of Psychiatry, 149,* 82-87.

Agras, W.S., Rossiter, E.M., Arnow, B., Telch, C.F., Raeburn, S.D., Bruce, B., Koran, L.M. (1994a). One-year follow-up of psychosocial and pharmacologic treatments for bulimia. *Journal of Clinical Psychiatry, 55,* 179-183.

Agras, W.S., Telch, C.F., Arnow, B., et al. (1994). Weight loss, cognitive behavioral, and desipramine treatments in binge eating disorder. An additive design. *Behavior Therapy, 25,* 225-238.

Beck, A.T., Hollon, S.D., Young, J.E., Bedrosian, R.C., & Budenz, D. (1985). Treatment of depression with cognitive therapy and amitryptiline. *Archives of General Psychiatry, 42,* 142-148.

Bellack, A.S., Hersen, M., & Himmelhoch, J. (1981). Social skills training compared with pharmacotherapy and psychotherapy in the treatment of unipolar depression. *American Journal of Psychiatry, 138,* 1562-1566.

Blackburn, I.M., Bishop, S., Glen, A.I.M., Whalley, L.J., & Christie, J.E. (1981). The efficacy of cognitive therapy in depression: A treatment trial using cognitive therapy and pharmacotherapy, each alone and in combination. *British Journal of Psychiatry, 139,* 181-189.

Brightwell, D.R., & Naylor, C.S. (1979). Effects of combined behavioral and pharmacologic program on weight loss. *International Journal of Obesity, 3,* 141-148.

Brownell, K.D., & Stunkard, A.J. (1981). Couples training, pharmacotherapy, and behavior therapy in the treatment of obesity. *Archives of General Psychiatry, 38,* 1224-1232.

Brownell, K.D., & Wadden, T.A. (1992). Etiology and treatment of obesity: Understanding a serious, prevalent, and refractory disorder. *Journal of Consulting and Clinical Psychology, 60,* 505-517.

Carlson, C., Pelham, W. E., Milich, R., & Dixon, J. (1992). Single and combined effects of methylphenidate and behavior therapy on the classroom performance of children with attention-deficit hyperactivity disorder. *Journal of Abnormal Child Psychology, 20,* 213-232.

Clum, G.A. (1989).Psychological interventions vs. drugs in the treatment of panic. *Behavior Therapy, 20,* 429-457.

Cohen, J. (1977). *Statistical power analysis for the behavioral sciences.* New York: Academic Press.

Consumer Reports. (1995, November). Mental health: Does therapy help? 734-739.

Covi, L., & Lipman, R.S. (1987). Cognitive-behavioral group psychotherapy combined with imipramine in major depression. *Psychopharmacology Bulletin, 23,* 173-176.

Craighead, L.W. (1984). Sequencing of behavior therapy and pharmacotherapy for obesity. *Journal of Consulting and Clinical Psychology, 52,* 190-199.

Craighead, L.W., Stunkard, A.J., & O'Brien, R. (1981). Behavior therapy and pharmacotherapy of obesity. *Archives of General Psychiatry, 38,* 763-768.

DeRubeis, R. J., Evans, M. D., Hollon, S. D., Garvey, M. J., & Tuason, V. B. (1990). How does cognitive therapy work? Cognitive change and symptom change in cognitive therapy and pharmacotherapy for depression. *Journal of Consulting and Clinical Psychology, 58,* 862-869.

Fichter, M. M., Leibl, K., Reif, W., Brunner, E., Schmidt-Auberger, S., & Engel, R. R. (1991). Fluoxetine versus placebo: A double-blind study with bulimic inpatients undergoing intensive psychotherapy. *Pharmacopsychiatry, 24,* 1-7.

Green, M.A. & Curtis, G.C. (1988).Personality disorders in panic patients: Response to termination of anti-panic medication. *Journal of Personality Disorders, 2,* 303-314.

Hersen, M., Bellack, A. S., Himmelhoch, J. M., & Thase, M.E. (1984). Effects of social skill training, amitriptyline, and psychotherapy in unipolar depressed women. *Behavior Therapy, 15,* 21-40.

Hinshaw, S., Henker, B., & Whalen, C. (1984). Cognitive-behavioral and pharmacologic interventions for hyperactive boys: Comparative and combined effects. *Journal of Consulting and Clinical Psychology, 52,* 739-749.

Hollon, S. D. & DeRubeis, R. J. (1981). Placebo-psychotherapy combinations: Inappropriate representation of psychotherapy in drug-psychotherapy comparative trials. *Journal of Consulting and Clinical Psychology, 90,* 467-477.

Hollon, S. D., DeRubeis, R. J., Evans, M. D., Weimer, M. J., Garvey, M. J., Grove, W. M., & Tuason, V. B. (1992). Cognitive therapy and pharmacotherapy for depression: Singly and in combination, *Psychological Bulletin, 9,* 774-781.

Hollon, S. D., DeRubeis, R. J., & Evans, M. D. (1987). Causal mediation of change in treatment for depression: Discriminating between nonspecificity and noncausality. *Psychological Bulletin, 102,* 139-149.

Jansson, L. & Ost, L. (1982). Behavioral treatment for agoraphobia: An evaluative review. *Clinical Psychology Review, 2,* 311-336.

Klein, D.F. (1964). Delineation of two drug-responsive anxiety syndromes. *Psychopharmacologia, 5,* 397-408.

Klein, D.F. (1980). Anxiety Reconceptualized. *Comprehensive Psychiatry, 21*, 411-427.

Lipsedge, M.S., Hajioff, J., Huggins, P., Napier, L., Pearce, J., Pike, D.J. & Rich, M. (1973). The management of severe agoraphobia: A comparison of iproniazid and systematic desensitization. *Psychopharmacologia, 32*, 667-80.

Marcus, M.D., Wing, R.R., Ewing, L., Kern, E., McDermott, M., & Gooding, W. (1990). A double-blind, placebo-controlled trial of fluoxetine plus behavior modification in the treatment of obese binge-eaters and non-binge-eaters. *American Journal of Psychiatry, 147*, 876-881.

Marks, I. M., Swinson, R. P., Basoglu, M., Kuch, K., Noshirvani, H., O'Sullivan, G., Lelliott, P. T., Kirby, M., McNamee, G., Sengun, S., & Wickwire, K. (1993). Alprazolam and exposure alone and combined in panic disorder with agoraphobia. A controlled study in London and Toronto [see comments]. *British Journal of Psychiatry, 162*, 776-87.

Marks, I.M. (1983). Are there anticompulsive or antiphobic drugs? Review of evidence. *British Journal of Psychiatry, 143*, 338-347.

Marks, I.M., Gray, S., Cohen, D., Hill, R., Mawson, D., Ramm, E. & Stern, R.S. (1983). Imipramine and brief therapist-aided exposure in agoraphobics having self-exposure homework. *Archives of General Psychiatry, 40*, 153-162.

Marks, I.M., Swinson, R.P. (1990). Results of London/Toronto comparative studies: Alprazolam and exposure for panic disorder with agoraphobia. *Journal of Psychiatric Research, 24 (Suppl.)*, 100.

Mavissakalian, M. & Perel, J. (1985). Imipramine in the treatment of agoraphobia: Dose-response relationships. *American Journal of Psychiatry, 142*, 1032-1036.

Mavissakalian, M., & Michelson, L. (1986). Agoraphobia: Relative and Combined Effectiveness of therapist-assisted in vivo exposure and imipramine. *Journal of Clinical Psychiatry, 47*, 117-122.

Michelson, L.& Mavissakalian, M.(1985).Psychophysiological outcome of behavioral and pharmacological treatments of agoraphobia. *Journal of Consulting and Clinical Psychology, 53*, 229-236.

Middleton, (1991). Psychology and pharmacology in the treatment of anxiety disorders: Co-operation or confrontation. *Journal of Psychopharmacology, 5*, 281-285.

Mitchell, J.E., Pyle, R.L., Eckert, E.D., Hatsukami, D., Pomeroy, C., Zimmerman, R.(1990). A comparison study of antidepressants and structured intensive group psychotherapy in the treatment of bulimia nervosa. *Archives of General Psychiatry, 47*, 149-157.

Mountjoy, C.Q., Roth, M., Garside, R.F. & Leitch, I.M. (1977). A clinical trial of phenelzine in anxiety depressive and phobic neuroses. *British Journal of Psychiatry, 131*, 486-492.

Murphy, G.E., Simons, A.D., Wetzel, R.D., & Lustman, P.J. (1984). Cognitive therapy and pharmacotherapy. *Archives of General Psychiatry, 41*, 33-44.

Noyes, R., Reich, J., Christiansen, J., Suelzer, M., et al. (1990).Outcomes of panic disorder: Relationship to diagnostic subtypes and comorbidity. *Archives of General Psychiatry, 47*, 809-818.

Otto, M. W., Pollack, M. H., & Sabatino, S. A. (1996). Maintenance of remission following cognitive behavior therapy for panic disorder: Possible deleterious effects of concurrent medication treatment. *Behavior Therapy, 27*, 473-482.

Otto, M. W., Pollack, M. H., Sachs, G. S., Reiter, S. R., Meltzer, B. S., & Rosenbaum, J. F. (1993). Discontinuation of benzodiazepine treatment: efficacy of cognitive-behavioral therapy for patients with panic disorder. *American Journal of Psychiatry, 150*(10), 1485-90.

Pelham, W. E., Carlson, C., Sama, S. E., Vallano, G., Dixon, M. J., Hoza, B. (1993). Separate and combined effects of methylphenidate and behavior modification on boys with attention deficit-hyperactivity disorder in the classroom. *Journal of Consulting and Clinical Psychology, 61*, 506-515.

Reich, J.H. & Green, A.F. (1991). Effect of personality disorders on outcome of treatment. *Journal of Nervous and Mental Disease, 179*, 74-82.

Rodin, J., Elias, M., Silberstein, L.R., & Wagner, A. (1988). Combined behavioral and pharmacologic treatment for obesity: Predictors of successful weight maintenance. *Journal of Consulting and Clinical Psychology, 56*, 399-404.

Schwartz, J.M., Stoessel, P.W., Baxter, L.R., Martin, K.M., et al. (1996). Systematic changes in cerebral glucose metabolic rate after successful behavior modification treatment of obsessive compulsive disorder. *Archives of General Psychiatry, 53*, 109-113.

Sheehan, D.V. (1982). Panic attacks and phobias. *New England Journal of Medicine, 307*, 156-158.

Sheehan, D.V., Ballenger, J., & Jacobsen, G. (1980). Treatment of endogenous anxiety with phobic, hysterical, and hypochondriacal symptoms. *Archives of General Psychiatry, 37*, 51-59.

Solyom, C., Solyom, L., LaPierre, Y., Pecknold, J., & Morton, L. (1981). Phenelzine and exposure in the treatment of phobias. *Biological Psychiatry, 16*, 239-247.

Solyom, L., Heseltine, G.F.D., McClure, D.J., Solyom, C., Ledwidge, B., Steinberg, G. (1973). Behaviour therapy versus drug therapy in the treatment of phobic neurosis. *Canadian Psychiatric Association, 18*, 25-31.

Taylor, C.B., King, R., Margraf, J., Ehlers, A., Telch, M.J., Roth, W.T., & Agras, W.T. (1989). Use of medication and in vivo exposure in volunteers for panic disorder research. *American Journal of Psychiatry, 146*, 1423-1426.

Telch, M. J., Brouillard, M., Telch, C. F., Agras, W. S., & et al. (1989). Role of cognitive appraisal in panic-related avoidance. *Behaviour Research & Therapy, 27*, 373-383.

Telch, M.J. (1991). Beyond sterile debate. *Journal of Psychopharmacology, 5*, 296-298.

Telch, M.J., Agras, W.S., Taylor, C.B., Roth, W.T., & Gallen, C. (1985). Combined pharmacological and behavioral treatment for agoraphobia. *Behaviour Research and Therapy, 23*, 325-335.

Telch, M.J., Tearnan, B.H., & Taylor, C.B. (1983). Antidepressant medication in the treatment of agoraphobia: A critical review. *Behaviour Research and Therapy, 21,* 505-517.

Telch, M.J. & Lucas, R. Combined pharmacological and psychological treatment of panic disorder: Current Status and Future Directions. In J. D. Maser & B. E. Wolff (Eds.) *Treatment of Panic Disorder: A consensus development conference* (pp. 177-197). Washington D.C.: American Psychiatric Press.

Tyrer, P. & Steinberg, D. (1975). Symptomatic treatment of agoraphobia and social phobias: A follow-up study. *British Journal of Psychiatry, 127,* 163-168.

Tyrer, P., Candy, J., & Kelly, D. (1973). Phenelzine in phobic anxiety: A controlled trial. *Psychological Medicine, 3,* 120-124.

Weissman, M.M., et al. (1979). The efficacy of drugs and psychotherapy in the treatment of acute depression episodes. *American Journal of Psychiatry, 136,* 555-558.

Zitrin, C.M., Klein, D.F., & Woerner, M.G. (1978). Behavior therapy, supportive psychotherapy, imipramine, and phobias. *Archives of General Psychiatry, 35,* 307-316.

Footnotes

[1]At first glance, assumption 1 appears quite reasonable. It would seem that even advocates of prescription privileges view psychotherapy as highly desirable, if not necessary. Few if any proponents of prescription privileges argue for the use of drugs in place of psychotherapy. However, we ought to keep in mind that the match between behavioral intentions and subsequent behavior is often poor. This may be particularly true for those prescribing psychologists working in clinical settings for which monetary incentives favor treatment with medications only.

Discussion of Telch, Sloan, and Beckner

Comment on Current Status of Combined Treatments

William G. Danton, Ph.D.
*University of Nevada School of Medicine
and Department of Veterans Affairs Medical Center*

Some psychologists are excited about the prospect of gaining prescription privileges. They argue that the authority to dispense medications to our patients will enable us to provide more effective treatments and be more competitive in the marketplace. They downplay concerns that psychology might abandon psychotherapy in favor of seemingly more time efficient and lucrative drug therapies. They believe that, as a more science-based discipline, we are inoculated against drug company seduction.

There may be considerable arrogance in the assumption that psychology will apply scientific rigor in judging the effectiveness of its treatments. In clinical practice, we certainly have not exercised such rigor in selecting effective psychotherapies; why would the case be different with pharmacotherapy? Nonetheless, this chapter by Telch, Sloan, and Beckner is an admirable attempt to present a scientific analysis of combination treatments for anxiety, depression, obesity, bulimia, and ADHD. They correctly surmise that many psychologists who support prescription privileges believe that they will not be abandoning psychotherapy for pharmacotherapy. Rather, these practitioners believe that they will combine the two treatments to the benefit of their patients. The core question then, is whether this combination is in fact effective.

Sadly, for those who advocate prescription privileges and at the same time argue that science will drive practice, the authors' analysis of current research literature suggests that there is little support for the notion that combined treatments provide greater benefit than single modality treatments. Telch, Sloan, and Beckner conclude that combined treatments outperformed single modality treatment in the short-term treatment for panic disorder and for obesity. At follow-up, combined treatments were not significantly more effective than single-modality treatments for any of the disorders studied.

In the treatment of panic disorder, for example, the authors argue that their analysis shows a significant overall, short-term advantage for combined treatment, consistent across five assessment domains. They found no evidence supporting combined treatment on follow-up. Drugs are effective at short-term suppression of anxiety, but they aren't as effective as psychotherapy in the long haul. Clum, Clum, and Surls (1993) and Gould, Otto, and Pollack (1995) have drawn similar conclusions. Gold, Otto, and Pollack also point out that well-controlled studies show that treatment using cognitive restructuring and interoceptive exposure have been associated with panic-free rates of 71 to 80 percent for short-term treatment in individual and group format, compared to 50 to 70 percent for benzodiazepine and antidepressant treatment.

The effectiveness of drug therapies in combination with psychotherapy is not impressive. However, simply comparing published research outcomes on these treatments individually, and in combination, does not tell the whole story. Although the authors made an attempt to select scientifically rigorous studies, some of the flaws associated with drug mono therapy and combination therapies are ubiquitous. First, there are problems with the integrity of the blind in so-called double blind studies. These studies often use an inert placebo and the treatments are not blind to the patient or the researcher. There are additional problems associated with placebo washout procedures, which may bias the selection of the subject pool. Most importantly, there are problems with industry-funded research, the so-called "file drawer problem," where negative findings are delayed or not published at all. The pool of drug studies, replete with these problems, may reflect an inflated efficacy before selected treatment comparisons are ever made.

For those who remain unconvinced that marketplace pressures would sway treatment providers, what about its influence on treatment research itself? Marks, et al. (1993), commenting on Upjohn Company's support of their anxiety study, lamented, "Monitoring and support stopped abruptly when the results became known. Thereafter, Upjohn's response was to invite professionals to critique the study they had nurtured so carefully before. The study is a classic demonstration of the hazards of research funded by industry."

The authors conclude with a number of suggestions for future research on combined treatments. Particularly appropriate are their calls to improve the generalizability of randomized clinical trials by using more diverse patient groups and to eliminate confounding of drug and placebo with psychotherapy treatment effects. They also make appropriate recommendations for learning more about treatment sequencing and selection protocols for different treatments.

These authors present an excellent review of the efficacy literature as it applies to combination treatments. They conclude that psychoactive medications given concurrently with psychosocial treatments do not enhance patients' clinical status for the diagnoses they studied. Similar conclusions have been drawn regarding the relative efficacy of medications and psychosocial mono-therapies in the treatment of anxiety and depression. Aaron Beck was once asked if he felt psychologists should be given prescription privileges. His answer was "What for?"

References

Beck, Aaron T. (1996) Personal communication.

Clum, G. A., Clum, G. A., & Surls, R. (1993). A meta-analysis of treatments for panic disorder. *Journal of Consulting and Clinical Psychology, 61* (2), 317-326.

Gould, R., Otto, M. W., & Pollack, M. H. (1995). A meta-analysis of treatment outcome for panic disorder. *Clinical Psychology Review, 15* (8), 819-844.

Marks, I. M., Swinson, R. P., Basoglu, M., Kuch, K., Noshirvani, H., O'Sullivan, G., Lelliot, P. T., Krrby, M., McNamee, G., Sengun, S., & Wickwire, K. (1993). Alprazolam and exposure alone and combined in panic disorder with agoraphobia. *British Journal of Psychiatry, 162,* 776-787.

Chapter 8

Antidepressant Medications: A Review of Their Potential for Toxicity

Melissa Piasecki, M.D.

University of Nevada School of Medicine

Ever since the tricyclic antidepressants were found to be effective in the treatment of Major Depressive Disorder (Kuhn, 1958), medication therapy has been an important treatment option for MDD and other depressive disorders. With the advent of Prozac in 1987 and the other serotonin reuptake inhibitors (SRIs) in following years, the number of prescriptions for antidepressant medication by psychiatrists and other physicians has increased to over 20 million per year (Wall Street Journal, 5/9/96). As the population of patients taking antidepressants grows, more individuals are at potential risk for adverse effects from these medications. The safety profiles vary dramatically among the different classes of antidepressants and even the newer, "safer" antidepressants present potential toxicities. This chapter reviews the side effects of antidepressant medications, emphasizing our growing understanding of clinically significant drug interactions with the SRIs.

Antidepressant Medications: A Review of Their Potential for Toxicity

The use of antidepressant medications for the treatment of Major Depressive Disorder and related depressive conditions has soared in recent years to a multibillion dollar industry (Wall Street Journal, 5/9/96). Many factors have contributed to this increase in medication use, including the development of newer drugs with fewer side effects and improved safety profiles in the case of overdose. Despite the advances in newer antidepressants, safety considerations remain important, particularly as our understanding of potential toxicities and drug interactions improves and as the population of patients receiving these medications continues to grow. This chapter will focus on the antidepressant medications which are most used at this time: serotonin reuptake inhibitors (SRIs), several other newer drugs which have recently been approved by the FDA for use in treatment of depression, and the cyclic antidepressants (TCAs).

Neurotransmitters and Depression

The use of medications for the treatment of depressive disorder is based on the theory that neurotransmitters regulate mood. Neurotransmitters are the chemical messengers which allow neurons to communicate. Those of greatest interest in the treatment of mood disorders include norepinephrine and serotonin.

The catecholamine theory of mood disorders suggests that depression is secondary to a relative deficiency of norepinephrine in areas of the brain. Drugs which enhance the action or concentration of norepinephrine are therefore thought to be therapeutic for the treatment of a depressive disorder. The serotonergic theory of depression similarly suggests that depression is secondary to a decrease in the amount of serotonin in the central nervous system required for mood stability. Drugs which increase the activity or concentration of serotonin are currently the focus for research and for the clinical treatment of depression (Cooper, Bloom and Roth, 1996).

Adverse Effects

A medication may adversely affect a patient in a number of ways. In this chapter, the different classes of medication will be discussed in terms of safety and side effects in different populations, as well as in terms of the different classes of adverse effects. These include intentional overdose by a patient, side effects due to the action of the drug on receptors in the central nervous system (such as anxiety or insomnia), and side effects due to the action of the drug in other parts of the body (such as diarrhea or constipation). Other side effects may result from the interactions of an antidepressant with another drug. Teratogenicity, the adverse effects of an antidepressant on a fetus, is another safety concern with the use of antidepressants.

Serotonin Reuptake Inhibitors

The SRIs have had an unprecedented popularity for the treatment of depression. After fluoxetine (Prozac) was introduced in December of 1987, its sales reached $350 million in 1989, (more than was spent on all classes of antidepressants two years earlier) (Cowley, 1990). In 1994, nearly a million prescriptions a month were written for Prozac, most by nonpsychiatric physicians. (Cowley, 1994). Other SRIs on the market for the treatment of depression include paroxetine (Paxil), and sertraline (Zoloft). Fluvoxamine (Luvox) is an SRI which has an FDA indication for obsessive compulsive disorder and which has been used for treatment of depression in other countries.

The action of the SRIs is indicated by their name: they selectively inhibit the reuptake of serotonin into the neuron. This inhibition, or blockage, of the serotonin transporter increases the amount of serotonin in the neural synapse within the central nervous system. Congruent with the serotonergic hypothesis of affective disorders, the increase in the serotonin concentration directly or indirectly acts to stabilize depressed mood (Cooper, Bloom and Roth, 1996).

The success of the SRIs lies partly in their safety profile. In contrast to the TCAs, they have different side effects, are less worrisome in cardiac and elderly patients, and are "suicide safe," or relatively non-toxic in the case of overdose. Initially, clinicians believed that SRIs had fewer adverse effects than the TCAs because they acted more selectively, with the effect localized to the serotonin reuptake receptor on the presynaptic neuron. Over time, clinical and research observations have documented a number of side effects as well as potentially serious drug interactions.

The most commonly documented side effects from the SRIs stem from non-selectivity. Although the SRIs appear to be selective for serotonin receptors, they act upon the serotonin receptors of other groups of cells in addition to the neurons in the brain which mediate mood. They may also affect subtypes of serotonin receptors other than the receptor which is the reuptake transporter. As a result of the increased serotonin concentrations in other areas of the brain, some patients experience anxiety, restlessness, and headaches. Increased serotonin concentrations in other parts of the body may result in gastrointestinal disturbances (nausea or diarrhea), tremor, sexual dysfunction (decreased libido, inhibited arousal and/or anorgasmia), dry mouth, sweating, and weight change. Of note, the rate of sexual dysfunction in men taking fluoxetine has been estimated to be as high as 75% (Potter, Manji and Rudorfer, 1995; Patterson, 1993).

In addition to the SRIs' more common adverse effects, there are numerous case reports of other potentially severe side effects in the literature. The SRIs may indirectly alter the functioning of the dopamine neurotransmitter system, thereby causing patterns of abnormal muscle tone or movements known as extrapyramidal reactions and tardive dyskinesia. Some case reports involve patients on other drugs who developed worsening of their extrapyramidal symptoms when an SRI was added; other reports associate the muscle or movement disturbance with the SRI alone (Chong, 1995; Sandler 1996). By 1991, 35 cases of tardive dyskinesia had been reported to the manufacturer of fluoxetine as an associated symptom, although some or all of these patients may have been exposed to other drugs which put them at risk for this complication (Gelenberg, 1996).

Another rare but potentially serious complication of SRI use is the syndrome of inappropriate ADH secretion, which can lead to abnormal electrolyte balances. This has been associated with all three SRIs currently approved for depression (Leung and Remick, 1995; Bluff and Oji, 1995; Flint, Crosby and Genik, 1996).

Drug interactions among the SRIs and other classes of drugs is an important and evolving area for understanding potential toxicities which may be more serious than those from direct drug effects. The SRIs can change the blood levels of many other medications and substances through enzyme inhibition in the liver, and through competitive protein binding.

Most medications are metabolized by a complex of enzymes in the liver known as the cytochrome p450 oxidase system. These enzymes allow for the biotransformation of drugs to other forms which allows the drug to be excreted or further broken down and eventually eliminated from the body. The cytochrome system is a group of related enzymes which are technically grouped into clusters, or isoenzymes, according to how many common features they share. Drugs that are metabolized by these enzymes are said to be substrates of the enzyme. The SRIs (and other drugs) inhibit the function of many of the p450 enzymes and can put patients at risk for clinically significant problems when another medication they take is a substrate. In effect, the p450 enzymes can be "shut down," limiting the metabolism of the substrate drug, resulting in increased blood concentrations of that drug (Nemeroff, DeVane and Pollack, 1996).

Over the last 20 years, pharmacologists and clinicians have developed a more detailed understanding of the drugs which inhibit or are substrates of enzymes. Some of this information comes from laboratory work, where enzyme inhibition is studied in test tubes. Most clinically relevant have been the observations made in patients who exhibit increased blood levels of substrate drugs when another drug inhibits enzyme function. An illustration of a p450 drug interaction is the inhibition of the p450 2D6 isoenzyme by fluoxetine. This SRI and its metabolite, norfluoxetine, are potent inhibitors of the 2D6 enzyme as well as several other cytochrome p450 enzymes. Substrates for the 2D6 enzyme include the tricyclic antidepressants, cardiac drugs (encainide, flecainide), antipsychotic drugs (clozapine, haloperidol), narcotics and even other SRIs (paroxetine). A patient on a cyclic antidepressant, for example, may experience a dramatic increase in the blood level of the TCA if fluoxetine were added because the metabolism of the cyclic antidepressant is thereby decreased.

In a study by Vandel et al. in 1992, patients experienced up to a five fold increase in imipramine (a TCA) plasma levels after 20 mg/day of fluoxetine was added. Increases in imipramine levels were variable in the twenty patients studied and some serious side effects were noted (delirium, seizures), although they were not consistently associated with the greatest plasma changes in TCA level (Vandel S., Bertschy, Bonin, Nezelof, Francois, Vandel, Sechter, and Bizouard, 1992).

Variability in individual response to enzyme inhibition is partly due to genetic differences—some individuals are "poor metabolizers" (and therefore at even greater risk for drug interactions through enzyme inhibition), where others are "extensive metabolizers". Although certain ethnic groups may be predisposed to decreased metabolism at a genetic level, there are no clinically useful means at present to screen for baseline metabolic abilities to minimize or avoid side effects from drug interactions. For the SRI paroxetine, the metabolism of the drug by the p450 system is significantly impaired for 7% of Caucasians, and 1% of Asians due to genetic deficiencies in one of the isoenzymes (Gibaldi, 1993). At present, clinicians are limited to careful medication histories and close monitoring of blood levels, when available, and other clinical tools to monitor for toxicities from these types of drug interactions. Because the different SRIs have different patterns of enzyme inhibition, and because our knowledge of these drug interactions is growing, this will be an evolving area in psychopharmacology in upcoming years (Nemeroff, DeVane and Pollack, 1996).

In the blood, some drugs are partially bound to plasma proteins. The non-bound portion of the drug is "available" to be clinically active. There are a limited number of binding spots in the bloodstream proteins, and some drugs "compete" for these spots. Competetive protein binding may lead to changes in another drug's level for patients also taking an SRI antidepressant. The SRIs are tightly bound to protein in circulation (77 to >97%), and will displace other drugs which have looser binding. This is relevant in the case of drugs like digoxin or warfarin, which can achieve toxic levels or cause significant medical complications when displaced by a more tightly bound drug (De Vane, 1992).

The SRIs also carry the risk of serotonin syndrome, which can occur in patients taking more than one serotonergic drug. This is a potentially life threatening syndrome consisting of at least three of the following ten symptoms: mental status changes, agitation, myoclonus, hyperreflexia, sweating, shivering, tremor, diarrhea, incoordination and fever (Sternbach, 1991). The most common reports of serotonin syndrome result from the coadministration of an SRI and an antidepressant from the class of monoamine oxidase inhibitors (MAOIs), although there is a case report of the syndrome following monotherapy with an SRI (Fischer, 1995). The syndrome has also been reported in patients treated with combinations of SRI' s and lithium or carbemazepine (Muly, McDonald, Steffens, and Book, 1993).

The long half life of the SRI fluoxetine can lead to serotonin syndrome if another serotonergic drug in initiated before the fluoxetine (and its active metabolites) have "washed out"–a minimum of five weeks after discontinuing the fluoxetine. The MAOIs (an older and rarely used class of antidepressants) also need a waiting period of at least several weeks after discontinuation prior to starting another serotonergic drug to avoid serotonin syndrome. The TCA clomipramine is also highly serotoneric and may act like an SRI in precipitating the syndrome in a patient exposed to a MAOI or another serotonergic drug (Sternbach, 1991).

Cyclic Antidepressants

Historically, our ability to treat depression with effective medication dates from the advent of the tricyclic antidepressant imipramine hydrochloride in the late 1950s. Before this, electroconvulsive therapy was the only biological treatment available (Kuhn, 1958). Over the next two decades, nine related compounds were developed and found to be effective in the treatment of depression. Chemically, these compounds are all made of two to four benzene rings, and so have been termed the "cyclic antidepressants" or TCAs (Baldessarini, 1990).

The action of cyclic antidepressants supports the catecholamine hypothesis of affective disorders. These medications increase the amount of noradrenaline in the neural synapse by blocking the cell's reuptake mechanism for noradrenaline. The mechanism acts via a type of transporter in the cell membrane which is specific for noradrenaline. Cyclic antidepressants also have some action on the reuptake transporter for serotonin (Cooper, Bloom and Roth, 1996).

Despite the adverse effects detailed below, cyclic antidepressants remain in use for several reasons. They have been in clinical use almost forty years and have been studied and used extensively not only in the treatment of depression, but also in the treatment of anxiety disorders and pain disorders. Many patients tolerate these medications well, and some of the side effects can be used to advantage. One example is the use of a cyclic antidepressant in a patient with major depressive disorder who suffers from difficulty falling asleep. The sedating qualities of the antidepressant help the patient fall asleep if the medication is taken near bedtime. Another reason for continued use of these medications is cost. Cyclic antidepressants, in their generic form, cost a fraction of the price of the newer drugs. Although the side effect profiles differ among the classes of antidepressants, efficacy in the antidepressant effects are similar.

Soon after the introduction of TCAs into clinical practice, they were found to have multiple side effects. Kuhn, in his landmark article, noted sixteen different side effects in the first 500 patients treated with imipramine (Kuhn, 1958). Since his publication, the adverse effects of the cyclic antidepressants have been studied in very large patient populations and are noted to stem from three different limitations: narrow therapeutic window resulting in high toxicity with overdose, lack of receptor specificity, and interactions with other drugs.

Overdose with cyclic antidepressants can be lethal and may represent the most common life-threatening drug overdose in the U.S. (Katholo and Henn, 1983). The safety margin for tricyclics is narrow, with a therapeutic dosage of 4 mg/kg and a potentially lethal dose of 20 mg/kg. (Preskorn, 1982). Symptoms of serious overdose include seizures, coma, hypotension, arrhythmias and cardiorespiratory arrest. (Frommer, Kulig, Marx and Rumack, 1987).

The cyclic antidepressants have been considered "dirty drugs" because they lack specificity for the neuroreceptors which mediate their clinical effect. The therapeutic effect of this class of drugs lies in their ability to block the uptake of endogenous biogenic amines (norepinephrine, serotonin, and dopamine). The clinical effect lags behind this blockade by several weeks, suggesting that a cascade of events within the central nervous system mediates the antidepressant activity (Baldesserini, 1990). Cyclic antidepressants affect other receptor systems, yielding various side effects without producing additional therapeutic effects. These include the blockade of the muscarinic cholinergic receptors both centrally and peripherally. Central blockade of these receptors may lead to memory impairment, confusion or delirium, especially in older patients who may be more sensitive (Pollack and Rosembaum, 1987; Potter, Manji and Rudorfer, 1995). Peripheral muscarinic blockade may lead to side effects whose severity can range from annoyance to medical emergency. These include dry mouth (which can lead to dental problems), blurred vision from impaired accommodation, increased heart rate, constipation (which can lead to severe bowel inactivity in at-risk patients), and urinary hesitation or retention (especially problematic in older men with enlarged prostates). Patients with narrow angle glaucoma are at risk for an acute crisis on cyclic antidepressants, and these drugs are contraindicated for this group of patients. (Ritch, Krupin, Henry and Kurata, 1994; Potter, Manji and Rudirfer, 1995; Pollack and Roenbaum 1987).

Cyclic antidepressants also affect the histamine and alpha 1 and 2 receptor systems. Histamine blockade can lead to sedation and significant weight gain—one survey found that patients on amitriptyline gained over seven kilograms during six months on the drug (Berken, Weinstein and Stern, 1984). Alpha 1 blockade can cause postural hypotension which produces dizziness or even fainting. This side effect sometimes limits the use of these medications in patients who are unable to effectively compensate for the decrease in blood pressure (Pollack and Rosenbaum 1987).

Cardiac patients are at special risk for adverse events with the use of cyclic antidepressants. These medications slow the intraventricular conduction system, and heart block (pathologic slowing of the heart's electrical impulse) can be directly related to the plasma concentration of a TCA. In addition, cyclic antideressants can be antiarrhythmic or proarrthymic (preventing or promoting arrhythmias), although the clinical implications for these findings in cardiac patients is still unknown. At present, patients with cardiac conduction abnormalities who are taking cyclic antidepressants should be monitored with serial EKGs and serum antidepressant levels (Glassman and Preud'homme, 1993; Dietch and Fine, 1990; Preskorn and Irwin, 1982).

Cyclic antidepressants can also have adverse effects on a patient through pharmacokinetic and pharmacodynamic interactions with other drugs. Pharmacokinetic interactions were discussed above with the SRIs. Pharmacodynamic interactions, in which one drug changes the effect of another drug at its site of action, can occur when cyclic antidepressants are used in conjunction with other medications such as cardiac and antiseizure drugs. With digoxin, for example, the alpha 1 blockade of the TCA can affect the left ventricle's function; with lidocaine or other antiarrythmics in its class, the cardiodepressant effects of the TCAs can be additive; and with the anti-seizure drugs carbamazepine and phenytoin the inhibition of sodium fast channels by tricyclics may decrease the seizure threshold and the effectiveness of the anticonvulsants (Preskorn and Irwin, 1982; Preskorn, 1996).

The variety of side effects and drug interactions which can occur with the cyclic antidepressants mandate a careful medical history and medication review for all patients who may take these medications. In addition, EKG monitoring and serial serum levels are indicated for selected patients on TCAs. Moreover, due to the high toxicity and lethality of cyclic antidepressant overdose, patients who are at risk for overdose need particularly careful management on these medications, such as dispensing only small amounts of the medication at one time.

Newer Antidepressants

Three structurally novel antidepressants have been introduced over the last four years: venlafaxine, nefazodone and mirtazapine. Unrelated chemically to the SRIs or the TCAs, these medications were developed to provide effective antidepressant treatment with minimal side effects. The potential toxicities of side effects and drug interactions with these newer drugs bears examination and comparison with the older, better known TCAs and SRIs.

Venlafaxine inhibits the reuptake of serotonin similar to the action of the SRIs, as well as the reuptake of norepinephrine. In addition, it weakly affects dopamine reuptake. Early studies suggested that venlafaxine's antidepressant effect may occur sooner (after two to four weeks of drug treatment) compared with the four to six week delay experienced with other drugs such as fluoxetine. Potential side effects of venlafaxine include sweating, headache, nervousness, nausea, abnormal ejaculation, and a sustained increase in diastolic blood pressure. It has a short half life (3–5 hours) which provides a prompt "wash out" after discontinuation and protein binding is low, at 27-30%. Although the antidepressant is an inhibitor of the p450 enzyme 2D6, it is also a substrate of that enzyme. Concomitant administration of a more potent inhibitor (such as the SRI paroxetine) would result in higher plasma levels of of the drug (Holliday and Benfield, 1995). Venlafaxine has the potential to cause serotonin syndrome and a case has been reported in a patient who was rapidly switched from an MAOI to venlafaxine (Heisler, 1996). As with the SRIs, venlafaxine has the potential for complications with drug interactions from the p450 system as well as from serotonin syndrome. The sustained increase in diastolic blood pressure noted in some patients requires monitoring and possible discontinuation of the medication for some patients (Feighner, 1995; Otton, 1996).

Nefazodone, the second of the three newer antidepressants, has both action on the serotonin reuptake receptor (inhibiting reuptake) as well as action on another serotonin receptor. It has a weak action at two other neurotransmitter sites (alpha adrenergic receptors and norepinephrine reuptake). Side effects from the medication include headache, dry mouth, somnolence, nausea, insomnia, constipation, and light headedness. Sexual dysfunction appears to be less frequent compared to the TCAs and SRIs. Impotence, libido, anorgasmia and abnormal ejaculation were noted at rates only slightly higher than for placebo control patients. The half life is short (2-4 hours) and the drug is extensively protein bound (although this has not been noted to result in clinically significant drug-drug interactions) (Robinson, D. S., Roberts, D. L., Smith, J. M., Stringfellow J. C., Kaplita, S. B., Seminara, J. A., and Marcus, R. N. 1996).

The major safety concern with nefazodone is its potent inhibition of the p450 enzyme 3A4. This enzyme metabolizes many drugs including the nonsedating antihistamines astemizole and terfenadine and the benzodiazepines triazolam and alprazolam. When these medications are co-administered with nefazodone, their metabolism may be inhibited and their plasma levels may reach toxic levels (Robinson, D. S., Roberts, D. L., Smith, J. M., Stringfellow, J. C., Kaplita, S. B., Seminara, J. A., and Marcus, R. N. 1996). Other inhibitors of the p450 3A4 enzyme have been implicated in severe cardiac complications, and one fatality with terfenadine toxicity secondary to P450 inhibition has been documented (Honig, Wortman and Zamani, 1993). Another prominent potential toxicity is that of serotonin syndrome if nefazodone were to be used in combination with another serotonergic drug or if appropriate wash out periods were not observed.

Mirtazapine is a new and structurally novel antidepressant which recently became available in late 1996. It has action at multiple receptors including serotonin, adrenergic and histamine receptors and it has some activity at the muscarinic cholinergic receptor as well. The antidepressant effect of mirtazapine is thought to be related to its effects on noreadrenalin through increased cell firing and noradrenalin release. Serotonin concentrations may be affected through a secondary mechanism. Side effects reported by the pharmaceutical company include somnolence, dizziness, weight gain, elevations in plasma cholesterol and liver enzymes, dry mouth, and constipation. It does not appear to have significant effects on sexual functioning. Three subjects of the three thousand patients involved in premarketing trials suffered from severe neutropenia (decreased white blood cell counts) which required discontinuation of the drug and careful monitoring (de Boer, T., 1996, Physician's Desk Reference, 1997).

The half life of mirtazapine is 20 to 40 hours and its protein binding is 85%. It is a substrate for several of the p450 enzymes but has not been noted from in- vitro tests to be a significant inhibitor of the enzymes. As with venlafaxine and nefazodone, it has the potential to cause serotonin syndrome and the pharmaceutical company posts a contraindication for use within fourteen days of an MAOI in the Physician's Desk Referenence (Physician's Desk Reference, 1997).

Although the newer antidepressants distinguish themselves with different side effect profiles, they share the potential toxicity of serotonin syndrome. In addition, these drugs may present new and significant toxicities with potential blood pressure elevations, neutropenia and p450 drug interactions. The newest antidepressants have not been tested in pregnant humans and are in the FDA pregnancy category C.

Discussion

As physicians prescribe antidepressants medications in record numbers, larger populations of patients are exposed to potential risks. Safe and effective prescribing becomes complicated by the potential adverse effects of the drugs and by medically complex patients. Side effects may occur through overdose, competetive protein binding, pharmacodynamic interactions, inhibition of the p450 enzymes system or serotonin syndrome. Some patients may be more vulnerable to drug side effects or drug interactions because of a genetic predisposition or, in the case of elderly patients, from the decreased metabolic capacity because of age related changes in their livers. Clearly, clinicians who prescribe antidepressants need to consider all of the above when diagnosing and treating patients with depression.

Another special population to consider regarding safety is women of childbearing age. Prescribing antidepressants to pregnant women may present risk to the fetus (there is currently scant safety information on most antidepressants and pregnancy). Routine history of menstrual cycles and pregnancy tests whenever indicated allow the clinician and the patient to make informed decisions early in a patient's pregnancy.

The first step in safe and effective prescribing is an accurate diagnosis. Clinicians must rule out underlying medical disorders which can present with depressive symptoms such as hypothyroidism, Cushing's disease and carcinomas. Substance abuse or dependence must be addressed as alcohol, stimulants, steroids and other substances can lead to symptoms which are similar or overlapping with a Major

Depressive Disorder. Some medications, such as beta blockers used for hypertension, have been implicated in depression and are described as "depressogenic."

An accurate psychiatric diagnosis is the cornerstone to effective drug prescribing. Major Depressive Disorder (MDD) has overlapping syptoms with other psychiatric disorders such as Adjustment Disorder, Bipolar Disorder (especially regarding a "mixed" or dysphoric manic state), or schizophrenia. An antidepressant medication may not yield benefits in patients who do not have MDD, and bipolar patients may experience new or worsening manic symptoms if treated with an antidepressant instead of a mood stabilizer such as lithium.

Another element of safe and effective use of antidepressants is a complete record of all current medications, including over the counter preparations. Publications, such as the Drug Newsletter, Aug. 1995, have tables which list potential interactions from the p450 enzyme system. Many medications (most cyclic antidepressants, theophylline, digoxin etc.) can be monitored via blood levels if a patient is at risk for a change in drug level from protein binding or from inhibited metabolism. This is particularly relevant for the medically ill or for known "poor metabolizers." A full medical history is also important in order to identify patients at risk for complications such as urinary retention or cardiac dysrhythmia.

Education is a key component to safe prescribing. Many of the side effects described by drug manufacturers are based on clinical studies with younger, healthy patients exposed to the drug for six or twelve week trials. As a drug becomes more widely used in the general patient population, new side effects and interactions are noted—such as the p450 interactions which were first widely described in 1993. Clinicians need to have a sound understanding of the limits of pharmaceutical company reporting as well as of the basis for potential drug interactions. Updates on new safety information may come in several forms: "Dear Doctor" letters from the pharmaceutical companies, self-directed learning, or Continuing Medical Education courses. Another important resource for education is consultation with "treatment team" members, which may include a pharmacist. Pharmaceutical companies can be helpful resources as well. Many provide toll-free numbers with medical information specialists to answer questions and provide references.

General guidelines can help decrease the risk of toxic events when prescribing antidepressants. The use of more than one psychotropic can be very helpful to many patients such as in the treatment of depression resistant to a single drug but responsive to combined treatment of an antidepressant plus lithium as an augmenting agent (Montigny, Cournoyer and Blier, 1981). Polypharmacy does, however, increase the risk of side effects and interactions and clinicians need to proceed cautiously and to monitor blood levels whenever possible.

All patients benefit from discussions of risks, benefits, side effects and expectations of treatment with medications so that they may actively participate in treatment choices and may give as fully informed consent as possible. Some patients may find the side effects or risks of certain antidepressants unacceptable and wish to avoid certain drugs. Others may wish avoid all antidepressants and prefer treatment with psychotherapy or other non-drug treatments for depression.

References

Baldessarini, R. J. (1990). Drugs and the treatment of psychiatric disorders. In A. G. Gilman, T. W. Rall, A. S. Nies & P. Taylor (Eds.) *Goodman and Gilman's The Pharmacological Basis of Therapeutics* (pp. 383-435). New York, New York: Pergamon Press.

Berken, G. N., Weinstein, D. O., & Stern, W. C. (1984). Weight gain: A side effect fo tricyclic antidepressants. *Journal of Affective Disorders, 7*, 133-138.

Bluff, D. D. & Joi, N. (1995). SIADH in a patient receiving sertraline, letter to the editor. *Annals of Internal Medicine, 123*, 811.

Chong, S. A. (1995). Fluvoxamine and mandibular dystonia. *Canadian Journal of Psychiatry, 40*, 430-431.

Cooper, J. R., Bloom, F. E., & Roth, R. H. (1996), *The Biochemical Basis of Neuropharmacology*, New York, New York: Oxford University Press.

Cowley, G., Springen, K., Leonard E. A., Robins, K. & Gordon, J. (March 26, 1990). The promise of Prozac. *Newsweek*, 39-41.

Cowley, G., Holmes, S., Lauerman, J. F. & Godon, J. (February 7, 1994). The culture of Prozac. *Newsweek*, 41-42.

de Boer, T. (1996). The pharmacologic profile of mirtazapine. *Journal of Clinical Psychiatry, 57*, 19-25.

de Montigny, C., Grunberg, F., Mayer, A., & Deschenes, J. P. (1981). Lithium induces rapid relief of depression in tricyclic antidepressant non-responders. *British Journal of Psychiatry, 138*, 252-256.

DeVane, C. L. (1992). Pharmacokinetics of the selective serotonin reuptake inhibitors. *Journal of Clinical Psychiatry, 53* (suppl), 13-20.

Dietch, J. T. & Fine, M. (1990). The effect of nortriptyline in elderly patients with cardiac conduction disease. *Journal of Clinical Psychiatry, 51*, 65-67.

Feighner, J. (1995). Cardiovascular safety in depressed patients: Focus on Venlafaxine. *Journal of Clinical Psychiatry, 56*, 574-579.

Fischer, P. (1995). Serotonin syndrome in the elderly after antidepressant monotherapy. *Journal of Clinical Psychopharmacology, 15*, 440-442.

Flint, A. J., Crosby, J. & Genik, J. L. (1996) Recurrent hyponatremia associated with fluoxetine and paroxetine. *American Journal of Psychiatry, 153*, 134.

Frommer, D. A., Kulig, K. W., Marx, J. A. & Rumack, B. (1987). Tricyclic antidepressant overdose: A review. *Journal of the American Medical Association, 23*, 521-525.

Gelenberg, A. J. (1996). SSRIs and EPS. *Biological Therapies Newsletter, 19*, 8.

Gilbaldi M. (1993). Ethic differences in the assessment and treatment of disease. *Pharmacotherapy, 13*, 170-176.

Gilman A. G., Goodman, L. S., Rall, T.W., Murad, F. (1985) *Goodman and Gilman's The Pharmacological Basis of Therapeutics*, (7th ed.). New York: Macmillan.

Glassman, A.H. & Preud'homme, X. A. (1993) Review of the cardiovascular side effects of heterocyclic antidepressants. *Journal of Clinical Psychiatry, 54* (2) (suppl.), 16-22.

Heisler, M. A., Guidry, J. R., Arnecke, B. (1996). Serotonin syndrome induced by administration of venlafaxine and phenelzine (letter). *Annals of Pharmacotherapy, 30*, 84.

Holliday, S. M. & Benfield, P. (1995). Venlafaxine: A review of its pharmacology and therapeutic potential in depression. *Drugs, 49*, 280-294.

Kathol, R. G. & Henn, F. A. (1983). Tricyclics–the most common agent used in potentially lethal overdoses. *The Journal of Nervous and Mental Disease, 171*, 250-252.

Langreti, R. (May 9, 1996). High anxiety: Rivals threaten Prozac's reign. *Wall Street Journal*, B1.

Leonard, B. E. (1993). The comparative pharmacology of new antidepressants. *Journal of Clinical Psychiatry, 54*, 3-15.

Kuhn, R. (1958). The treatment of depressive states with G 22355 (imipramine hydrochloride). *American Journal of Psychiatry, 115*, 459-464.

Muly, E. C., McDonald, W., Steffens, D., & Book, S. (1993). Serotonin syndrome produced by a combination of fluoxetine and lithium (letter). *American Journal of Psychiatry, 150*, 1565.

Nemeroff, C. B., DeVane, C. L., & Pollock, B. G. (1996). Newer antidepressants and the cytochrome p450 system. *American Journal of Psychiatry, 153*, 311-320.

Otton, S. V. (1996), Venlafaxine in vitro is catalysed by CYP2D6. *British Journal of Clinical Pharmacology, 41*, 149-159.

Physician's Desk Reference (1997). Montvale, New Jersey: Medical Economics Inc.

Pollack, M. H. & Rosenbaum, J. F. (1987). Management of antidepressant-induced side effects: A practical guide for the clinician. *Journal of Clinical Psychiatry, 48*, 3-8.

Potter, W. Z., Manji, H. K., & Rudorfer, M. V. (1995). Tricyclics and tetracyclics. In A. F. Schatzberg & C. B. Nemeroff (Eds.) *The American Psychiatric Press Textbook of Psychopharmacology* (pp. 141-182). Washington D.C.: American Psychiatric Press.

Preskorn, S. H. (1996). Reducing the risk of drug-drug interactions: A goal of rational drug development. *Journal of Clinical Psychiatry, 57*, 3-6.

Preskorn, S.H. & Irwin, H.I. (1982). Toxicity of tricyclic antidepressants–kinetics, mechanism, intervention: A review. *Journal of Clinical Psychiatry, 43*, 151-156.

Rickels, K & Schweizer, E. (1990) Clinical overview of serotonin reuptake inhibitors. *Journal of Clinical Psychiatry, 51*, 9-12.

Ritch, R., Krupin, T., Henry, C. & Kurata, F. (1994). Oral imipramine and acute angle closure glaucoma. *Archives of Opthalmology, 112*, 67-68.

Robinson, D. S., Roberts, D. L., Smith, J. M., Stringfellow, J. C., Kaplita, S. B., Seminara, J. A. & Marcus, R. N. (1996). The safety profile of nefazodone. *Journal of Clinical Psychiatry, 57*, 31-38.

Sandler, N. H. (1996). Tardive dyskinesia associated with fluoxetine. *Journal of Clinical Psychiatry, 57*, 91.

Sternbach, H. (1991). Serotonin syndrome. *American Journal of Psychiatry, 148*, 705-713.

Sugrue, M. F. (1983). Chronic antidepressant therapy and associated changes in central monoaminergic function. *Pharmacologic Therapy, 21*, 1-37.

Vandel, S., Bertschy, G., Bonin, B., Nezelof, S. Francois, T. H., Vandel, B., Sechter, D., Bizouard, P. (1992). Tricyclic Antidepressant plasma levels after fluoxetine administration. *Neuropsychobiology, 25*, 202-207.

Discussion of Piasecki

Diving into the Chemical Soup

Gregory J. Hayes, M.D., M.P.H.
University of Nevada School of Medicine

There is no topic better than the side effects and potential drug interactions of psychoactive medications to dramatize the complexity of the chemical soup into which psychology stands poised to dive. Psychologists are relatively inexperienced with the polydrug world of modern medicine. The reality of this world, as Dr. Piasecki has described, should give any thoughtful psychologist pause: do you really want to deal with all this?

My first experience of the complexities of drug use came during my third year of medical school. On the wards for extended periods for the first time, I one day came face to face with a time bomb. The time bomb I speak of was an older gentlemen, accompanied by his helpful wife, who entered the hospital with pains and other symptoms potentially related to heart, intestine, several other organ systems, and/or drugs. His mental status was questionable as well and his wife served as the primary historian. As I proceeded with my history and physical, I inquired about what medications my patient was using. His wife, ever helpful, held out a large brown paper bag. Peering inside I found a multitude of bottles, fourteen in all. I felt completely overwhelmed. He takes all of these? Oh yes, his wife replied. And I am careful he takes them correctly, she added. It was then the image of a time bomb appeared. I imagined I was in a nitroglycerin factory and that my patient would blow up if I made one false move. I felt almost paralyzed by the difficulty of the situation. Contemplating the possible interactions between these drugs and the side effects of each, I realized that collectively they might well be the primary reason for my patient's admission. But really I could not be sure; the potential combinations were simply too complex for someone with only a biology under-graduate degree and two years of medicine under his belt. And just imagine if my patient's helpful wife had been absent from the equation! What if there was only this patient of questionable mental abilities and the bag of medications was simply not available? What if this gentleman was the sole person in charge of deciding when and if he took a particular medication—and how much he felt like taking? The time bomb may well have exploded before the patient ever reached the hospital.

Such cases are not uncommon. The use of multiple physicians, both generalists and specialists, can create an unanticipated chemical mix inside a patient who then seeks help or is brought in for acute or chronic mental health problems. For reasons of mental illness alone this person may be a poor historian, and only a fraction of his medical history may be clearly known. Yet in this environment there is the pressure to add yet other drugs—anti-depressants, anti-psychotics, and the like—to treat the diagnosed mental condition. And as in my example above, even if all the medications are known, the consideration of potential interactions and side effects can be extraordinarily difficult.

This reality must also be coupled with the cultural forces which strongly pressure for doing everything which might be helpful. Such pressures are particularly strong in our own culture. One of the reasons, for example, why Great Britain's health care costs per capita are one-third those of the United States is that society's willingness to "let time heal" and "nature take its course." In the United States we are much more likely to treat, treat, treat—overusing medications of all types. That is not simply a function of the professionals who prescribe them, but of the consumers—patients, clients—who demand them. As psychology considers the possibility of granting prescribing privileges to its members, the sobering impact of the forces that will be unleashed must be carefully contemplated.

The aggressive nature of the U.S. health care system, especially that portion functioning within the medical model, is a product of the culture in which it is embedded. More importantly it is no passing fancy. Medical anthropologists can trace these aggressive tendencies far into the past. Even a 150 years ago, for example, physicians were often believers in "more is better." In the United States physicians were more likely than their European counterparts to say: I don't have any idea what is wrong with you, but I have 10 ideas of what we could try, so let's try them all. In Europe the strategy was more conservative: I don't have any idea what is wrong with you, and until I do I really don't think we should do anything. This aggressive U.S. stance lead to treatments which were sometimes much worse than ineffective, causing temporary or lasting illness, injury or even death.

Drug interactions and side effects for psychoactive drugs are more complex and convoluted than almost any other class of drug. As Dr. Clark previously pointed out, medical training is insufficient for the proper use of such medications. Even among psychiatrists, only the most conscientious will come close to understanding and considering the potential problems which might arise, especially when a patient/client is on multiple medications, psychoactive and otherwise. If psychologists are to handle such new duties responsibly and ethically, an extraordinary amount of training and continuing education will be required. That is possible, but is it really desirable?

In my view, the time-consuming impact of responsibly using psychoactive drugs will almost unavoidably render prescribing psychologists "junior psychiatrists" over time. Psychotherapeutic skills will of necessity diminish as more and more time is spent on the chemistry of mental illness. An effort any less time consuming will lead to the increasing misuse of these potent medications, especially in the face of a growing number of clients who will to demand such drugs even when their scientific efficacy is marginal. Either way the costs will far exceed the benefits, I believe.

Should psychologists enter into this murky chemical world? In my view they should not. Granting the ability to prescribe to psychologists will lessen the quality of psychotherapy they deliver, just as it did to psychiatrists 40 years ago. That would be a disaster for the nation's health where psychology's contribution stands as an important and effective alternative to the drug use of the medical model. Anything which threatens this contribution should be avoided at all cost.

If psychologists must become involved in the use the psychoactive drugs, a more productive way to do so would be through participation on a multidisciplinary treatment team. Here the psychologist could represent the values of his or her profession by lobbying for the use of effective non-drug treatment strategies, the use of drugs only in those circumstances of demonstrated efficacy, and the careful evaluation of potential drug interactions and side effects—all without having to take on the extraordinary burden of primary responsibility for prescribing the medications used.

Chapter 9

A Cost-effectiveness Model:
Is Pharmacotherapy Really Less Expensive than Psychotherapy for Depression?

David O. Antonuccio, Ph.D.
*University of Nevada School of Medicine
and Department of Veterans Affairs Medical Center*
Michael Thomas, Ph.D., M.B.A.
University of Nevada Dept. of Accounting and CIS
William G. Danton, Ph.D.
*University of Nevada School of Medicine
and Department of Veterans Affairs Medical Center*

The point prevalence of unipolar depression is estimated to be between 3% and 13% with as much as 20% of the adult population experiencing at least some depressive symptoms at any given time (Amenson & Lewinsohn, 1981; Oliver & Simmons, 1985; Kessler, McGonagle, Zhao, Nelson, Hughes, Eshleman, Wittchen, & Kendler, 1994). The lifetime incidence of depression is estimated to be between 20% and 55%. Women are consistently found to have rates of depression twice as high as men. In 1990, at least 11 million Americans experienced an episode of depression, costing the U.S. economy an estimated $44 billion in increased accident rates, increased substance abuse, increased medical hospitalization, and increased somatic illnesses and outpatient medical utilization (Greenberg, Stiglin, Finkelstein, & Berndt, 1993). Antidepressant drug treatment (Morris & Beck, 1974) and cognitive behavior therapy (Antonuccio, Ward, & Tearnan, 1989) are empirically based treatments for depression that have established clinical efficacy (Antonuccio, Danton, & DeNelsky, 1995). In the era of managed care and limited resources, depression treatments must demonstrate their cost-effectiveness as well as their clinical effectiveness. The current paper addresses the relative clinical effectiveness and cost-effectiveness of drugs and cognitive behavior therapy (CBT) in the treatment of unipolar depression. The outcome literature is briefly reviewed and three particularly well-controlled long-term comparative studies from the psychiatric literature are closely examined. Several meta-analyses comparing drugs and psychotherapy for depression are also reviewed. A cost-effectiveness model is generated from this outcome literature.

Clinical Outcome of CBT Compared with Pharmacotherapy

One approach to treating depression involves addressing the cognitions that mediate the impact of events in patients' lives (e.g., Beck, Rush, Shaw, & Emery, 1979; Beck & Young, 1985). The proponents of this approach assert that it is not necessarily aversive events that lead to depression, but rather cognitions about those events. Some examples of common thinking patterns that can lead to depression include overgeneralized thinking, perfectionistic thinking, and the tendency to catastrophize.

Many studies have shown cognitive therapy to be more effective than antidepressant medication (Blackburn, Bishop, Glen, Whalley, & Christie, 1981; Evans, Hollon, DeRubeis, Piasecki, Grove, Garvey, & Tuason, 1992; Kovacs, Rush, Beck, & Hollon, 1981; Rush, Beck, Kovacs, & Hollon, 1977; Rush, Beck, Kovacs, Weissenburger, & Hollon, 1982). Some studies have shown cognitive therapy to be as effective as antidepressant medication (Elkin, Shea, Watkins, Imber, Sotsky, Collins, Glass, Pilkonis, Leber, Docherty, Fiester, & Parloff, 1989; Hollon, DeRubeis, Evans, Wiemer, Garvey, Grove, & Tuason, 1992; Murphy, Simons, Wetzel, & Lustman, 1984) or combined cognitive/drug treatment (Beck, Hollon, Young, Bedrosian, & Budenz, 1985; Blackburn, et al., 1981; Covi & Lipman, 1987; Evans et al., 1992; Hollon et al., 1992; Murphy et al., 1984). Yet other studies suggest that cognitive therapy adds to the efficacy of standard antidepressant drug treatment (Bowers, 1990; Dunn, 1979; Miller, Norman, Keitner, Bishop, & Dow, 1989; Teasdale, Fennell, Hibbert, & Amies, 1984).

Other studies have evaluated CBT treatments that emphasize the behavioral aspects (e.g., social skills and pleasant activities). Some studies found such behavioral interventions are more effective than medication alone (McLean & Hakstian, 1979; Miller et al., 1989), are as effective as combined treatment (Hersen, Bellack, Himmelhoch, & Thase, 1984; Stravynski, Verreault, Gaudette, Langlois, Gagnier, & Larose, 1994; Wilson, 1982), or add to the efficacy of standard drug treatment with drug-refractory depression (Antonuccio, Akins, Chatham, Monagin, Tearnan, & Ziegler, 1984). One study (Roth, Bielski, Jones, Parker, & Osborn, 1982) found that adding antidepressant medication to such a behavioral intervention speeded recovery somewhat, but the outcomes were equivalent at treatment termination.

Finally, the preponderance of the evidence suggests that drug treatments do less well than CBT during follow-up (e.g., Blackburn, Eunson, & Bishop, 1986; Evans et al., 1992; Hersen et al., 1984; Hollon et al., 1991; Kovacs et al., 1981; McLean & Hakstian, 1990; Rush et al., 1977; Shea, Elkin, Imber, Sotsky, Watkins, Collins, Pilkonis, Beckham, Glass, Dolan, & Parloff, 1992; Simons, Murphy, Levine, & Wetzel, 1986), and are not more effective than psychotherapy with endogenous (Blackburn et al., 1981; Zimmerman & Spitzer, 1989; Greenberg, Bornstein, Greenberg, & Fisher, 1992a), severe (Hollon et al., 1992; Shea et al., 1992; McLean & Taylor, 1992), chronic (Rush, Hollon, Beck, & Kovacs, 1978), or inpatient (Brugha, Bebbington, MacCarthy, Sturt, & Wykes, 1992) depression.

Murphy et al. (1984)

One particularly well-controlled study (Murphy, Simons, Wetzel, & Lustman, 1984) randomly assigned 87 moderately to severely depressed psychiatric outpatients to 12 weeks of cognitive therapy, nortriptyline, cognitive therapy plus nortriptyline, or cognitive therapy plus active placebo. The placebo was designed to have mild sedative and anticholinergic effects to simulate actual medication. The therapists in this study were 3 psychologists and nine psychiatrists. While the 70 patients who completed treatment showed significant improvement on the patient-rated Beck Depression Inventory (BDI; Beck, Ward, Mendelson, Mock, & Erbaugh, 1961) and the clinician-rated Hamilton Rating Scale for Depression (HRSD; Hamilton, 1960), the treatment conditions were not differentially effective at treatment termination or at one month follow-up. Inclusion of drop out patients' end point scores did not affect these results. Thus, cognitive therapy alone was as effective as nortriptyline, and there was no additive effect of the combined treatments. Notably, the investigators drew venous blood samples every other week to ensure that plasma nortriptyline levels were in the therapeutic target window of 50-150 ng/ml.

The recovered patients (N=44) from Murphy et al. (1984) were followed for one year after treatment termination (Simons, Murphy, Levine, & Wetzel, 1986). Patients who had received cognitive therapy, whether or not they also received nortriptyline, were less likely to relapse. Patients who had received nortriptyline, whether or not they had also received cognitive therapy, were more likely to relapse. These results suggested that not only was medication treatment more likely to result in relapse, but it actually may have interfered with the long-term efficacy of cognitive therapy.

The NIMH Collaborative Depression Study

The recent multi-site NIMH collaborative study on the treatment of depression (Elkin, Shea, Watkins, Imber, Sotsky, Collins, Glass, Pilkonis, Leber, Docherty, Fiester, & Parloff, 1989) has been cited to suggest that drugs are superior to CBT in the treatment of severe depression. This ambitious project compared Beck's version of cognitive therapy, Klerman and Weissman's interpersonal therapy, imipramine (median of 185 mg/day with a median plasma level of 231 ng/ml), and a pill placebo group. The authors concluded that there were no differences in overall effectiveness, but imipramine appeared to be more effective with severely depressed patients. The results of the analysis actually showed that imipramine did marginally better than the placebo condition with severely depressed patients at termination, but only on clinician-rated measures like the HRSD or the Global Assessment Scale (GAS; Endicott, Spitzer, Fleiss, & Cohen, 1976), and not on patient-rated measures like the BDI. Despite media reports to the contrary, drugs were not significantly better than either of the psychotherapies with severely depressed patients on any measures. Since the placebo was inert, clinician raters may have been inadvertently "unblinded" by side effects, a problem with many drug studies (Fisher & Greenberg, 1993). Also, the medication condition may have functioned more like a combined treatment condition because the clinical management provided "supportive psychotherapy." It is noteworthy that patients in the medication condition were still on medication when the termination assessments were done, while the comparison conditions were actually terminated prior to assessment. This is a common practice in studies utilizing a drug condition.

An 18 month follow-up (Shea, Elkin, Imber, Sotsky, Watkins, Collins, Pilkonis, Beckham, Glass, Dolan, & Parloff, 1992) of the original NIMH collaborative study was conducted. Although not statistically significant, the psychotherapies outperformed imipramine on almost every outcome measure. In fact, cognitive therapy was ranked best on 11 of the 13 outcome measures reported in the published tables. There was a slight advantage of the psychotherapies over drug treatment with the milder depressions. The treatments were not statistically different in outcome with severe depression. There did appear to be a reduced risk for relapse among the cognitive behavior therapy patients. Of all patients entering treatment, the cognitive behavioral condition had the highest percentage of patients recover, the highest percentage of patients recover without a subsequent major depressive relapse, and the highest percentage of patients recover without major depressive relapse or subsequent treatment. Patients who had received imipramine were most likely to seek treatment during the follow-up period, had the highest probability of relapse, and had the fewest weeks of minimal or no symptoms. These results are consistent with the relatively poor long-term drug outcomes reported in studies cited earlier.

Continuation Drug Treatment

Some investigators have argued that the relatively high relapse rate after drug treatment indicates that depression should be treated like a chronic medical disease, requiring ongoing, long-term, high dose medication treatment indefinitely (e.g., Frank, Kupfer, Perel, Cornes, Jarrett, Mallinger, Thase, McEachran, Grochocinski, 1990; Kupfer, Frank, Perel, Cornes, Mallinger, Thase, McEachran, & Grochocinski, 1992; Paykel, Dimascio, Haskell, & Prusoff, 1975; Reynolds, Frank, Perel, Imber, Cornes, Morycz, Mazumdar, Miller, Pollock, Rifai, Stack, George, Houck, & Kupfer, 1992). This logic is problematic: Drug treatment results in a higher relapse rate than cognitive behavior therapy, therefore, patients should be maintained on drugs to prevent relapse. These maintenance studies typically rely on clinician ratings of outcome, and all patients are initially given combined treatment or drug treatment only. The maintenance phase of treatment is conducted only with the responders. Since psychotherapy alone is not offered to patients initially, the maintenance phase of treatment is essentially restricted to drug responders and those patients who can tolerate the side effects. Therefore, the patient samples in these drug maintenance studies should not be considered representative of the general population of depressed patients.

A notable exception is a recent well-controlled study with two years of follow-up evaluating the impact of continuing medication (Hollon, et al., 1992; Evans, et al., 1992). These investigators randomly assigned 107 nonpsychotic, nonbipolar depressed patients to 12 weeks of cognitive therapy alone, imipramine hydrochloride alone (mean of 232 mg/day with plasma levels at least 180 ng/ml), or combined treatment. A total of 64 patients completed treatment with no differential attrition. Cognitive therapy and pharmacotherapy did not differ in terms of symptomatic response on patient-rated or clinician-rated measures, even among severely depressed patients. Initial severity predicted poorer response within the pharmacotherapy condition but not within cognitive therapy. The combined treatment was not significantly more effective than the single treatments. Two patients committed suicide with study medication and a third patient made a nonlethal attempt. Two other patients were withdrawn from pharmacotherapy alone because of severe suicidal risk. Three other patients were withdrawn from pharmacotherapy alone because of severe side effects. During follow-up, half of the patients treated with pharmacotherapy alone continued to receive study medications for the first year of follow-up. Among patients showing at least partial response, patients previously treated cognitively (with or without medications) showed a significantly lower relapse rate compared to imipramine patients from whom medications were withdrawn. Thus patients treated with three months of cognitive therapy (either alone or in combination with medications) had less than half the relapse shown by patients who received three months of medication alone. The relapse rate after 3 months of cognitive therapy did not differ from that of patients provided with 15 months of medication. Rather than supporting long-term drug treatment, these data support the cost effectiveness of treating depression with brief cognitive-behavior therapy.

Future studies also need to investigate whether, or how much, relapse might be further reduced if continuation CBT is offered. A preliminary investigation showed that when recovered drug treatment patients have CBT added to their drug regimen, they have a substantially lower relapse rate (35%) compared with routine clinical management (70%) over a 4 year period during which the medications are gradually discontinued (Fava, Grandi, Zielezny, Rafanelli, & Canestrari, 1996).

Meta-analytic Comparisons of Drugs vs. Psychotherapy

Isolated studies provide pieces of the puzzle, but meta-analyses, covering all available studies meeting specified criteria, help put the puzzle together. One such meta-analysis of 56 controlled outcome studies considered the relative effectiveness of drug therapy and psychotherapy for treating unipolar depression in adults (Steinbrueck, Maxwell, & Howard, 1983). Effectiveness was measured by the effect size of the treatment condition compared with the control condition; i.e., the treatment mean minus the control mean divided by the control standard deviation. The evidence suggested that, when compared to a control group, psychotherapy had a significantly larger impact (mean effect size = 1.22) than drug therapy (mean effect size = .61). Some of the difference in mean effect size may be due to the different blinding procedures and the different types of control groups. Drug studies were more likely to use a double blind placebo while psychotherapy studies were more likely to use a waiting list control group.

As part of a quantitative analysis, Dobson (1989) reviewed eight randomized studies (N=721) directly comparing Beck's cognitive therapy versus tricyclic medication in the treatment of depressed outpatients. This review suggested that cognitive therapy is superior to drug treatment as measured by the BDI. The average cognitive therapy recipient did better than 70% of the medication patients, with an average differential effect size of .53 in favor of cognitive therapy.

Another meta-analysis (Conte, Plutchik, Wild, & Karasu, 1986) investigated whether combined psychotherapy and pharmacotherapy is superior to either treatment alone for outpatients with unipolar depression. The researchers reviewed 17 controlled studies (N=1009) reported between 1974 and 1984. In the analysis, studies were given different weights based on the scientific quality of the design, which were multiplied by weights based on the outcome of the study. A preponderance of the weighted evidence (53%) indicated the combined active treatments (drug plus psychotherapy) were more effective than minimal contact plus placebo. A modest amount of evidence (29%) indicated the combined treatments were superior to pharmacotherapy alone. However, there was only slight evidence favoring the combination over psychotherapy plus placebo (19%), combination over psychotherapy alone (18%), or combination over pharmacotherapy plus minimal contact (15%). In other words, 82% of the weighted evidence indicated no advantage of combined treatment over psychotherapy alone. A close inspection of the data indicates that, of the four studies that employed a combined behavioral plus drug condition in comparison with a behavioral plus placebo medication, 97% of the evidence indicated no significant difference. Interestingly, 3% of the evidence favored the behavioral intervention when combined with the placebo rather than the tricyclic medication.

Robinson, Berman, and Neimeyer (1990) conducted a unique meta-analytic review of the controlled comparative outcome research on depression. After combining and weighting (based on sample size) the results of 8 well-controlled studies, psychotherapy had a statistically significant mean effect size that was .13 larger than that for drug therapy. Independent raters then judged investigator allegiance on a 5-point scale for each comparison between treatments by reviewing the introductory comments for each study included in the meta-analysis. After controlling for investigator allegiance through the use of regression procedures, the advantage of psychotherapy shrank to .07 and was no longer statistically significant. It should be noted that if investigator allegiance is correlated with a third variable such as scientific rigor or efficacy, statistically controlling for allegiance may disproportionately penalize studies that are well designed or show large effects of a particular treatment. This review also found no advantage to the combined treatment over psychotherapy (in 12 studies) or over drug therapy (in 5 studies).

Another meta-analysis (Hollon, Shelton, & Loosen, 1991) reviewed nine randomized controlled studies (N=542) which directly compared cognitive therapy and tricyclic medications in the treatment of nonbipolar depressed outpatients. Based on their analysis, these authors concluded that (1) cognitive therapy appears to be roughly comparable to medications in the treatment of the acute episode; (2)

combined cognitive therapy and drug treatment does not appear to be clearly superior to either modality alone, although trends of potential synergistic enhancement justify additional studies with larger samples; and (3) treatment with cognitive therapy (with or without drugs) during the acute episode appears to reduce the risk of subsequent relapse following termination. However, because of limitations in study design and execution, low power, and possible differential retention (i.e., drug conditions might be more likely to retain relapsers), the authors conservatively considered their conclusions to be tentative.

Wexler and Cicchetti (1992) conducted a meta-analysis of treatment success rates, treatment failure rates, and treatment dropout rates from 7 well-controlled studies (N=513) comparing psychotherapy and medication for depression. They concluded that combined treatment offers no advantage over treatment with psychotherapy alone, and only modest advantage over treatment with pharmacotherapy alone. They suggest that psychotherapy alone should usually be the initial treatment for depression rather than exposing patients to unnecessary costs and side effects of combined treatment. When dropout rate is considered together with the treatment success rates, the pharmacotherapy alone condition is substantially worse than psychotherapy alone or the combined treatment. Their review suggests that in a hypothetical cohort of 100 patients with major depression, 29 would recover with pharmacotherapy alone, 47 would recover if given psychotherapy alone, and 47 would recover if given combined treatment. Negative outcomes (i.e., drop-outs or no response) would occur in 52 pharmacotherapy patients, 30 psychotherapy patients, and 34 combined patients. Co-morbid personality disorder and substance abuse may further decrease treatment response (Wexler & Nelson, 1993).

In summary, several meta-analyses, reported in both psychiatry and psychology journals, covering multiple studies with thousands of patients, are remarkably consistent in supporting the perspective that psychotherapy is at least as effective as medication in the treatment of depression. These conclusions hold for both vegetative and social adjustment symptoms, especially when patient-rated measures are used and long-term follow-up is considered. Though there is some overlap of included studies, all of these meta-analyses were conducted independently. Except for the meta-analyses of Dobson (1989) and Hollon et al. (1991), which used only studies including cognitive-behavioral interventions, the meta-analyses combined all brands of psychotherapy for depression. This may obscure differences in outcome between the different brands of treatment. Different types of psychotherapy may have different outcomes (e.g., McLean & Hakstian, 1979). It should also be noted that Robinson et al. (1990) found psychotherapy outcomes to be robust on both self-report and clinician measures. In contrast, antidepressant drugs have not fared well compared with control conditions on patient-rated measures (Greenberg, Bornstein, Greenberg, & Fisher (1992b). Despite the foregoing evidence to the contrary, the conventional wisdom in medicine, among the lay public, in the media, and even within the mental health profession, continues to be that drugs are more effective and less expensive than psychotherapy for depression (e.g., Kramer, 1993), and that the combination treatment is superior to either one alone. There is also a tendency to minimize the side effects of antidepressant drugs.

Side Effects

If one accepts the data and the argument that drug treatment of depression may not be as effective as conventional wisdom would suggest, it does not necessarily follow that drugs should be relegated to a second class treatment status. Some patients prefer medications to psychotherapy and strongly believe in their efficacy. By prescribing medication, a clinician could take advantage of any nonspecific and placebo factors associated with drug treatment. However, some of the costs of medications may be underappreciated. Research suggests that antidepressants are the most common agent used in suicide by poisoning (Kapur, Mieczkowski, & Mann, 1992) and are involved in half of serious adult overdoses (Kathol & Henn, 1982). We are aware of no data about the relative risk of suicide in patients treated with drugs compared with those treated with psychotherapy. Although a suicidal patient treated with psychotherapy may commit suicide, the treatment itself does not become the cause of death.

Even at therapeutic levels there are many potential side effects of tricyclic antidepressants. The anticholinergic side effects include dry mouth, blurred vision, urinary retention, constipation, and delirium (Settle, 1992). There may also be sedative effects, cognitive deficits, speech blockage, excessive perspiration, weight gain, and dental caries (Settle, 1992). There is some evidence of risk for extrapyramidal symptoms, seizures, sleep disruption, and mania, depending on the type of antidepressant (Settle, 1992). The cardiovascular risks include heart failure (especially with bundle branch block), hypertension, hypotension, arrhythmias, and sudden death (Jefferson, 1992). Tricyclic antidepressants appear to increase the risk of sudden unexpected death by over 400% for patients diagnosed with cardiac disease (Moir, Crooks, Cornwell, O'Malley, Dingwall-Fordyce, Turnbull, & Weir, 1972). Sexual side effects have commonly included low libido, erectile disorder, orgasm or ejaculatory impairment, and less commonly, painful ejaculation, penile anesthesia, spontaneous orgasm, and even yawning combined with orgasm (Seagraves, 1992). There is a well-documented withdrawal phenomenon associated with tricyclic medication (Dilsaver & Greden, 1984). The most common withdrawal symptoms include general somatic or gastrointestinal distress with or without anxiety and agitation, sleep disturbance characterized by excessive and vivid dreaming and initial and middle insomnia, movement disorder, and psychic and behavioral activation extending on a continuum to mania. Use of antidepressants in medically ill inpatients has resulted in a 60% unfavorable response rate, and 32% had to be discontinued due to significant side effects, the most common of which was delirium (Popkin, Callies, & Mackenzie, 1985). There is even recent suggestive evidence implicating antidepressants in the development of breast cancer (Halbreich, Shen, & Panaro, 1995). Thus, there is much evidence that antidepressant medications are not benign treatments for many patients.

Newer antidepressants, the selective serotonin reuptake inhibitors (SSRIs), were developed on the theory that depression results from a deficiency in serotonin levels, despite the fact that studies have not shown that serotonergic activity is lowered in depressive states (Hallman & Oreland, 1989). The SSRIs theoretically increase the serotonin available to the brain by interfering with its reuptake. However, the brain quickly (as soon as two days in animal studies) compensates for this artificial intrusion of extra serotonin through a process called down regulation, and reduces the number of serotonin receptors (Breggin, 1994). It has been demonstrated that with other drugs, compensatory receptor changes can become permanent (Breggin, 1994), potentially creating serious long-term problems.

So far, the newer SSRIs appear to be a safer alternative to the tricyclic antidepressants. Although they appear to have about the same risk of overdose, death appears to be a less likely outcome with the SSRIs (Kapur et al., 1992). While the newer SSRIs may be safer when used alone, there are data to suggest that, when combined with other medications, they are more dangerous due to their pharmacodynamic and pharmacokinetic properties (e.g., Settle, 1992; Nemeroff, DeVane, & Pollock, 1996). For example, they can be lethal when combined with MAO inhibitors. Given the common use of multiple concurrent medications, it is not clear that the newer antidepressants will actually result in safer outcomes. Even when used alone, fairly common side effects of the SSRIs include agitation, sleep disruption, nausea, and sexual problems (Settle, 1992). They can also increase the risk of miscarriage and neonatal complications if used during the first trimester (Pastuszak, Schick-Boschetto, Zuber, Feldcamp, Pinelli, Sihn, Donnenfeld, McCormack, Leen-Mitchell, Woodland, Gardner, Horn, & Koren, 1993), a significant concern given that 70% of the antidepressants are prescribed for women (Olfson, & Klerman, 1993), many of child bearing age. For a minority of patients these new medications may carry a significant risk for suicide induction, mania, akathisia, and extrapyramidal effects (Lenhoff, 1994).

To be fair, one might legitimately ask about the side effects, i.e., the unintentional negative effects, of psychotherapy. Though controversial, there are apparently instances in psychotherapy of false memory syndrome caused by suggestions of abuse, or inappropriate hypnotic interventions under certain narrow conditions (Loftus, 1993). However, this syndrome is probably rare and irrelevant to most treatments of depression which typically do not utilize hypnosis or suggestions of abuse. McLean and Hakstian (1979) found that patients in the insight-oriented psychotherapy condition were more likely than those in the control condition to remain in the moderate to severe range of depression. This could be considered a negative side effect of this type of therapy if it is replicated in other studies. Compared with the medical risks associated with drug treatments, psychotherapy appears relatively benign. If malpractice rates are any indication, the risks associated with prescribing drugs are much higher than those associated with psychotherapy. Though side effects are important "costs" to consider, it is difficult to quantify them for inclusion in a cost-effectiveness model. It is especially difficult to quantify those side effects for which patients do not seek medical treatment.

Comparative Cost-Effectiveness of Drugs and Psychotherapy

Yates (1995) described several models for measuring cost-effectiveness and cost-benefit in clinical research, and for optimizing cost-effectiveness and cost-benefit in clinical practice. Traditional research only looks at how procedures are implemented and to what extent they lead to certain outcomes. Cost effectiveness analyses add data on treatment costs to find the least expensive way to achieve certain outcomes or the most effective way to deliver services within budget constraints.

Treatment Outcome Distribution

In the current model, three different treatment options are examined: 1) CBT alone, 2) fluoxetine alone, or 3) combination CBT and fluoxetine. Based on the outcome data from the Wexler and Cicchetti (1992) meta-analysis and the long-term outcome studies described in this paper, an estimate can be made regarding the percentage of patients who will recover, partially recover, remain depressed, drop out, or relapse in each of the three treatment options. All of the existing comparative studies use tricyclic antidepressants. Because the preponderance of the evidence suggests that SSRIs in general, and fluoxetine in particular, have similar efficacy (Greenberg, Bornstein, Zborowski, Fisher, & Greenberg, 1994) and overall drop-out rates when compared to tricyclic antidepressants (Song, Freemantle, Seldon, House, Watson, Long, & Mason, 1993; Anderson & Tomenson, 1995), the tricyclic outcome numbers are used. Of those depressed patients who start drug treatment alone, it is estimated that 29% will recover, 19% will have partial success, 17% will not respond, and 35% will drop out (Wexler & Cicchetti, 1992). For CBT alone, 47% will recover, 23% will have partial success, 11% will not respond, and 19% will drop out. For the combined condition, 47% will recover, 19% will have partial success, 8% will not respond, and 26% will drop out (Wexler & Cicchetti, 1992). These treatment outcome distributions are used in Figures 2 through 5.

Relapse Rates and Time Comparisons

Roughly 27% of the recovered CBT patients will relapse, 59% of the recovered drug only patients will relapse, and 29% of the recovered combined treatment patients will relapse (Simons et al., 1986; Evans et al., 1992; Shea et al., 1992). The average time to relapse could also be estimated from the studies reviewed. The average CBT patient who relapsed did so in about 12.1 months. Relapsing drug only patients took an average of 6.6 months. The average combination patient who relapsed did so in 9.6 months. Relapse costs are based on how much longer patients will experience depression in the drug and combination conditions (due to earlier relapse) compared with the CBT condition. All of the treatment studies looked at relapse in the recovered patients only. For the purposes of this model, we have assumed that partially recovered patients don't relapse, but that they incur half the costs to society of a depressed patient during the time period under investigation.

Drop-out Treatment Costs

Drop out costs were also calculated based on an estimate of the average time to drop out from the reviewed studies. The average CBT drop-out patient quit treatment after 6.58 months. The relative times to drop out in drug only and the combination treatment were 5.11 months and 3.83 months respectively.

Subsequent Treatment Rates

Kovacs et al. (1981) found that of all patients starting treatment, 50% of CBT patients and 76% of drug patients will reenter treatment. Shea et al. (1992) found that 12% of recovered CBT patients and 37% of recovered pharmacotherapy patients return to treatment during follow-up. We assumed the average of these return rates for relapsed patients, 31% for CBT and 57% for drugs alone. Because there are no data to guide us about the return rates for combination patients, we assumed the average return rate (44%) for the combination condition. Based on Shea et al. (1992), we assumed that of the relapsed CBT patients who return to treatment, 28% will seek CBT, 29% will seek drug treatment, and 43% will seek "any" treatment (assumed to be the average of the three treatment costs). Of the relapsed drug only patients who return to treatment, we assume 33% will seek CBT, 29% will seek drug treatment, and 38% will seek "any" treatment. The length of subsequent treatment following CBT and drug only treatment was 4.2 weeks and 20.3 weeks respectively (Shea et al., 1992). Subsequent treatment duration and rates for the combination treatment were assumed to be equivalent to the CBT condition. We assumed that drop-out patients do not return to treatment.

Figure 1 depicts the comparative cost analysis of CBT alone, fluoxetine alone, or the combination treatment. Three levels of analysis are included: 1) direct costs to patients or third party payers, 2) direct costs to the community, and 3) indirect costs to society. It can be seen that drug treatment is 87% more expensive than CBT when direct costs to the patient and third party payer costs are considered. The combination treatment is 114% more expensive than CBT alone. When costs to the community and costs to society are considered, the total treatment costs for fluoxetine alone and combination treatment are 31% and 33% more expensive for CBT, respectively. These treatment costs are used in Figures 2 though 5. Figure 2 depicts a time-line model for the expected socio-economic costs of CBT over the lifetime of a depressed patient. Figure 3 shows, by way of example, how those expected costs were calculated. Figure 4 depicts a timeline model for the expected socio-economic treatment costs of fluoxetine alone. Figure 5 depicts a timeline model for the expected socio-economic treatment costs of the combination treatment.

Comparative Cost Data

Figure 1 provides the treatment costs used in Figures 2 through 5. Assumptions and data for each line item of cost in Figure 1 follows.

Table 1: Comparative cost analysis of depression treatments

	TOTAL COSTS BY TREATMENT TYPE FOR 2-YEAR TREATMENT PLAN			COST DIFFERENCES COMPARED TO CBT	
	CBT	Pharmacological	Combination	Pharmacological	Combination
Direct patient/third party provider costs					
Health care provider charges	$1,475	$1,120	$2,800	<$355>	$1,325
Medication	0	3,629	3,629	3,629	3,629
Lost wages	401	214	356	<187>	<45>
Travel costs	60	72	84	12	24
Comorbidity costs	4,874	7,703	7,703	2,830	2,830
Total costs to the patient/third party provider	*$6,809*	*$12,738*	*$14,572*	*$5,929*	*$7,763*
Percentage cost difference from CBT				*87%*	*114%*
Direct costs to the community					
Economic multiplier effect from lost wages	$861	$459	$766	<$402>	<$96>
Reduced taxes due to lost wages	163	87	145	<76>	<18>
Reduced community service work by patients	400	400	400	0	0
Total costs to the community	*$1,424*	*$946*	*$1,310*	*<$478>*	*<$114>*
Percentage cost difference from CBT				*<34%>*	*<8%>*
Indirect costs to society					
Lost productivity during treatment	$3,729	$4,256	$3,781	$527	$53
Economic multiplier effect from lost productivity	8,017	9,150	8,130	1,133	113
Reduced taxes due to lost productivity	1,516	1,730	1,537	214	21
Lost income potential from suicide	1,913	1,913	1,913	0	0
Total costs to society	*$15,174*	*$17,049*	*$15,362*	*$1,874*	*$187*
Percentage cost difference from CBT				*12%*	*1%*
TOTAL TREATMENT COSTS	$23,408	$30,733	$31,245	$7,325	$7,837
Percentage cost difference from CBT				31%	33%

Table 2: CBT timeline model of expected treatment costs

Patient Categories	Birth and Pre-diagnosis	2-year treatment period	Potential relapse period (12.1 mo)	Remaining life and Death
Complete Treatment	ignore*	47% success @ $23,408 Tx cost 23% partial success @ $23,408 Tx cost 11% Fail @ $23,408 Tx cost	27% for 0 mo. @ cost to society of $1,230/mo all @ 1/2 of cost to society of $1,230/mo all @ cost to society of $1,230/mo	ignore*
Dropout before end of treatment	ignore	19% @ partial Tx cost of 17.42 months from dropout to end of Tx period $4,821 Plus @ $1,230 cost to society/mo		ignore
Return for subsequent treatment	ignore	ignore**	31% for an average 4.2 weeks = $956 treatment cost	ignore

EXPECTED SOCIO-ECONOMIC TREATMENT COST = $27,594

Notes:
* For the pre-diagnosis and post-diagnosis ("Remaining life") time periods, depressed people incur the same cost to society regardless of which treatment they received. Because costs during these times periods are not different between the treatments, they cannot affect the cost differences of the treatments. Therefore, they are ignored.
** Return for subsequent treatment during the initial 2-year treatment period: Ignore this possibility because only drop-outs could do this. We assume all patients receiving subsequent treatments do so only during the potential relapse period.

Table 3: Calculation of CBT expected treatment costs

Patient's expected outcome	Percentage of patients	Calculation	Expected Cost
Treatment success	47%	x $23,408 Treatment cost	= $11,002
	47%	x 27% Relapsing x $1,230 Post-treatment cost to society x 0 Months relapsed	= 0
Partial success	23%	x $23,408 Treatment cost	= 5,384
	23%	x 0.5 Post-treatment cost to society of $1,230 x 12.1 Month relapse period	= 1,712
Failures	11%	x $23,408 Treatment cost	= 2,575
	11%	x $1,230 Post-treatment cost to society x 12.1 Month relapse period	= 1,638
Drop-outs	19%	x $4,821 Partial treatment cost	= 916
	19%	x $1,230 Post-treatment cost to society x 17.42 Months to end of 2-year treatment period	= 4,072
Sum	100%		
Subsequent treatment	31%	x $956 Treatment cost	= 296
CBT EXPECTED TREATMENT COST			$27,594

Table 4: Pharmacological timeline model of expected treatment costs

Patient Categories	Birth and Pre-diagnosis	2-year treatment period	Potential relapse period (12.1 mo)	Remaining life and Death
Complete Treatment	ignore	29% success @ $30,733 Tx cost 19% partial success @ $30,733 Tx cost 17% Fail @ $30,733 Tx cost	59% for 5.5 mo. @ cost to society of $1,230/mo all @ 1/2 of cost to society of $1,230/mo all @ cost to society of $1,230/mo	ignore
Dropout before end of treatment	ignore	35% @ partial Tx cost of 18.89 months from dropout to end of Tx period $3,891 Plus @ $1,230 cost to society/mo		ignore
Return for subsequent treatment	ignore		57% for an average 20.3 weeks = $4,149 treatment cost	ignore

EXPECTED SOCIO-ECONOMIC TREATMENT COST = $36,942

Total cost difference from CBT $9,348
Percentage cost difference from CBT   34%

Table 5: Combination timeline model of expected treatment costs

Patient Categories	Birth and Pre-diagnosis	2-year treatment period	Potential relapse period (12.1 mo)	Remaining life and Death
Complete Treatment	ignore	47% success @ $31,245 Tx cost 19% partial success @ $31,245 Tx cost 8% Fail @ $31,245 Tx cost	29% for 2.5 mo. @ cost to society of $1,230/mo all @ 1/2 of cost to society of $1,230/mo all @ cost to society of $1,230/mo	ignore
Dropout before end of treatment	ignore	26% @ partial Tx cost of $5,020 Plus 20.17 months from dropout to end of Tx period @ $1,230 cost to society/mo		ignore
Return for subsequent treatment	ignore		44% for an average 4.2 weeks = $956 treatment cost	ignore

EXPECTED SOCIO-ECONOMIC TREATMENT COST = $34,323

Total cost difference from CBT $6,729
Percentage cost difference from CBT   24%

Health Care Costs

In the model, all treatments are delivered over a 2 year period. It is assumed that CBT is delivered weekly for 15 weeks, followed by 5 booster sessions over the remaining period. It is assumed that half of CBT patients are treated in group sessions, the rest in individual sessions. CBT sessions are costed at $100 per individual session or $30 per group session. Fluoxetine is costed at $2.49 per 20 mg pill (personal communication, Safeway Pharmacy, 6-7-96). It is assumed that the typical patient will take 2 pills per day and see a psychiatrist at least once every 6 weeks. It is assumed a psychiatrist charges $70 for a typical 30 minute medication check (personal communication, University of Nevada Mental Health Associates, 6-21-96).

The combination treatment is assumed to comprise 20 one hour sessions delivered in the same pattern as the CBT alone treatment. The assumption is made that the patient sees a psychiatrist individually who can prescribe the medication and provide the CBT in the combined treatment. It is assumed that the medication treatment is woven into the session. For the combination treatment, it is assumed that the prescription is phoned into the pharmacy when needed between therapy sessions, so no extra trips to the doctor are required. The psychiatrist is assumed to charge $140 per session in the combined treatment (i.e., double the half-hour rate). All three treatment protocols are based on models described in the studies reviewed in this chapter.

Lost Wages and Travel Costs

The opportunity cost (i.e., the differential money that could have been made by doing something else) for patients who receive treatment is assumed to be $8.90 per hour. This is the after-tax net pay based on a $15 per hour gross wage rate. It is assumed the average CBT individual session is an hour and the average group session is 2 hours. It is assumed that the average medication check with a psychiatrist lasts about 30 minutes. It is assumed that prescriptions are filled on site or after work if they are purchased at an off-site pharmacy. It is assumed that it takes 1 hour to get to and from all appointments. The 1995 IRS mileage rate of 30 cents per mile is used. The average round-trip to the doctor is assumed to be 10 miles while a round-trip to the pharmacy is assumed to be 5 miles.

Comorbidity Costs

Simon (1995) reported 1992 HMO medical costs for depressed and nondepressed patients. Depressed patients had a mean of $1,875 higher health care costs overall compared to nondepressed matched controls. Less than 20% of the difference between depressed and nondepressed patients was due to mental health costs. Among depressed patients treated with antidepressant drugs, the mean total health care costs were $2,035 higher than those for comparable nondepressed patients. Nonmedicated depressed patients had a mean of $1,287 higher health care costs than those for the comparison group. Cost differences between depressed and nondepressed patients are multiplied by 80% to negate the direct costs of mental health treatments. The cost differences are adjusted to current retail prices paid by patients or third party payers. It is assumed that some of the costs of side effects are captured here when patients seek treatment, resulting in higher overall treatment costs, for their side effects. To the extent that patients do not seek treatment for side effects, comorbity costs for fluoxetine are understated.

Economic Multiplier and Taxes

We used the Nevada state household spending multiplier as of 6-21-96. This measures the effect on the economy from spending $1.00 of household income. Household income is the net pay brought home by the income earners. Since the economic multiplier applies to net pay, it does not consider the effect of taxes from paychecks. Therefore, the lost taxes are separately calculated (federal and state income taxes at 28% and 5%, social security at 7.65%).

Community Service

We assumed the average adult donates 40 hours per year to community service. We also assumed the cost of providing these services, if not donated, is $10 per hour. We also assumed that depression causes a 50% reduction in donated time across all treatments.

Lost Productivity During Treatment

Greenberg et al. (1993) estimated that 7.8 million workers lost 290 million workdays in 1990 due to depression. This is 37 workdays per year per patient. We assumed an unrecovered patient loses 37 days per year during the 2 year period under consideration. It is assumed a recovered patient loses half that amount (18.5 days) and a partially recovered patient loses something in the middle, about 27.75 workdays. An expected number of days lost was calculated for a typical patient from each of the three treatments. The expected days lost was then multiplied by the average wage rate.

Lost Income Potential from Suicide

In 1990, there were an estimated 11 million depressed Americans, resulting in 18,400 suicides (Greenberg et al., 1993). Those suicides resulted in a lost income potential of $7.5 billion dollars for an average of $407,609 per suicide or $681.81 per depressed person. Adjusting for inflation, this is $1,913 per year per 2 year treatment period per depressed patient in lost income potential from suicide. Costs to society from suicide are post-treatment costs, and are estimated to be the same for all depressed patients regardless of treatment type.

Other Considerations

Because two of the authors practice CBT, a special attempt was made to bias against CBT in terms of costs where ever judgement was involved. For example, in the outcome studies of CBT, the treatment is usually delivered in 10 to 20 sessions over a period of 3 or 4 months. The average number of session in these studies is actually about 12 to 15. We purposely chose 20 sessions of CBT delivered over the

2 year period which is likely to inflate the cost of CBT somewhat.   All of the comparison studies offered a comparable number of drug sessions to match treatment intensity of the CBT. We purposely chose less frequent and less intense drug treatment in this analysis to reflect real world practices. The costs for drug treatments in our model are therefore likely to be less than the actual costs in most of the treatment outcome studies we reviewed. There is also some evidence that CBT can be delivered rather effectively in the form of a self-help manual (Jamison & Scogin, 1995). Such an option was not considered in our model. If it were, it would significantly reduce the direct cost of CBT treatment. The CBT outcome numbers inferred from the Wexler and Cicchetti (1992) meta-analysis are likely to underestimate actual CBT outcome because that meta-analysis included the inferior outcome for the insight oriented psychotherapy from McLean and Hakstian (1979). Also, our model does not incorporate new data indicating that health insurance costs increase for those who have a history of fluoxetine use (Protos, 1995). Finally, we were unable to develop a way to quantify the nonmedical treatment costs of side effects. Such costs are extremely important and are an issue for future consideration. It is quite likely that if side effects were somehow quantified they would overwhelm the model, with even greater advantages accruing to CBT.

Conclusions

As can be seen from the figures, CBT is the most cost-effective treatment, followed by combined treatment, followed by fluoxetine alone. Over the 2 year period under evaluation, fluoxetine alone will result in 34% higher expected costs than CBT alone and the combination treatment will result in 24% higher costs than CBT alone. Based on this cost-effectiveness model, CBT should be considered the treatment of first choice for unipolar depression. If the treatment fails, it can be supplemented by fluoxetine or another SSRI. Fluoxetine alone does not appear as cost-effective as the other two treatments. In this model, if fluoxetine is used, it should be used only in combination with CBT.

It is important to note that we are proposing a model. It is quite possible to debate the numerical values that are used for each of the cost variables. We have tried to incorporate available data on outcome, relapse, and drop out percentage, variables that may be overlooked in any analysis that considers only direct costs. However, we hope we have generated a fairly comprehensive model that can be used by others to evaluate the costs and benefits of these treatments in real world settings. Also, costs are not static. We expect the prices of medication and provider charges to change over time and vary with setting.

We have deferred any attempt to quantify the nonmedical costs of side effects. We encourage others to develop creative ways to quantify the costs associated with side effects that don't result in treatment seeking, so they can be incorporated into future models. Even though antidepressants are the most common agents used in suicide by poisoning, no attempt has been made to quantify differentially suicide for each treatment because there are no current data available to allow estimates of the relative risk of suicide for patients receiving CBT or fluoxetine.

Despite the outcome and cost data detailed in this chapter, antidepressant medication continues to be the most popular treatment in the U.S. (Narrow, Regier, Rae, Manderscheid, & Locke, 1993). These data and analyses suggest that treatment patterns for depression ought to be carefully reexamined. It appears that for depression, CBT is at least as clinically effective and more cost-effective than antidepressant medication.

Finally, we would like to note that we do not consider cost-effectiveness to be the ultimate criterion by which treatment options ought to be evaluated. When loved ones become depressed, we want them treated with the most clinically effective interventions. CBT currently offers an alternative that is both clinically effective and cost-effective, providing an easy choice.

References

Amenson, C. S., & Lewinsohn, P. M. (1981). An investigation into the observed sex difference in prevalence of unipolar depression. *Journal of Abnormal Psychology*, *90*, 1-13.

Anderson, I. M., & Tomenson, B. M. (1995). Treatment discontinuation with selective serotonin reuptake inhibitors comared with tricyclic antidepressants: a meta-analysis. *British Medical Journal*, *310*, 1433-1438.

Antonuccio, D. O., Akins, W. T., Chatham, P. M., Monagin, J. A., Tearnan, B. H., & Ziegler, B. L. (1984). An exploratory study: The psychoeducational group treatment of drug-refractory unipolar depression. *Journal of Behavior Therapy and Experimental Psychiatry*, *15*, 309-313.

Antonuccio, D. O., Danton, W. G., & DeNelsky, G. Y. (1995). Psychotherapy versus medication for depression: Challenging the conventional wisdom with data. *Professsional Psychology: Research and Practice*, *26*(6), 574-585.

Antonuccio, D. O., Ward, C. H., & Tearnan, B. H. (1989). The behavioral treatment of unipolar depression in adult outpatients. In M. Hersen, R. M. Eisler, & P. M. Miller (eds.), *Progress in Behavior Modification* (pp. 152-191). Newbury Park, California: Sage Publications, Inc.

Beck, A. T., Hollon, S. D., Young, J. E., Bedrosian, R. C., & Budenz, D. (1985). Treatment of depression with cognitive therapy and amitriptyline. *Archives of General Psychiatry*, *42*, 142-148.

Beck, A. T., Rush, A. J., Shaw, B. F., & Emery, G. (1979). *Cognitive Therapy of Depression*. New York: Guilford.

Beck, A. T., & Young, J. E. (1985). Depression. In D. H. Barlow (Ed.), *Clinical handbook of psychological disorders* (pp. 206-244). New York: Guilford.

Beck, A. T., Ward, C. H., Mendelson, M., Mock, J., & Erbaugh, J. (1961). An inventory for measuring depression. *Archives of General Psychiatry*, *4*, 561-571.

Blackburn, I. M., Bishop, S., Glen, A. I. M., Whalley, L. J., & Christie, J. E. (1981). The efficacy of cognitive therapy in depression: A treatment trial using cognitive therapy and pharmacotherapy, each alone and in combination. *British Journal of Psychiatry*, *139*, 181-189.

Blackburn, I. M., Eunson, K. M, & Bishop, S. (1986). A two-year naturalistic follow-up of depressed patients treated with cognitive therapy, pharmacotherapy, and a combination of both. *Journal of Affective Disorders, 10,* 67-75.

Bowers, W. A. (1990). Treatment of depressed in-patients: Cognitive therapy plus medication, relaxation plus medication, and medication alone. *British Journal of Psychiatry, 156,* 73-78.

Breggin, P. (1994). *Talking Back to Prozac.* New York: Saint Martin's Press.

Breggin, P. (1991). *Toxic Psychiatry.* New York: Saint Martin's Press.

Brugha, T. S., Bebbington, P. E., MacCarthy, B., Sturt, E., & Wykes, T. (1992). Antidepressants may not assist recovery in practice: A naturalistic prospective survey. *Acta Psychiatric Scandanavia, 86,* 5-11.

Carroll, K. M., Rounsaville, B. J., & Nich, C. (1994). Blind man's bluff: Effectiveness and significance of psychotherapy and pharmacotherapy blinding procedures in a clinical trial. *Journal of Consulting and Clinical Psychology, 62*(2), 276-280.

Conte, H. R., Plutchik, R., Wild, K. V., & Karasu, T. B. (1986). Combined psychotherapy and pharmacotherapy for depression: A systematic analysis of the evidence. *Archives of General Psychiatry, 43,* 471-479.

Covi, L., Lipman, R. S., Derogatis, L. R., Smith, J. E., & Pattison, J. H. (1974). Drugs and group psychotherapy in neurotic depression. *American Journal of Psychiatry, 131,* 191-198.

Covi, L., & Lipman, R. S. (1987). Cognitive behavioral group psychotherapy combined with imipramine in major depression. *Psychopharmacology Bulletin, 23*(1), 173-176.

Dilsaver, S. C., & Greden, J. F. (1984). Antidepressant withdrawal phenomena. *Biological Psychiatry, 19,* 237-256.

Dobson, K. S. (1989). A meta-analysis of the efficacy of cognitive therapy for depression. *Journal of Consulting and Clinical Psychology, 57,* 414-419.

Dunn, R. J. (1979). Cognitive modification with depression-prone psychiatric patients. *Cognitive Therapy and Research, 3,* 307-317.

Elkin, I., Shea, T., Watkins, J. T., Imber, S. D., Sotsky, S. M., Collins, J. F., Glass, D. R., Pilkonis, P. A., Leber, W. R., Docherty, J. P., Fiester, S. J., & Parloff, M. B. (1989). National Institute of Mental Health Treatment of Depression Collaborative Research Program: General Effectiveness of Treatments. *Archives of General Psychiatry, 46,* 971-982.

Endicott, J., Spitzer, R. L., Fleiss, J. L., & Cohen, J. (1976). The Global Assessment Scale: A procedure for measuring overall severity of psychiatric disturbance. *Archives of General Psychiatry, 33,* 766-771.

Evans, M. D., Hollon, S. D., DeRubeis, R. J., Piasecki, J. M., Grove, W. M., Garvey, M. J., & Tuason, V. B. (1992). Differential relapse following cognitive therapy and pharmacotherapy for depression. *Archives of General Psychiatry, 49,* 802-808.

Fava, G. A., Grandi, S., Zielezny, M., Rafanelli, C., & Canestrari, R. (1996). Four-year outcome for cognitive behavioral treatment of residual symptoms in major depression. *American Journal of Psychiatry, 153*(7), 945-947.

Fisher, S., & Greenberg, R. P. (1993). How sound is the double-blind design for evaluating psychotropic drugs? *Journal of Nervous and Mental Disease, 181*, 345-350.

Frank, E., Kupfer, D. J., Perel, J. M., Cornes, C., Jarrett, D. B., Mallinger, A. G., Thase, M. E., McEachran, A. B., & Grochocinski, V. J. (1990). Three-year outcomes for maintenance therapies in recurrent depression. *Archives of General Psychiatry, 47*, 1093-1099.

Greenberg, P. E., Stiglin, L. E., Finkelstein, S. N., & Berndt, E. R. (1993). The economic burden of depression in 1990. *Journal of Clinical Psychiatry, 54*, 405-418.

Greenberg, R. P., Bornstein, R. F., Greenberg, M. D., & Fisher, S. (1992a). As for the kings: A reply with regard to depression subtypes and antidepressant response. *Journal of Consulting and Clinical Psychology, 60*, 675-677.

Greenberg, R. P., Bornstein, R. F., Greenberg, M. D., & Fisher, S. (1992b). A meta-analysis of antidepressant outcome under "blinder" conditions. *Journal of Consulting and Clinical Psychology, 60*, 664-669.

Greenberg, R. P., Bornstein, R. F., Zboroswski, M. J., Fisher, S., & Greenberg, M. D. (1994). A meta-analysis of fluoxetine outcome in the treatment of depression. *The Journal of Nervous and Mental Disease, 182*(10), 547-551.

Hamilton, M. (1960). A rating scale for depression. *Journal of Neurology, Neurosurgery, and Psychiatry, 12*, 56-62.

Halbreich, U., Shen, J., & Panaro, V. (1996). Are chronic psychiatric patients at increased risk for developing breast cancer? *American Journal of Psychiatry, 153*(4), 559-560.

Hall, R. C., Popkin, M. K., Devaul, R. A., Fallaice, L. A., & Stickney, S. K. (1978). Physical illness presenting as psychiatric disease. *Archives of General Psychiatry, 35*, 1315-1320.

Hallman, J., & Oreland, L. (1989). Serotonergic mechanisms and psychiatric disorders. *Nordisk Psykiatrisk Tidsskrift, 43*(20), 53-59

Hersen, M., Bellack, A. S., Himmelhoch, J. M., & Thase, M. E. (1984). Effects of social skill training, amitriptyline, and psychotherapy in unipolar depressed women. *Behavior Therapy, 15*, 21-40.

Hollon, S. D., DeRubeis, R. J., Evans, M. D., Wiemer, M. D., Garvey, M. J., Grove, W. M., & Tuason, V. B. (1992). Cognitive therapy and pharmacotherapy for depression: Singly and in combination. *Archives of General Psychiatry, 49*, 774-781.

Hollon, S. D., Shelton, R. C., & Loosen, P. T. (1991). Cognitive therapy and pharmacotherapy for depression. *Journal of Consulting and Clinical Psychology, 59*, 88-99.

Jamison, C. & Scogin, F. (1995). The outcome of cognitive bibliotherapy with depressed adults. *Journal of Consulting and Clinical Psychology, 63*(4), 644-650.

Jefferson, J. W. (1992). Treatment of depressed patients who have become nontolerant to antidepressant medication because of cardiovascular side effects. *Journal of Clinical Psychiatry Monograph, 10*, 66-71.

Kapur, S., Mieczkowski, T., & Mann, J. J. (1992). Antidepressant medication and the relative risk of suicide attempt and suicide. *Journal of the American Medical Association, 268,* 3441-3445.

Kathol, R. G. & Henn, F. A. (1982). Tricyclics: The most common agent used in potentially lethal overdoses. *Journal of Nervous and Mental Disease, 171,* 250-252.

Kessler, R. C., McGonagle, K. A., Zhao, S., Nelson, C. B., Hughes, M., Eshleman, S., Wittchen, H., & Kendler, K. S. (1994). Lifetime and 12-month prevalence of DSM-III-R psychiatric disorders in the United States. *Archives of General Psychiatry, 51,* 8-19.

Koranyi, E. D. (1979). Morbidity and rate of undiagnosed physical illnesses in a psychiatric clinic population. *Archives of General Psychiatry, 36,* 414-419.

Kovacs, M., Rush, A. J., Beck, A. T., & Hollon, S. D. (1981). Depressed outpatients treated with cognitive therapy or pharmacotherapy: A one-year follow-up. *Archives of General Psychiatry, 38,* 33-39.

Kramer, P. (1993). *Listening to Prozac.* New York: Viking.

Kupfer, D. J., Frank, E., Perel, J. M., Cornes, C., Mallinger, A. G., Thase, M. E., McEachran, A. B., & Grochocinski, V. J. (1992). Five-year outcome for maintenance therapies in recurrent depression. *Archives of General Psychiatry, 49,* 769-773.

Lenhoff, M. (1994). Potential complications of fluoxetine. *VA Practitioner, 11*(3), 33-41.

Loftus, E. F. (1993). The reality of repressed memories. *American Psychologist, 48*(5), 518-537.

McLean, P. D., & Hakstian, A. R. (1979). Clinical depression: Comparative efficacy of outpatient treatments. *Journal of Consulting and Clinical Psychology, 47,* 818-836.

McLean, P. D., & Hakstian, A. R. (1990). Relative endurance of unipolar depression treatment effects: Longitudinal follow-up. *Journal of Consulting and Clinical Psychology, 58,* 482-488.

McLean, P. D., & Taylor, S. (1992). Severity of unipolar depression and choice of treatment. *Behavior Research and Therapy, 30*(5), 443-451.

Miller, I. W., Norman, W. H., Keitner, G. I., Bishop, S. B., & Dow, M. G. (1989). Cognitive-behavioral treatment of depressed inpatients. *Behavior Therapy, 20,* 25-47.

Moir, D. C., Crooks, J., Cornwell, W. B., O'Malley, K., Dingwall-Fordyce, I, Turnbull, M. J., & Weir, R. D. (1972). Cardiotoxicity of amitriptyline. *Lancet,* September 16, 561-564.

Morris, J. B., & Beck, A. T. (1974). The efficacy of antidepressant drugs: A review of research (1958 to 1972). *Archives of General Psychiatry, 30,* 667-674.

Murphy, G. E., Simons, A. D., Wetzel, R. D., & Lustman, P. J. (1984). Cognitive therapy and pharmacotherapy: Singly and together in the treatment of depression. *Archives of General Psychiatry, 41,* 33-41.

Narrow, W. E., Regier, D. A., Rae, D. S., Manderscheid, R. W., & Locke, B. Z. (1993). Use of services by persons with mental and addictive disorders: findings from the National Institute of Mental Health Epidemiological Catchment Area Program. *Archives of General Psychiatry, 50*, 95-107.

Nemeroff, C. B., DeVane, C. L., & Pollock, B. G. (1996). Newer antidepressants and the cytochrome P450 system. *American Journal of Psychiatry, 153*(3), 311-320.

Oliver, J. M., & Simmons, M. E. (1985). Affective disorders and depression as measured by the diagnostic interview schedule and the Beck Depression Inventory in an unselected adult population. *Journal of Clinical Psychology, 41*, 469-477.

Olfson, M. D. & Klerman, G. L. (1993). Trends in the prescription of antidepressants by office-based psychiatrists. *American Journal of Psychiatry, 150*(4), 571-577.

Pastuszak, A. Schick-Boschetto, B., Zuber, C., Feldcamp, M., Pinelli, M., Sihn, S., Donnenfeld, A., McCormack, M., Leen-Mitchell, M., Woodland, C., Gardner, A., Horn, M., & Koren, G. (1993). Pregnancy outcome following first-trimester exposure to fluoxetine (Prozac). *Journal of the American Medical Association, 269*, 2246-2248.

Paykel, E. S., Dimascio, A., Haskell, D., & Prusoff, B. A. (1975). Effects of maintenance amitriptyline and psychotherapy on symptoms of depression. *Psychological Medicine, 5*, 67-77.

Popkin, M. K., Callies, A. L., & Mackenzie, T. B. (1985). The outcome of antidepressant use in the medically ill. *Archives of General Psychiatry, 41*, 469-477.

Protos, J. (1995). Jagged little pills: The financial side effects of Prozac can be unnerving. *Smart Money*, December, 83.

Reynolds, C. F., Frank, E., Perel, J.M., Imber, S.D., Cornes, C., Morycz, R. K., Mazumdar, S., Miller, M. D., Pollock, B. G., Rifai, A. H., Stack, J. A., George, C. J., Houck, P. R., & Kupfer, D. J. (1992). Combined pharmacotherapy and psychotherapy in the acute and continuation treatment of elderly patients with recurrent major depression: A preliminary report. *American Journal of Psychiatry, 149*(12), 1687-1692.

Robinson, L. A., Berman, J. S., & Neimeyer, R. A. (1990). Psychotherapy for the treatment of depression: A comprehensive review of controlled outcome research. *Psychological Bulletin, 108*(1), 30-49.

Roth, D., Bielski, R., Jones, M., Parker, W., & Osborn, G. (1982). A comparison of self-control therapy and combined self-control therapy and antidepressant medication in the treatment of depression. *Behavior Therapy, 13*, 133-144.

Rush, A. J., Beck, A. T., Kovacs, M., & Hollon, S. D. (1977). Comparative efficacy of cognitive therapy and pharmacotherapy in the treatment of depressed outpatients. *Cognitive Therapy and Research, 1*, 17-37.

Rush, J., Beck, A. T., Kovacs, M., Weissenburger, J., & Hollon, S. D. (1982). Comparison of the effects of cognitive therapy and pharmacotherapy on hopelessness and self-concept. *American Journal of Psychiatry, 139*(7), 862-866.

Rush, A. J., Hollon, S. D., Beck, A. T., & Kovacs, M. (1978). Depression: Must psychotherapy fail for cognitive therapy to succeed? *Cognitive Therapy and Research, 2*, 199-206.

Seagraves, R. T. (1992). Sexual dysfunction complicating the treatment of depression. *Journal of Clinical Psychiatry Monograph, 10,* 75-79.

Settle, E. C. (1992). Antidepressant side effects: Issues and Options. *Journal of Clinical Psychiatry Monograph, 10,* 48-61.

Shea, M. T., Elkin, I., Imber, S. D., Sotsky, S. M., Watkins, J. T., Collins, J. F., Pilkonis, P. A., Beckham, E., Glass, D. R., Dolan, R. T., & Parloff, M. B. (1992). Course of depressive symptoms over follow-up: Findings from the National Institute of Mental Health treatment of depression collaborative research program. *Archives of General Psychiatry, 49,* 782-787.

Simons, A. D., Murphy, G. E., Levine, J. L., & Wetzel, R. D. (1986). Cognitive therapy and pharmacotherapy for depression: Sustained improvement over one year. *Archives of General Psychiatry, 43,* 43-48.

Song, F., Freemantle, N. Sheldon, T. A., House, A., Watson, P., Long, A., & Mason, J. (1993). Selective serotonin reuptake inhibitors: meta-analysis of efficacy and acceptability. *British Medical Journal, 306,* 683-687.

Steinbrueck, S. M., Maxwell, S. E., & Howard, G. S. (1983). A meta-analysis of psychotherapy and drug therapy in the treatment of unipolar depression with adults. *Journal of Consulting and Clinical Psychology, 51,* 856-853.

Stravynski, A., Verreault, R., Gaudette, G., Langlois, R., Gagnier, & Larose, R. (1994). The treatment of depression with group behavioral-cognitive therapy and imipramine. *Canadian Journal of Psychiatry 39*(7), 387-390.

Teasdale, J. D., Fennell, M. J. V., Hibbert, G. A., & Amies, P. L. (1984). Cognitive therapy for major depressive disorder in primary care. *British Journal of Psychiatry, 144,* 400-406.

Wexler, B. E., & Cicchetti, D. V. (1992). The outpatient treatment of depression: Implications of outcome research for clinical practice. *The Journal of Nervous and Mental Disease, 180* (5), 277-286.

Wexler, B. E. & Nelson, J. C. (1993). The treatment of major depressive disorders. *International Journal of Mental Health, 22*(2), 7-41.

Wilson, P. H. (1982). Combined pharmacological and behavioural treatment of depression. *Behaviour Research and Therapy, 20,* 173-184.

Yates, B. (1995). Cost-effectiveness analysis, cost-benefit analysis, and beyond: Evolving models for the scientist-manager-practitioner. *Clinical Psychology: Science and Practice, 2*(4), 385-398.

Zimmerman, M., & Spitzer, R. L. (1989). Melancholia: From DSM-III to DSM-III-R. *American Journal of Psychiatry, 146,* 20-28.

Discussion of Antonnucio, Thomas, and Danton

Neither Simple Nor Easy: Psychotherapy and Cost-Benefit Analysis

Robert F. Peterson, Ph.D.
University of Nevada

The use of cost-benefit analysis as social policy in the United States goes back to 1902 (Campen, 1986), when the government required the Corps of Engineers to evaluate the outcomes of federal expenditures for navigation. Since cost-benefit analysis involves the evaluation of alternative courses of action (Levin, 1983), the usefulness of such an approach has become increasingly apparent and has been embraced by decision makers in business, education, and government. Given the rate of increase in the costs of medical care over the last decade, it should be no surprise that a cost-benefit analysis would also be extended to health expenditures, and to psychological and behavioral treatment.

The analysis of benefit is certainly not new to psychology and the other behavioral sciences. Methodologies for outcome evaluation are well known and well developed. Hundreds of journals report results comparing alternative learning or clinical treatment procedures. Some contrast treatment and no treatment control groups, some different treatments, and some the same treatment at different times, places and under different conditions. As a result, many psychological and behavioral approaches have reached the point where considerable data now exist on their efficacy.

Cost-Benefit and Treatment Evaluation

The term "psychotherapeutic" includes a multiplicity of approaches ranging from simple reinforcement for specific behaviors, to complex verbal and interpersonal interactions. There are over 230 different techniques used with children and adolescents alone (Kazdin, 1988). The number of adult psychotherapies may be even larger. In addition to therapy techniques, there is a host of non-procedural elements as well. They include the type of disorder, client and therapist characteristics, therapist skill and training, length of treatment, research design, assessment methods, and many others.

This plethora of variables leads to some interesting possibilities. Parloff (1982) pointed out that a comparison of only 250 therapies with 150 types of disorders would require about 47 million separate evaluations. And such an analysis has yet to consider costs! Bambi has indeed met Godzilla. Nevertheless, given a culture where competition is continuously waged over quality and price, a cost-benefit analysis of psychotherapy appears inescapable. As Yates said: "We can no more claim that the cost-effectiveness or cost-benefit of clinical services are unassessable than we can assert that the outcomes of our services are unmeasurable" (Yates, 1995, p. 385).

Since the number of possible treatments is very large, all treatments can not be compared. The question then becomes which treatment techniques are to be evaluated? This decision is likely to hinge on variables such as popularity or frequency of use, relative ease and cost of evaluation, existence of prior research suggesting efficacy, the importance and severity of the disorder targeted by the treatment, and subjective notions of treatment cost. Political and economic factors will also play a role in determining what to evaluate. This is especially true when potential outcomes are likely to influence the differing economic interests of psychotherapy providers, pharmaceutical companies, and physicians.

Cost Analysis

Cost is a very powerful change agent. Consider the current social experiment in "managed care." Managed care developed because of unacceptable increases in the cost of health services. This change occurred despite the fact that the potential benefits of managed care were uncertain. The success of managed care will hinge upon whether lower or stable costs (benefit 1) can be achieved while maintaining or improving health care services and outcomes (benefit 2). Psychological treatment is in a similar situation. The availability, utilization, and growth of psychotherapy will also depend upon constraints in cost while maintaining or improving benefits.

It would make little sense to evaluate a therapeutic approach in terms of cost until its benefits are known. Thus cost analysis should follow or, at the very least, be carried out at the same time as benefit analysis. One recent study did both. Shapiro, et al. (1994) conducted a study of two psychotherapy approaches while also evaluating the treatment "dose" (number of therapy sessions) and interactions with the severity of the disorder. They found that cognitive-behavioral treatment was marginally better than psychodynamic-interpersonal treatment, and that 16 sessions showed slightly better results than 8. The most interesting finding however, was an interaction between level of depression and length of treatment. Severely depressed clients did much better after 16 sessions of treatment than when given 8; moderately depressed clients did not show greater improvement with longer treatment. While this study evaluated specific treatment approaches for a particular disorder, more general information on the dose-response relationship can be found in a meta-analysis of over 2,000 patients (Howard, Kopta, Krause, and Orlinsky, 1986). This analysis covered a 30 year period and included a variety of therapies and disorders. Results showed that about half the patients demonstrated improvement by the eighth session, with 75% improved after 26 sessions.

The evaluation of therapy type and length as important psychotherapeutic variables assumes that psychotherapists are interchangeable. Such an evaluation also assumes that similarly diagnosed clients are likewise interchangeable. These are questionable assumptions. As Butler and Strupp (1986) have pointed out, techniques "gain their meaning and, in turn, their effectiveness from the particular interaction of the individuals involved" (p.33). Studies have demonstrated that different therapists using the same treatment show different rates of treatment success (Luborsky, McLellan, Woody, & O'Brien, 1985). There is evidence that therapist variables and the collaborative bond between client and therapist also play a role in pharmacological therapy (Krupnick, et al, 1996). Those who advocate a cost-benefit analysis of procedures must show that differences in the effectiveness of individual therapists, or variations in client characteristics have not confounded conclusions about the value of particular treatments, whether they be interpersonal or pharmacological.

Cost Perspectives and the Problem of Assumptions

A central issue in a cost-benefit analysis is the question of who pays and who benefits. Effects on clients, of course, are primary. Clients need to receive the best possible treatment at reasonable costs. However, cost-benefit analysis should also evaluate impacts on others as well. These would include practitioner costs of delivering treatment and the monetary, professional, and personal benefits which result. When a treatment involves medication, pharmaceutical industry costs and benefits of developing drugs should be considered along with those of the physicians who prescribe them. The insurer, whose primary interests are more likely to focus on cost containment, has an obvious interest in a cost-benefit analysis and wants effective treatments and patient satisfaction both in the shortest possible time period.

Insurance policy holders, families, employers, legislative bodies and society at large also have a stake in psychological treatment. A key question is how to select which groups or interests are most relevant and how to measure outcomes which affect them. Appropriate, accurate measures are fundamental and may differ depending on the consequences for each group. Policy holders for example, will be interested in the costs of insurance, while families will be sensitive to improvements in interpersonal relationships. Employers are likely to be concerned with job stability and productivity. Legislative bodies, acting for society at large, might focus on subsequent hospital or medical utilization and suicide or divorce rates, to mention only a few possibilities. While a variety of measures will be needed to assess these changes, most of them can be translated into monetary costs which will remain a central criterion. The specific set of cost-benefit outcome measures selected will be crucial since the use of any particular set of assessment tools can influence the conclusions drawn.

Evaluation of different treatments for psychological disorders is enormously complex. Even when procedural and relationship variables are minimized, it is a difficult undertaking at best. The study presented by Antonuccio, Thomas, and Danton is a valuable attempt to compare the cost-effectiveness of psychological and pharmacological treatment. Many more such studies are needed. And they are likely to be controversial. Given the difficulty of agreement on what variables should be included in comparisons of treatment effectiveness, as well which assumptions and measures are basic to a cost-benefit analysis, it is obvious that the search for what works, and whether it is worth it, is just beginning.

References

Butler, S. F., & Strupp, H. H. (1986). Specific and nonspecific factors in psychotherapy: A problematic paradigm for psychotherapy research. *Psychotherapy, 26,* 303-313.

Campen, J. T. (1986). *Benefit, cost and beyond: The political economy of benefit-cost analysis.* Cambridge, MA: Ballinger Publishing Company.

Kazdin, A. E. (1988). *Child psychotherapy: Developing and identifying effective treatments.* Elmsford, NY: Pergamon.

Krupnick, J. L., Sotsky, S. M., Simmens, S., Moyer, J., Elkin, Watkins, J. & Pilkonis, P. A. (1996). The Role of the Therapeutic Alliance in Psychotherapy and Pharmacotherapy Outcome: Findings in the National Institute of Mental Health Treatment of Depression Collaborative Research Program. *Journal of Consulting and Clinical Psychology, 64,* 532-539.

Levin, H. M. (1983). *Cost-effectiveness: A primer.* Beverly Hills, CA: Sage Publications.

Howard, K. I., Kopta, S. M., Krause, M. S., & Orlinsky, D. E., (1986). The dose-effect relationship in psychotherapy. *American Psychologist, 41,* 159-164.

Luborsky, L., McLellan, A. T., Woody, G. E., O'Brien, C. P., & Auerback, A. (1985). *Archives of General Psychiatry, 42,* 602-611.

Parloff, M. B. (1982). Psychotherapy research evidence and reimbursement decisions: Bambi meets Godzilla. *American Journal of Psychiatry, 139,* 817-727.

Shapiro, D. A., Barkham, M., Rees, A., Hardy, G., Reynolds, S., and Startup, M. (1994). Effects of treatment duration and severity of depression on the effectiveness of cognitive-behavioral and psychodynamic interpersonal psychotherapy. *Journal of Consulting and Clinical Psychology, 62,* 522-534.

Yates, B. T. (1995). Cost-effectiveness Analysis, Cost-Benefit Analysis, and Beyond: Evolving Models for the Scientist-Manager-Practioner. *Clinical Psychology: Science and Practice, V2 N4,* 385-398.

Chapter 10

The Role of Professional Psychology in the Era of Health Care Reform: Psychology's Battle to Survive in the Market Place

Kirk Strosahl

Group Health Cooperative of Puget Sound

As the different perspectives presented in this book amply demonstrate, the debate over whether psychologists should be granted prescriptive authority continues to grow in both the complexity of issues involved, and the degree of polarization that is emerging among the "pro" and "con" factions. While both sides no doubt have absolute confidence in the validity of their positions, much of the debate seems to generate more heat than light, as to how psychology as a discipline will move forward to resolve this growing schism. This author believes that a framework for resolution is possible, but only to the extent that both sides operate from a common contextual gestalt. Specifically, the prescription privileges controversy is not a "freak of nature," but the logical conclusion to a series of fundamental changes in the evolution and role of psychology in response to the demands of health care reform and managed care.

In this paper, I will attempt to show where psychology has been, where it is now as a discipline, and what the future holds for both professional and academic psychologists. To do this, it will be necessary to touch upon the following topics: 1) the evolution of the mental health industry in general over the last half century; 2) how psychology has matured from a cottage industry to a professional guild; 3) how health care reform and managed health care have fundamentally changed the clinical practice and economic context of psychology; 4) understand the contemporary economic forces which are threatening the viability of professional psychology; 5) how the prescription privileges movement is but one of several ways psychology is trying to re–engineer itself to maintain financial viability. My hope is to show that psychology is facing a major challenge that it may well not survive, at least in anything resembling its current form. In this context, the prescription privileges debate, like other professional psychology initiatives (i.e., parity legislation, regulatory functions over managed care, anti-trust lawsuits over use of clinical practice guidelines) can be evaluated for what it is, rather than what the rhetoric suggests it is.

Position On Prescription Privileges

Before beginning, I would like to state that I am neither a staunch advocate for, nor a staunch opponent of, prescriptive authority for psychologists. There are certainly practice settings where psychologists would be better equipped if they had prescriptive authority. In my clinical practice as an on site behavioral health consultant for two medical practice groups with over 25 physicians, I routinely encounter medical patients who have been placed on psychoactive medicines. Not uncommonly, the medicines used are not appropriate for the condition being treated or, if they are appropriate, they are prescribed at inadequate dosages. While I can generally get any needed changes accomplished by consulting with the prescribing physician, this process is not as efficient as simply being able to make the adjustments myself on the spot.

While prescriptive authority certainly would have its benefits for some practicing psychologists, I have little confidence in the American Psychological Association and its ability or commitment to managing appropriately the dissemination of prescriptive privileges among its members. I am convinced that this is primarily an economic and industry initiative and, for that reason, reckless, self serving decision making may override a cautious, common sense approach. Given psychology's demonstrated lack of ability to maintain quality control over its training institutions, I shudder when I think of APA taking control over the training of psychologists in prescriptive practices.

On the other hand, I am not convinced that the opponents of prescriptive authority are in touch with the demands of the health care market place, nor do I believe that any group (even training institutions and academic faculties) can lay claim to the final definition of what psychological practice is supposed to be. I am concerned when I hear claims that prescriptive authority will ruin the core values and processes of psychological practice. It assumes that some group "owns" the core definition and has been mandated to protect it, an oligarchic theme to say the least. So, I'm sitting on the fence with respect to this issue, and I'm deeply disappointed in what I perceive to be the lack of meaningful dialogue or good faith negotiation between the opposing sides. I hope that this conference might be a jumping off point for such a constructive, conciliatory process.

Psychology: Where We Have Been

It is fair to say that the origins of clinical psychology were quite modest, yet some of the values that gave birth to psychological practice back in the 1950s are still influential today. As you know, psychology really began as a "cottage industry," that was almost completely subsidized by customers who paid out of pocket for services (Strosahl, 1994). This resulted in psychological services being accessible to only a small percentage of the population. In that context, psychology's key business partner was the fee paying client. Because a relatively small percentage of the population could afford such services, there was not a great demand for professional psychologists. Indeed, the profession had only a limited number of training sites and the number of graduates was small. Even in those years however, the dominant training model was to graduate "generalists" who could succeed in an office based private practice setting. There was very limited competition from other professional groups, leaving psychology with a fairly well defined industry niche. Most psychologists did psychological testing and conducted a generalist private practice, and did fare well financially. There was very little guild consciousness at this point. Although APA existed, it was primarily a scientific organization. This reflected the overall fact that academic/scientific psychologists were the dominant group in defining the values and purposes of psychological science and practice. Since academic institutions were also the professional training facilities, it was natural that the academic image of psychology would be promoted above all others. For many in the academy, these were the "golden years" of psychological science and practice. Life was simple; the rules of the road were straightforward and could be followed without any major paradigm shifts.

Psychology: Where We Are Now

As an industry matures, it naturally seeks to expand its product line and market share. Such was the case with psychology, commencing in the late 1960s. There were a number of key developments in American society that made this expansion. First, the federal government, with the birth of the "Great Society" philosophy, created the Medicaid and Medicare insurance systems. People often forget that before that time, health care coverage was viewed as a privilege, not a right. People also forget that the United States government is the largest insurance company in the world, and that the precedents it sets usually have a domino effect into business, industry, and insurance practices. This is exactly what happened after the formation of the Medicare/Medicaid payment systems. Employers and unions became increasingly interested in providing health care coverage for their workers. At first, mental health benefits were limited or non-existent, but that too changed over the years. At the end of the 1970s, most health care in this country was covered either by the government or by employer purchasers.

It is staggering to think about where we are now. Nearly 165 million people in this country have employer subsidized health care; nearly 26 million of these people are in Health Maintenance Organizations. The federal governments is responsible for about 40% of the health care coverage, primarily in its Medicare and Medicaid products.

The second major factor was the success psychology had in legal anti-trust challenges against psychiatry. Whereas psychiatry initially was the major beneficiary of the movement toward insured mental health care, psychology soon began to participate as well. By the early 1980s, the vast majority of a professional psychologist's income was being generated from insurance reimbursed mental health care. There were very few utilization management or managed care philosophies in play then, so seeing an insured client was "like money in the bank." The financial incentives available at the time favored developing long term therapy arrangements with clients. There were no doubt rampant abuses of this unrestricted flow of insurance dollars, the self righteous claims of psychologists not withstanding. It would be fair to say that all clinical problems were viewed as requiring long term therapy and the notion of time limited, evidence based treatment had little or no influence. The main problem facing psychology at this juncture was there weren't enough psychologists to meet the growing demand for services.

The third major factor was the American Psychological Association's decision to initiate the professional training schools and to increase the number of APA approved training programs in clinical and counseling psychology. This was an understandable response to the short supply of psychologists at the time, but it had some unintended negative consequences and, due to the serendipity of the market place, came at exactly the wrong time. The unintended consequence was that enlarging our training capacity resulted in a significant increase in professional psychologists, with a corresponding loss of quality control in training. In short, psychology flooded the market place with marginally trained providers whose primary identity was as clinical practitioners, not as scientific practitioners. In a fundamental way, Psychology began to lose its distinctive identity both internally and in the market place as well. The serendipitous market place occurrence was the concurrent rapid expansion of masters level providers, who came to the market place to compete for their share of insurance dollars. This resulted eventually in a dramatic oversupply of mental health providers, especially in urban areas, which would allow the predatory pricing strategies of early managed care to have such an impact. The health and mental health care feeding frenzy of the late 1970s and early 1980s not only triggered health care reform, it left the mental health industry with a badly tarnished image in the eyes of business, industry, and insurance. Internally, the advent of the professional psychology model would change the political complex of the American Psychological Association. No longer would it be a haven for scientific psychologists, but instead would evolve into a well funded guild association with long political, social, and economic agendas. This change was formally signaled by the creation of the American Psychological Society, as a separate organization, although in truth the transformation to a professional guild had been in process for several years.

The fourth and most contemporary factor is the evolution of the industry toward managed care. While the professional guilds would have us believe that managed health care is a conspiracy hatched in a cigar smoke filled room by a group of money hungry insurance executives, the fact is that the health and mental health professions produced the managed care movement because of their economic success, or what skeptics have termed largesse. This largesse can be measured by looking at the escalating cost of insurance premiums which are generally based in actual utilization experience. From 1975 to 1985, health insurance premiums were increasing by 25% a year; from 1985 to 1990, 19% a year (Strosahl, 1994). Recall that in 1981, the United States entered into a severe economic recession. Companies that formerly had been increasing profits by 20-30% a year and could integrate increased fringe benefits costs into their overhead now began to search for ways to control or reduce costs. One area that fairly well jumped out at corporate financial officers were the staggering annual increases in their health care premiums. After numerous futile attempts to engage the health care disciplines in a dialogue to develop better self-regulatory practices, the decision was made on a company by company basis to out-source utilization management and cost control functions to managed care organizations. As students of industry will attest, successful business practices are quickly disseminated and there was little doubt that employing managed care solutions did radically reduce costs. Industry journals produced story after story of managed care strategies reducing costs by as much as 40% in a one to two year period.

This brings us to the present day environment, and if we look at the changes from the early years of psychology collectively, it has been a very successful ride indeed. Psychology is now a mature service industry in nearly every respect. We have a long list of specialized services such as health psychology, industrial psychology, behavioral medicine, neuropsychology and so forth. We have a very potent guild organization with political action arms that are run not by scientists, but by attorneys. Socially, we are looking at the very real possibility of parity legislation that will essentially unlock mental health benefits and make them comparable to health benefits. Psychological services are now accessible to the majority of the population and psychology now has new business partners: the managed care industry and purchasers of mental health care who ordinarily are not the client.

We also have more than our share of problems. Internally, the schism between scientific and applied psychology has grown more vitriolic. The definition of psychology has become confused because of the tremendous diversity of psychological service products available. This makes discussions about changes in products or core roles even more difficult. In the market place, psychology at the same time is facing tremendous competitive pressures. Due to the oversupply of mental health providers in general, the competition for industry niches is vicious. This problem is compounded by the loss of quality control in the training of professional psychologists. In contemporary managed care systems, psychologists are commonly viewed as overpaid masters level providers. Our penchant for training generalist private practice oriented providers has backfired badly. The research as this point does not point to superior outcomes being obtained by doctoral level providers, and managed care administrators have capitalized on this information by adopting a "lowest capable provider" approach in practice networks. Specifically, the assumption is that masters level providers are just as effective as psychologists with the majority of clinical problems. This means many fewer psychologists are needed in clinical practice settings at the same time professional schools are graduating literally thousands of psychologists every year. Many of these new professionals will "die on the vine" waiting for non-existent practice network openings, which, if they do occur, will be filled with lower priced providers. The irony is that the managed care market place as a whole seems to moving toward purchasing the specialty psychological products (i.e., behavioral medicine, neuropsychology, program development and evaluation, administration) while the guild keeps training providers who provide general services. Whatever one's stance on the prescriptive authority issue is, this much can be said that is positive: It does signal that psychology's guild leaders now recognize that the main way to stay financially viable is to offer a fairly unique and restricted set of services.

Psychology: Where We Are Headed

If the changes that have occurred in the last decade are any indication, psychology is headed into a period of unparalleled turbulence both internally and in the market place. I have written elsewhere about Generation One and Generation Two of managed health care (Strosahl, 1995). Generation One has been focused on cost containment through supply side management strategies. This involved using the oversupply of providers to ratchet down session costs to unrealistically low levels, while at the same time aggressively managing and truncating services. However, getting the cheapest therapists you can, and then requiring abnormally short lengths of care across the board eventually creates quality problems. At this point, business, industry, and the government are well aware of the limitation of all out cost containment strategies. At some point, they begin to pay for the costs of the poor quality that emanates from overly zealous cost containment practices.

Currently, my assessment is that we are in a transition to Generation Two of managed care. This movement will be characterized by an emphasis on clinical quality, consumer satisfaction, and providing services in the most efficient manner possible. Outcomes based management will become the dominant method. Clinicians who produce good clinical outcomes, satisfy clients, and do it efficiently will be the big winners. However, the average line clinician will not be a psychologist. Instead, psychologists will be used to treat complex, difficult cases, or cases that clearly require training in a special clinical procedure. There will be many fewer psychologists in the market place in the next 5-10 years, and those that do make it will be providing some type of specialized psychological service (i.e., chronic pain, occupational medicine, behavioral medicine, neuropsychology). Many of the psychologists that are being trained now will never be able to practice and will leave the discipline. For those who manage to survive, a significant proportion will revert back to fee for service clients only, because of the inaccessibility of managed care provider networks.

There is an often overlooked implication of this evolution, if it turns out to be true, namely that the supply of psychologists will shrink drastically and many psychology training programs will disappear. I think the academic environment will undergo a radical downsizing as state and federal funds are shifted into applied training and service delivery settings. Many training clinics I know of are already facing financial insolvency because most managed care systems will not reimburse for services provided by interns or trainees. Particularly in medical school settings, the enormous profit margins realized during the era of unmanaged insurance reimbursement have disappeared. Without this pot of service dollars to rely on, many such facilities will be forced radically to downsize faculty and training services, simply to avoid bankruptcy.

The managed care market place will also undergo a radical transformation. I believe that we will see the development of huge regional delivery systems, that result from merger after merger. In the end, there may only be five or six mega-companies that will compete for the mental health dollar. At this point, the "industrialization" of mental health will have been completed. Terms like "supplier," "vendor," "customer," and "purchaser" will be commonplace in the parlance of psychologists. This new market place will be an "at risk" environment. Capitation, or pre-paid health care, will become the dominant financing mechanism. Practice groups will be "at risk" for managing their pre-paid premiums, while the purchasers will set the rules for what services must be delivered, how quality and consumer satisfaction must be demonstrated and so forth. It will not be possible, as it is now, for a practice group to "play games" with capitated moneys by simply denying services. I fully expect that there will be a long list of contractual requirements and a mechanism for determining whether those requirements are met. Practice groups that come in under budget, but have poor clinical quality, poor customer satisfaction and insufficient penetration of services will go by the way side. The groups that will emerge victorious will be the high performance behavioral health care groups.

What will characterize high performance behavioral health care groups? First, they will be committed to a population based model of service delivery. Often in association with medical practice groups, they will use consistent, evidence based care processes to address high volume and/or high impact. This will include critical pathways for disorders such as depression, panic, substance abuse, chronic pain, and ADHD, to name a few. These pathways will be supported by clinical practice guidelines, which are systematically developed decision rules that are to be applied by clinicians in their treatment of a particular patient with a particular condition. All clinical services will be supported by such guidelines and results will be measured using standard, universally applied outcomes assessment packages. Psychologists in these groups will not be used primarily as line clinicians, but rather as clinical specialists (for difficult or complicated cases) or in "provider extender" roles such as consultation for and training of masters level providers. I also believe that appropriately trained psychologists will be a highly prized commodity in the arena of program development, evaluation and administration.

A second aspect of high performance behavioral health care groups will be the ability to deliver integrated psychological services in primary care and specialty medicine settings. Psychology could well become a "medical" discipline because of the established value of psychological services in reducing medical costs and increasing health and mental health outcomes (Strosahl & Sobel, 1996). Whereas the specialty mental health market place looks bleak in terms of job growth, I believe there is an enormous opportunity for psychology to thrive and prosper as a legitimate medical service. With the possible advent of parity legislation and captitation as the dominant financing method, the transition into primary care could be an extremely effective economic growth strategy. This will require some modifications in the way psychologists are trained, particularly with respect to delivering consultation services to medical providers and their patients (Strosahl, 1996).

Within the profession of psychology, I only see a strengthening of the guild oriented mentality that has become so dominant in these last several years. This means that the rift between scientific psychologists and professional psychologists will continue. This will produce a collection of good and bad outcomes. The good outcomes will be the growing influence psychology will exert in the creation of legislation and progressive health care policy. I think this makes it unlikely that mental health benefits will ever be removed as part of the health care reform process. Believe it or not, there is still a minority sector of business and industry that is firmly opposed to continuing any mental health benefits. We need to acknowledge the positive impact our guild has had upon the general policy discussions about the legitimacy of mental health issues in public health, and on the need to address those issues as a matter of public health.

The bad outcomes will essentially be generated by the same processes; specifically, a self serving interest orientation that may lead to reckless decision making. One contemporary example of this is the threats of anti-trust lawsuits from divisions within APA in response to the guideline template committee's report. Another is the APA's nearly suicidal stance with respect to managed mental health care. The rhetoric notwithstanding, the anti-managed care stance of our guild is being driven by the economic interests of the dominant constituency, and it has backfired badly. Rather than capitalizing on the opportunity to create a collaborative partnership with managed care (which would allow us to influence their policies and decision making process), we have chosen to join the ranks of the resistant. In doing so, we have missed a golden opportunity to shape the process of health care reform.

The Prescription Privileges Debate In Context

It is now possible for us to examine the prescription privileges debate within a context more meaningful than the rhetoric laced discussions that typically take place. As the preceding analysis of the role of psychology in the current era of health care reform suggests, our future is anything but assured. Professional psychologists are facing intense competitive pressures, which include being undercut by a vast pool of master's level trained providers without a particularly strong market place identity to counter-act this encroachment. This problem is compounded by the general perception in behavioral health care that all forms of psychotherapy work equally well and can be administered by any competent provider. In short, our claims that psychologists generate superior treatment outcomes have fallen on deaf ears. What hasn't eluded the attention of behavioral health administrators are the large variations in clinical competence and repertoire among psychologists, a fact which when combined with the higher price of psychological providers, leaves us in a very precarious position indeed.

Unfortunately, the one potential advantage of being a guild industry has not materialized; specifically, the ability of the guild to promote a unique "core" definition of psychology which cannot be encroached upon by other disciplines. Instead, our guild organization has spent millions of dollars fighting managed care and health care reform initiatives, while dues paying professional members are being squeezed out of practice networks and facing financial extinction. Lest we feel we are in a unique dilemma, it is important to note that these same forces have decimated psychiatry, as well as other high priced medical specialties. Indeed, the health care market place has shifted almost completely to a "mid-level" and "lowest capable provider" mentality that threatens virtually every medical and behavioral health specialty discipline. We are truly faced with perhaps the most serious economic shakedown in the history of health care.

It is no coincidence that the prescription privilege movement has popped up as the effects of managed care have become a paramount industry issue. What is unique is that, whereas prior paradigmatic shifts in psychology have largely been driven by the scientific community, this shift is being driven by the market place. For better or for worse, scientific psychology has not been meaningfully impacted by these market place developments. This fact, combined with scientific/academic psychology's sense of "ownership" over the definition of psychology as a discipline largely explains the fierce opposition to prescription privileges in the scientific community. Given the growing rift between professional and scientific psychology, this difference of perspective easily devolves into a, "Yes I will . . . No you won't" political firestorm.

How Would Psychology Be Effected: A Market Place View

My purpose in this presentation has been to examine the prescription privilege controversy from a managed care, market place perspective. I am not going to speak to the more esoteric, yet fundamental questions of how psychology as an intellectual enterprise will be advantaged or disadvantaged. From the market place perspective, there is little doubt in my mind that prescription privileges would give psychology an enormous advantage in the behavioral health care industry.

First, it would give psychology a tremendous competitive advantage over psychiatry. Psychologists would have the unique identity of being the only non-medical providers who come armed with psychotherapy and psychopharmacology competencies. Recall that organized psychiatry, in its drive to create a monopoly based upon a biological and medical emphasis in treatment, largely abandoned its psychotherapy training emphasis. It is not unreasonable to say that the weakest psychotherapists in today's managed care systems are practicing psychiatrists. This movement away from psychotherapy has become institutionalized to the point that many managed care systems refuse to let their psychiatrists provide psychotherapy, and instead define their role as dispensers of medication. The point here is that psychology, armed with prescription privileges, would not simply become "miniature psychiatry," as some have argued. This of course could happen if psychology lost its training focus in the conversion to a prescribing profession. If it didn't, psychology easily could supplant psychiatry and prescribing nurse specialists as the pre-

ferred provider for dispensing medication while concurrently delivering psychotherapy.

Second, prescription privileges would separate psychology from the encroaching masters level behavioral health disciplines, such social work, masters level
psychology, counseling and so forth. In my opinion, we really have little hope of
forestalling this onslaught of lower trained providers, unless there is some stunning
demonstration that using lower price providers leads to less clinical quality. Thus,
psychology will either be severely downsized as a discipline (with a resulting
backlash into the academic/scientific institutions), or it will find specialized roles
to play. Prescriptive authority is one of several specialized roles that conceivably
could insure that the industry will grow, not shrink. Some opponents of prescription
privileges argue that this separation wouldn't last long, because masters level providers would simply follow psychology and seek prescriptive authority. I have reason
to doubt this prediction would come true. I don't believe the typical masters level
provider has the interest or the desire to be a practicing pharmacotherapist. I do think
the three additional years of training that doctoral level psychologists receive makes
them more comfortable addressing medical issues in general. In other words, I do
think that there will be some self-regulation among the behavioral health disciplines, and there will not be a mad dash once the prescriptive authority door is
opened.

I now want to turn to the most fundamental development that is occurring in
health care reform. Specifically, this is the movement toward integrated delivery
systems in the attempt to meet consumer preferences for "one stop shopping" of
health and behavioral health services, to increase coordination of care and to reduce
costs. The third advantage that psychology would enjoy as a prescribing discipline
would involve its role as a "mid level provider" in the integrated health care systems
of the future. Recall that nearly 70% of all psychotropic agents are prescribed by
general medical practitioners in primary care (Beardsley et. al., 1988). As behavioral
health services are folded into primary health care, prescribing psychologists would
have a unique competitive position.

Unlike current mid-level providers in health care settings (Physician Assistant,
ARNP), psychologists would specifically be licensed to provide psychopharmacology services, in addition to their existing behavioral medicine intervention repertoire. I believe this would lead to literally thousands of new job opportunities for
psychologists, if the current explosion in other mid level health care provider
disciplines is any indication.

Finally, we must not forget that by obtaining prescription privileges, psychology
would enter into a de facto partnership with the pharmaceuticals industry. This
partnership up to now has largely been dominated by psychiatry, with extremely
potent political and financial results. This is one area where scientific psychology
also could be a huge beneficiary. As psychology evolves into a mainstream prescribing discipline, academic/scientific institutions would become targets for drug company training grants, drug certification trials and so forth. Psychology is already a

potent guild and likely would become the predominant guild in the behavioral health industry, given this new business partner. At the same time, opponents rightfully point to the pitfalls associated with new business relationships that potentially can create conflicts of interest, or worse, can influence the core definition of a discipline such as happened with psychiatry over the last several decades.

Summary: An Eco-System Analogy

Elsewhere in this volume, Dr. McFall presents a very elegant eco-system analogy to show that seemingly innocuous changes can have a dramatic domino effect in eco-systems. He applies this to the issue of prescription privileges, to show that such a change may have dramatic unintended consequences for the discipline of psychology. Being from a state (Washington) that has endured its share of vitriolic debates over environmental protection versus economic stability, I would like to offer my own contretemps.

As you know, the debate over environmental protection versus economic stability came into sharp focus as a result of the Spotted Owl controversy. In short, protectionists claimed to have irrefutable data showing the Spotted Owl pairs would only nest in old growth forest. To continue to log old growth would result in the extinction of the bird, which was already on the endangered species list. The majority of old growth forest in Washington is federally owned land, and the decision (made with all good intention) to restrict logging practices became part of a complex of economic influences that devastated the forestry industry in this state. The basis of this decimation was a simple scientific "fact": Spotted Owls could only mate in old growth forest. As the years wore on and the commercial locus of the timber industry shifted away from Washington, scattered reports began to emerge that Spotted Owl pairs had been observed nesting in second growth (replanted) forests as well. This, of course, would refute the need to restrict logging in old growth forests, but by that time, most of the timber industry infrastructure in the state had disappeared and the economic focus of the state had been fundamentally changed. Within months, protectionists filed new "scientific" claims about the danger of extinction to other species if the government were to open up old growth forests to traditional logging practices.

This analogy may be interpreted differently, depending upon which side of the prescription privileges debate one happens to be. For me, this analogy illustrates both the good and the bad of hotly contested issues, where the strength of personal convictions becomes confused with "scientific fact." The truth at this point is that no one has solid evidence about what impact prescriptive privileges will have on the discipline of psychology. We are reading tea leaves, and out of consideration for those on both sides of the fence, we should acknowledge that we are speaking based on our individual values as psychologists. One further extension of the analogy is called for here. As the citizens of the state of Washington are learning, decisions based upon polarized reasoning seldom end up addressing the common good. As we are finding out, we have to find a balance between our economic well-being and the protection of an endangered species.

References

Beardsley, R., Gardocki, G., Larson, D. & Hidalgo, I. (1988) Prescribing of psychotropic medication by primary care physicians and psychiatrists. *Archives of General Psychiatry, 45,* 1117-1119.

Strosahl, K. (1996). Confessions of a behavior therapist in primary care: The odyssey and the ecstasy. *Cognitive and Behavioral Practice, 3,* 1-28.

Strosahl, K. (1995). Behavior therapy 2000: A perilous journey. *The Behavior Therapist, 18,* 130-133.

Strosahl, K. (1994). Entering the new frontier of managed mental health care: Gold mines and land mines. *Cognitive and Behavioral Practice, 1,* 5-23.

Strosahl, K. & Sobel, D. (1996). Behavioral health and the medical cost offset effect: Current status, key concepts and future applications. *HMO Practice, 10,* 156-162.

Discussion of Strosahl

On Professional Psychology's Battle to Survive in the Marketplace

Robyn D. Walser, M.A.

University of Nevada

There can be little doubt about the significance of the plan to pursue prescription privileges for psychologists. Strosahl's chapter on "The Role of Professional Psychology in the Era of Health Care Reform: Psychology's Battle to Survive in the Marketplace" points squarely at some of the issues confronting psychology today. Psychologists find themselves in a time when the very foundation of what psychology has to offer is being challenged. Given this bold statement, I believe it is fair to say that the prescription privileges issue extends beyond the simple notion of whether psychologists should prescribe or not, and casts us into the question of what is the fabric of psychology?

The application of psychological principles to problems in living has been identified as one of the major roles of psychologists. However, the move to gain prescription privileges reflects an identity crisis, and realigns the field with psychiatry and the application of medicine in treatment. We currently have well developed principles of psychology, theory, and practice, and we continue to progress in both a scientific and useful fashion, particularly as the science relates to the treatment of the human condition and the understanding of human behavior. Furthermore, developing these issues will not inherently change the focus of psychology, on the one hand, as they are already largely a part of the profession. On the other hand, a move to prescribe may fundamentally change the field.

It may be true that many psychologists are responding to the issue of prescription privileges based on their own values rather than fact. And I believe that responding from this position has contributed to the heat of the debate among those who are "pro" and "con" with respect to the prescription privileges issue. However, operating on one's own values does not preclude the existing evidence as to the impact that prescription privileges might have on the discipline of psychology. Strosahl explains that we do not have any "solid evidence" as to the effect that privileges might have on our field. Nevertheless, evidence is available, and we should use historical precedence to inform our decisions. We don't need to look too far to see what has happened to the practice of psychiatry; the core definition of that discipline has been influenced and changed. Psychiatrists have become well-paid drug dispensers, and the "couch" has been missing from their bag of interventions for quite some time. We as psychologists are very likely to be subject to the same contingencies as psychiatrists, should we gain prescriptive authority.

Furthermore, the Department of Defense's prescription authority training program for psychologists also gives us an idea of the type of changes we are likely to face should psychologists prescribe. We should not ignore these compelling words. Tim Adams, one of the first participants in the Department of Defense project, describes his training and experience:

> The program at USUHS emphasizes recognition of what are normal physical findings with an understanding of normal organ functioning . . . In the inpatient psychiatry rotation, I am responsible for recognition of physical and psychological pathology, and appropriate treatment for my patients. This points out that as a psychologist prescribing medications and being responsible for the physical wellbeing of a patient, *the role is no different from* the psychiatrist. (p. 30, DeLeon, 1995, emphasis added)

And with respect to the psychologist's changing role once prescriptive authority is attained, another participant in the Department of Defense project states:

> As a psychologist, I have always tried to be sensitive to patient concerns about physical touch, personal space, and the personal relationship between therapist and patient ... When I first began doing physical examinations, I felt my identity as a psychologist being challenged. (p. 30, DeLeon, 1995)

We should not take this evidence for granted. Preparing ourselves to conduct physical examinations is perhaps preparing us for a fundamental change in our training. Allowing privileges may have "dramatic unintended consequences," just as rubber stamping Professional Schools of Psychology did. Furthermore, if the prescription privileges issue is truly driven by industry and economics, again we might find ourselves left with a "badly tarnished image in the eyes of business, industry and insurance." If we add to the above the notion of quality control in training, we may find ourselves in an even greater predicament. Quality control implies some type of underlying values and philosophy in practicing psychology that should be upheld. Hopefully these values are based on both ethical and scientific practice. Strosahl maintains, however, that psychology has demonstrated a lack of ability to exercise quality control over its training institutions, more specifically professional schools. This is one of the reasons for the loss of the unique "core" definition of psychology and for the encroachment of other disciplines upon the field. Prescriptive practices will only blur the lines among disciplines even further. Additionally, opposers of prescription authority, usually of the academic sort, who are trying to maintain a core set of values and processes of psychological practice, who are trying to define the "core" of the field, are being accused of employing oligarchy as a result of their efforts. No wonder the fabric of applied psychology is coming unraveled.

There have been many interesting twists and turns in psychology's history as a developing profession, the advent of the professional school not withstanding. Strosahl states, in response to APA's approval of professional schools and the subsequent significant increases in professional psychologists and loss of quality control: "In a fundamental way, psychology began to lose its distinctive identity both internally and in the marketplace as well." The race to prescription privileges throws us into nearly the same dilemma—loss of a distinctive identity. Issues and concerns about the direction the field of psychology is taking in relation to prescription privileges may be contributing to the plight of our identity. Some of the specific concerns involved include possible dramatic changes in training in clinical psychology, and the straying of the field from scientifically based psychotherapy treatment approaches. In addition, prescription authority may permit psychologists to compete financially in the current managed care dominated market place, but it is possible that it will do so not on the basis of the traditional core of the scientific discipline but by splicing some other profession on to psychology (Hayes, Walser, & Follette, 1995). There is a finer course of action: to show that we can serve consumers, and that we can assist in the development and evaluation of applied programs that are both effective and proficient through a strong science orientation of applied psychology. Instead, we find ourselves advocating for, and arguing about, something in which psychologists have little expertise.

I agree with the notion that we as psychologists need to be more flexible in terms of our future and the types of professional positions we are willing to be trained in and accept. It is to our benefit to create evidenced-based care that addresses high volume and high impact driven systems. To be flexible in our roles and to build our training in consultation services and program development, evaluation and administration, are *a few* of many ways that we can adjust to a changing system and develop a niche in the managed care arena.

Furthermore, increasing our product line and market share is an admirable goal, and one that I believe those who oppose prescription privileges want to attain. However, those opposing prescription privileges would like to attain this goal by staying within their own field of practice. That is, to focus on science based intervention and a level of analysis that is distinct from other fields of study (Hayes et al., 1995). This position supports the notion of psychology as a science in its own right.

It is clearly true that the field of mental health is changing and adaptation, by psychologists and training institutions, to a managed health care system is appropriate. However, the question of whether prescription privileges is a part of that adaptation is at best unclear, and at worst, a redefinition and changing of the field to a medical science. Perhaps the final outcome of prescribing psychologists is unknown, and a move to civilized debate may prove useful. Psychology would do well to reflect on the possible outcomes and any unintended consequences of the rush to prescription privileges, for, as Voltaire once observed, "History never repeats itself, man always does."

References

DeLeon, P. K (1995). Prescription privileges: Exciting federal developments, *The Independent Practitioner, 15,* 30-3 1.

Hayes, S. C., Walser, R. D., & Follette, V. M. (1995). Psychology and the temptation of prescription privileges. *Canadian Psychology, 36,* 313-320.

Chapter 11

Creating an Honorable Alternative to Prescription Privileges in the Era of Managed Care

Steven C. Hayes, Ph.D. and John T. Blackledge

University of Nevada

The prescription privilege movement is a response to real and important forces impinging upon the practice of psychology. While adding drug prescription authority is one logical reaction to some of these forces, it ignores others and responds in a fashion that creates notable dangers for the discipline and profession. Opponents and proponents of prescription privileges alike must take seriously, however, the great demands being placed upon the profession of psychology. The profession is clearly going through a difficult transition, and it is irresponsible to ignore the challenges. An honorable alternative must be created in order responsibly to oppose the movement towards prescribing authority.

Factors Leading to the Prescription Privilege Movement

The prescription privilege movement is not occurring in a vacuum. It is a reflection of professional and economic developments. In an earlier article (Hayes & Heiby, 1996) we argued that five factors were driving this movement. We will review them briefly here.

Practicing Psychology as Psychotherapy Delivery

When psychology in general and clinical psychology in particular expanded during the post-war era it was spurred by a changing role for psychologists in the healthcare delivery system. The Veterans Administration and others had an interest in seeing a successful challenge to the domination of psychiatry over psychotherapy. As a result, there was a gradual transition from training that emphasized assessment, consultation, and limited work in institutional settings to training that emphasized psychotherapy and more independent practice.

In the 1970s and 1980s, third party payments began to flow to clinical or counseling psychology on a fee-for-service basis. For a time, only psychiatry and psychology could be so reimbursed. This produced tremendous economic success for hard working psychological practitioners, and psychology became increasingly dedicated to psychotherapy training. Having linked its wagon to the actual delivery of psychotherapy, however, the practice of psychology became vulnerable to any

262   Steven C. Hayes and John T. Blackledge

forces of supply and demand that influence the practice of psychotherapy. Unfortunately, there was and is little evidence that psychotherapy need be delivered by a doctoral-level professional to be effective (Christensen & Jacobson, 1994; Dawes, 1994). Thus, practicing psychology became dedicated to a method in which expertise did not directly translate into healthcare impact.

Oversupply of Psychotherapists and the Expansion of Insurance Reimbursement

Doctoral level psychologists doing psychotherapy are increasingly in competition with other providers. Just as psychiatry could not keep psychology out of psychotherapy, psychology could not keep others out. The list is quite long, including social work, nursing, marriage and family therapy, counseling and guidance, drug and alcohol counseling, sex therapy, biofeedback, and many others. Initially, these professionals did not have access to third party payments, but soon enough many of them did. The number of available psychotherapists soared. Many of these providers were master's level, and were willing to accept lower fees.

The psychotherapy boom fed growth within psychology as well. The rise of tuition dependent professional schools of psychology created a training structure in which schools cannot admit small classes and survive. The combination of increased supply and lower cost competition is having a predictable economic impact: psychologists are being squeezed.

The Rise of Managed Care

Over the last ten years healthcare delivery has become managed healthcare delivery (Strosahl, 1994). Indemnity insurance has virtually disappeared. We will discuss this trend in great detail below, but this is the single biggest force leading to the prescription privilege movement, primarily because it has put lower payments to doctoral level psychologists and has restricted patient access.

All of this has put the practice of psychology, as it has existed over the last few decades, under tremendous pressure. By itself this would not lead to an interest in prescription privileges, however. Two other developments have prepared the ground intellectually and practically for this change.

The Hegemony of Syndromal Classification

Psychology has adopted the psychiatric nosology. The double whammy of third party indemnity insurance reimbursement systems linked to syndromal classification, and federal grant funding organized in terms of these categories overwhelmed the psychological opposition. Today even many former opponents of syndromal and disease oriented classification systems have accepted these practices, and psychologists in training are carefully schooled in the diagnostic nuances of psychiatry's classification system (Riley, Elliott, & Thomas, 1992). With this adoption of psychiatry's underlying model into clinical psychology (Hayes & Follette, 1992; Follette, Houts, & Hayes, 1992) has come a preparedness to adopt psychiatry's approach to human problems as part of psychology itself.

The Medical Guild and Drug Company Interests

Finally, the ability of the medical guild to control access to medications is weakening in area after area. To contain costs, physicians in practice are often turning to the very professions (e.g., Nurse Practitioners) that are encroaching on the traditional practice of medicine. This dilution of medical resistance means that it is not as big of a step to imagine that psychology could gain access to pharmacotherapy methods.

Drug companies have seized on this opportunity. Drug company sponsored symposia are now all over national and state psychological associations (see chapter by Sanua, this volume).

Wrong Solution, Right Problem

These factors show that applied psychology has a problem and that prescription privileges are intellectually acceptable to a large group of psychologists. But is this the right solution? There are several academic reasons to think not (Hayes & Heiby, 1996). But there are also practical reasons. The single biggest practical problem is this: Prescription privileges will not solve the problem psychology has with managed care.

It will not do so for several reasons. First, we now know that prescription privileges for psychologists will not be won in the state legislatures without substantial training programs, at least initially. But if these training programs take, say, two years, then the existing practice base cannot practically take advantage of them. Thus, at best the beneficiaries will be students in training or new professionals will access the training and will use it to compete against the existing practitioners. It will be of small comfort that these new competitors go under the label "psychologist" if the economic impact on existing psychologists is negative.

Second, we also now know that prescription privileges for psychologists will not come quickly. Managed care is changing so fast that we do not have time to wait for ten years to respond to it. If existing practitioners attempt to join their prescribing colleagues, not by shutting down their practice but by gradually do training over several years, by the time they finish the entire field may have moved on. Prescription privileges cannot be an immediate solution, and we need one.

Third, if the training required is substantial, managed care companies will have to pay a premium over existing prescribers. In managed care, prescribing is being moved out of specialty care into primary care. This does not just mean MD general practitioners, but also nurse practitioners and physician's assistants, both of whom would require much less training than a Ph.D. psychologist with a two year prescribing post doc.

Fourth, consumer confusion will increase and pressure will build to define psychology as a prescribing field, which will further disenfranchise the existing practitioners. Managed care companies themselves may accelerate this process. If so, however, it seems clear that university-based programs will resist these trends, while professional schools will not, thus very quickly, the practice of psychology

may be almost entirely based on professional school graduates. This could significantly reduce the reputation of psychology as a profession and thus the stature and
financial rewards of being a professional psychologist.

Finally, in the longer term if psychologists obtain prescription privileges the
gates will be opened for other non-medical mental health practitioners to also
obtain them. It would only be a matter of time before prescription privileges would
be available to the many rather than the few and yet another class of competition
will have been created. Managed care companies would exploit this and push
salaries lower, despite the additional training.

Psychology must have a more effective and more immediate response to the
challenge of managed care. We will argue that such an alternative exists: the full
participation of doctoral level psychologists in an industrialized system of evidence-
based health care. In this approach, the solution to managed care is finding a way
to use the skills possessed by psychologists to help managed care companies compete and win in the marketplace. Before we present an approach that we believe
would work, we will discuss the managed care context so that the challenge is clear.

The Nature of Managed Care

The first phase of the managed care movement was characterized by a wide
variety of strategies designed to save medical costs by reducing the demand for
health services, while retaining sufficient quality to succeed in the market place
(Mechanic, 1996). This phase seems now to be ending. Several factors are limiting
the ability of managed care organizations to reduce costs by the strategies used in
the first wave of healthcare delivery system industrialization.

First, within the managed care industry there has been a strong process of
shakeout and consolidation. Hardly a week passes in which companies do not
combine, buy out large hospitals, create joint ventures, and so on. Consolidation
is leading to huge MCOs. For example, in 1997 the top five PPOs covered over
85,000,000 lives (The National Psychologist, 1997). In late 1997 a large company
(Magellan) was in the process of consolidating enough smaller companies through
buy-outs to put almost 60,000,000 lives—a quarter of the population in the United
States—into a single firm. It is easy to foresee a day only a few years in the future in
which most large metropolitan areas will have four to five very large managed care
firms controlling 80 to 90% of the health care delivery within their geographical
area. This trend towards consolidation means that it is no longer possible to deny
services to individuals with high levels of need with the expectation that that individual will soon move on to some other plan covered by some other company.

The change in thinking produced by consolidation is profound. Health care
managers are intimately aware of the average length of time participants stay with
a given firm, since that figure is directly related to the financial success of the
company. As participant permanence increases, the original vision of the operating
characteristics of managed care organizations—that they would have a built in
economic incentive for prevention, early intervention, and effective treatment—is
finally beginning to be realistic in the marketplace. Consider, for example, what

happens if a panic disordered person is denied treatment or if the treatment is ineffective. When that person eventually shows up in the emergency room with a "heart attack" hundreds or even thousands of dollars will be spent needlessly. It would be cheaper to pay for several more sessions of psychotherapy, provided the treatment is effective.

A second force leading to change is the rapid rise of the fully capitated and fully integrated managed care organizations, either full health maintenance organizations (HMOs), or provider organizations that assume financial risk and benefits based on the number of covered lives (Giles, 1993; Quirk et al., 1995; Strosahl, 1994). Full capitation provides incentives for efficiency, while full integration (in which behavioral healthcare is seen as part of a larger system of healthcare delivery) prevents advantages for cost offsets from one sector to another.

Cost offset was a rampant problem so long as coverage for behavioral health services was provided by a separate company that was not held accountable for the total cost of healthcare delivery–the so-called "carve out" firms. But the trend is now moving away from carve outs and toward what are being called "carve ins" (Strosahl, 1994). In integrated systems when the panic disordered person above shows up in the emergency room, the costs of the reduced mental health services are felt directly.

When the cost of services is tracked on a per member per month basis, and cost offset strategies are rendered ineffective, the role of providers begins to change. Providers have to be guided, not merely reimbursed. In staff model systems, where providers are salaried employees, companies have long been willing to change how providers practice. In provider panel MCOs more and more companies are beginning to do the same in the interests of quality. This essentially treats providers as staff. Staff model or staff model equivalent organizations set up the system for many forms of management that would otherwise be impossible.

A third factor that is moving managed care from "Generation I" to "Generation II" is that there is a competitive cost to arbitrary limits on health care utilization. Neither employees nor employers are happy when session limits are reached, and yet a significant behavioral health problem remains. Of the two, employers exert the most pressure for change. In order to be adopted as a health care provider, a managed care company must first be adopted by business and industry as an alternative to provide to their employees. Without access to employer provided health care, managed care organizations cannot compete and succeed. Yet arbitrary limits can cost companies directly. For example, an alcoholic receiving treatment for a substance abuse problem is likely to produce costs to an employer if treatment is terminated before the problem is solved. For that reason, in mature managed care environments arbitrary session limits produce a competitive disadvantage.

A fourth factor is the rapid increase in legislation, litigation, accreditation, regulation, and quality ratings (Mechanic, 1996). Evidence for these changes can be found in the daily newspaper in the form of disputes over "drive by deliveries" or lawsuits over denial of services. Several states have modified their laws to allow MCOs to be sued more readily, hoping that litigation will cut back on abusive practices (Verhovek, 1997). Accreditation by the National Committee for Quality Assurance (NCQA) has emerged over a period of a very short few years to be one of the most important competitive advantages that a managed care organization can have. Originally a creation of the managed care industry, NCQA has instituted very strict quality standards. For example, by 1998 behavioral healthcare MCOs will have to implement at least two empirically-based clinical practice guidelines. These changes have altered the business landscape. Managed care firms cannot count on economic success for themselves and their stock holders merely by limiting service access. Indeed, excessive limits of that kind can cost them business and shrink profits.

As a result of all these changes we are entering into a new era in managed care health delivery. This new era is characterized by a kind of accountability that is driven by the economics of the market place.

If we imagine a world both where it is not possible to deny services to persons in need, and where there is a set and limited amount of money available to meet those needs, service delivery must be linked to client needs, and must be effective and efficient. Effectiveness is important because it makes it more likely that the client will not return for additional demands for service delivery with a given problem. Each demand for a service delivery carries with it some significant cost. Efficiency is important because this treatment goal must be met at the minimal possible cost. This is the only way that the overall costs can be kept down, and the services offered in the competitive market place by the managed care corporation can be competitively priced compared to other vendors. This is the world that we are in fact entering. It is a world that opens up tremendous opportunities for scientifically oriented applied psychologists.

Science is the best method for making the decisions that are required in the world we have described. There simply has been no better method devised in human history to guide the development of effective and efficient technologies. Thus, managed care corporations can succeed in this stage of development in part by turning to psychosocial science to help develop effective and efficient services carefully linked to the actual needs of clients.

The era we are entering in psychosocial interventions is much like the era biology entered when biotechnology became of economic importance. Basic and applied science has been enormously supported in biology because of the capacity of biological science to produce drugs, agents, and materials that are valued in health care delivery. Similarly, psychosocial science is now of economic importance to an industry that controls a significant portion of the gross domestic economy. We are already seeing many signs that, as a result, applied psychological science is becoming commercial.

Advances in Psychological Science

The changes in health care delivery systems that are leading to evidence based care in behavioral health would not by themselves be enough to change the way that behavioral health services are provided, nor to open a new world of practice up to psychology, were it not for significant advances in applied psychological science. If these changes in the health care industry had happened forty years ago, psychology would be predominately silent when asked how best to deliver effective and sufficient services to populations that most need them. At that time we did not know how to divide client populations into treatment responsive groups, nor how to evaluate the effectiveness and efficiency of treatment technologies. Much has changed since then. We know how to manualize psychosocial interventions, to access important processes of change, to fit treatment technologies to specific client groups, and how to evaluate overall clinical outcomes. Much more remains to be done in all of these areas, of course, but the amount of knowledge that has been generated is nevertheless substantial.

A variety of evidence exists for that view. The interest in meta-analysis is an example. This methodology will only make sense in the context of a substantial scientific literature that can be summarized by it. Similarly, the development of lists of empirically validated treatments, such as the list generated by division twelve of the American Psychological Association (Chambless et al., 1996), is another example.

There are still weaknesses, however. Perhaps the weakest single link in psychological science in these areas is the need to triage clients on the basis of the likelihood of improvement for specific kinds of clinical interventions. We do not yet know very much about how to match treatments to clients beyond crude categories of target behaviors or measures of chronicity or severity. Similarly, effectiveness research has lagged behind efficacy research, and there are few well-established methods for conducting effectiveness research (Strosahl, Hayes, Bergan, & Romano, in press).

Scientifically Based Practice Guidelines

The glue that binds scientific psychology to the success of the healthcare delivery system is empirically-based practice guidelines. Every large managed care firm has already developed, and is continuing to develop, practice guidelines for the guidance of their health practitioners. The interests behind the development of practice guidelines are economic and proprietary within the managed care industry. A system that is able to deliver efficient and effective services better than a competitor is a system that will be able to survive in competition with that competitor. But to enter into a quality improvement cycle, unexplained variability must be reduced among the providers within a given system. When variability is contained, systematic improvement is possible. By generating practice guidelines health care delivery systems can hope to improve over time in the quality and cost effectiveness of their delivery systems. Even if the guidelines are largely mistaken, their specificity allows them to be evaluated and developed over time.

What distinguishes practice guidelines from lists of empirically evaluated treatments is that practice guidelines provide a clinical decision tree, or an outline of clinical decision making. Many of the forks in the decision tree can be addressed only by expert opinion, or by extension of psychological knowledge from other domains. There is much that we still do not know. But practice guidelines attempt to specify a sequence of decisions and to sensitize the clinician to variables that might predict better outcomes.

Scientific societies are beginning to generate these practice guidelines as well. The American Psychiatric Association already has five guidelines completed and is in the process of rapidly developing many more. Division 12 of the American Psychological Association has developed a template for practice guidelines.

In the current environment no one has yet determined how to generate empirically based practice guidelines in a fashion that is not proprietary or based on fairly narrow disciplinarian interests. It is not surprising, for example, that the psychiatric practice guidelines tend to emphasize the delivery of pharmacotherapy. Similarly, it is not surprising that the proprietary guidelines being generated by managed care organizations, or by the several independent corporations that sell practice guidelines to the industry, tend to emphasize the treatment modalities that are best represented in the existing health care system. At one time, the federal government would be looked to to generated nonproprietary and valid practice guidelines. The Agency for Health Care Policy Research, a federally mandated arm of the government, generated several practice guidelines in areas of health care delivery. Unfortunately, some of the disciplines and professions that were not treated as well as they expected to be treated prevailed upon Congress to remove funding for AHCPR. For example, back surgeons were very angry that AHCPR has stated that there was little evidence for the efficacy of back surgery in the reduction of minor back pain. Such political effects shows how difficult it will be to generate practice guidelines that are widely respected and fair minded. It seems clear that the government will not be able to fill this gap. It is not yet clear how it will be done, but the public need suggests that eventually a system will be produced that will allow the generation of responsible multidisciplinarian and multiassociation practice guidelines that can be linked to the managed care industry.

The American Association of Applied and Preventive Psychology and the Association for the Advancement of Behavior Therapy have made progress toward such a system in their sponsorship of the Practice Guidelines Coalition (PGC). PGC is worth a description, because its bold goals lay out one possible future that might lay ahead.

The central mission of the Practice Guidelines Coalition is the development of a multi-disciplinary, multi-organizational partnership that is dedicated to better behavioral health care through the dissemination and implementation of nonproprietary clinical practice guidelines for behavioral health providers, that are based on a broad consensus about the best available evidence. The PGC was based on two meetings of over fifty representatives from managed care associations, other behavioral health care provider groups, behavioral science associations, professional groups, and consumer groups that the government held in 1996-97. The representatives met to consider how best to work together to promote better behavioral health care delivery through evidence-based practice guidelines. The Coalition intends to develop clinical practice guidelines that are brief, evidence-based, readily understandable by practitioners, focused on core clinical processes and measurable outcomes, nationally disseminated, multi-disciplinary, and available in the public domain. The coalition intends to construct processes of review and development that are empirically sound, efficient, open, and participatory. Participants generally agreed that credible non-proprietary practice guidelines are best fostered through a broad, consensus building process based on a working partnership among all the key constituencies in behavioral health, avoiding any hint of disciplinary, professional, corporate, or guild bias. During 1997-98 two pilot guidelines projects will be developed (in the area of panic disorder and chronic pain), to be concluded by summer of 1998. If the process is perceived to be successful, the Practice Guidelines Coalition will then be formally constituted.

An Integrated Model of Science Based Practice

What would the world of clinical practice look like if it were based on a systematic attempt to create value in an industrialized system of behavioral healthcare delivery? We have described one possible model elsewhere (Hayes, Barlow, and Nelson-Gray, in press). We will provide a brief overview of that model here because it describes many, many areas where psychologists could provide services that few or no other professions could provide.

An integrated model of science based practice is shown in Figure 1. The circles at the bottom of the figure represent portions of the community affected by health care issues. The largest, outer, circle represents the total community and all its potential and actual health care concerns. Within that larger circle lies a smaller circle which has been labeled prevention. This circle represents that portion of the total community whose potential health care concerns could be eliminated by preventive efforts. Prevention is the first component of this integrated model.

Prevention

It has long been recognized that primary prevention—the prevention of a disorder prior to its occurrence (Kessler & Albee, 1975)—could sometimes save human and economic costs as compared to even fairly effective intervention after the fact. For example, solving drug problems after they occur is difficult, expensive, and time consuming (Rice, Kelman, & Miller, 1991), while some drug prevention programs are known to reduce the incidence of this difficult to treat problem (e.g., Botvin & Toru, 1988). There is a significant role for psychology in prevention. Psychology has been in the forefront of developing preventive models, evaluating those models, disseminating them and training others in various aspects of health care. As the managed care industry matures, the economics of prevention for the first time are such that successful prevention efforts can be supported by a private industry because of the costs that they ultimately save.

Consumer Awareness

The next circle is labeled "awareness of a problem," and represents that portion of the total community that is currently aware of their health care problems. When

An Integrated System of Science-Based Practice

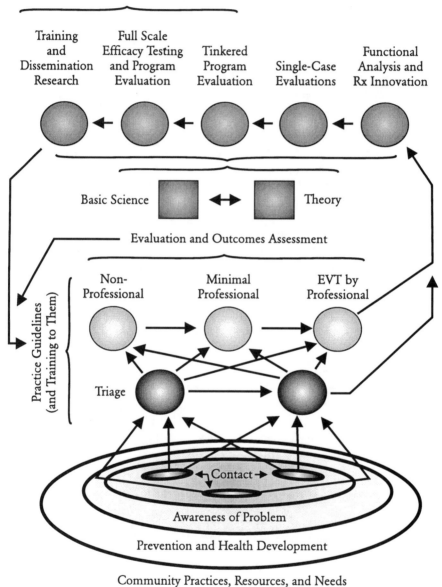

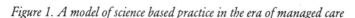

Figure 1. A model of science based practice in the era of managed care

problems are not prevented, someone must first become aware of the existence of the problem before any formal contact will occur with a change system. The person becoming aware of the problem might be the person who has the problem, or significant others, teachers, friends, parents, and so on.

There is a significant role for psychologists in this aspect of a science based model of health service delivery. Psychologists should be involved in the design and development of media and educational programs that will allow the public and various agents to properly detect the existence of problems that can be successfully treated. In the new world of computers, cd roms, interactive television, the internet, and so on, it is not unreasonable to expect that more and more health care detection and remediation will occur through self help sources formed by the best available scientific evidence, and disseminated through technological outlets. A brief excursion on the internet will reveal that almost every detectable kind of health problem has support groups, information systems, treatment networks, and so on, available electronically.

In an era of managed care, early detection and awareness is not just the sensible and humane thing to do, it may also be the less costly thing to do. For example, untreated depression is known to lead to much higher healthcare utilization and costs (Von Korff & Marshall, 1992). Yet even extremely limited interventions for depression are known to have great benefits, provided the program is delivered early in the depressive process (Robinson, Wischman, & DelVento, 1997). In order for treatment to occur early, however, the community must know and understand something about the nature of behavioral disorders and their treatment. Community and media programs to improve awareness of behavioral health issues are known to have a significant and lasting positive impact (Barker, Pistrang, Shapiro, Davies, & Shaw, 1993).

Points of Contact

A third component of this model refers to that portion of the population that is both aware of their health care problems and makes initial contact with a formal change system. When someone has become aware that they or someone they care about has a problem, they may refer to or seek out these formal change systems. These points of contact include the primary medical care setting, the schools, community agencies, or the church, among others.

Psychologists have been remarkably slow in integrating their services with these initial contact sources, even if there exists any evidence that such integration can have great benefits. For example, when a depressed person comes to a primary care setting they tend to be more responsive to short term treatment and advice as to how to deal with their depression, and this can have more of an impact than even much larger infusion of mental health care after the depressive episode has worsened (Robinson et al., 1997).

Psychologists have a long history of involvement in primary care (Cummings, 1992). Yet this early involvement did not lead to a more integrated delivery system. The failure to integrate behavioral healthcare into the larger system of healthcare delivery has had major negative consequences in providing proper care to the many behavioral health problems that present in primary care (Spitzer, Williams, Kroenke, Linzer, deGruy, Hahn, Brody, & Johnson, 1994). It has also restricted patients' access to help with the behavioral aspects of physical health problems (for a good example, see Cockburn, Thomas, McLaughlin, & Reading, 1995).

Churches and synagogues provide another good example of a neglected point of contact. They provide a traditional source of counsel and comfort in dealing with behavioral problems, with greatly reduced stigma and resistance to psychological suggestions (Pargament, Falgout, Ensing, Reilly, Silverman, Van Haitsma, Olsen, & Warren, 1991). Churches may be an especially important way to reach minority groups, such as African-Americans (Thomas, Crouse Quinn, Billingsley, and Caldwell, 1994) with preventative, educational, detection, or early intervention programs.

Triage

The fourth component of this model is triage. When a problem has been detected and referred to an initial contact with a formal change system, someone must decide where the person with their particular need should be sent. For example, many problems can be dealt with directly by community agencies, the church, school, or primary care. No referral elsewhere may be needed. The particular treatment components that would be applied, however, could range from very minimal to very intensive intervention. In other cases, the person will be referred to other systems or agencies to make the decision about how best to help the individual. Thus, as is shown in the figure, there are multiple triage agencies serving the multiple points of contact with a formal change system. Within each of these triage components, various decisions have to be made about the nature of the person's problem and how it best can be ameliorated. Psychology has many tasks within this component. Psychology has a long history of the development and the evaluation of assessment systems, but a relatively short history with the development of assessment systems that are tightly linked to treatment decisions (Hayes, Nelson, & Jarrett, 1987). The establishment of assessment systems with treatment utility and the training and supervision of accessors who can apply these systems is a large area of work for which psychology has special skills.

Stepped Care

After triage, a stepped care model is employed. Based on client needs, various kinds of services may be delivered from nonprofessional preventions, to those with minimal professional input, to empirically validated treatments delivered by professionals. The nonprofessional interventions may include audio- or video-tapes, self help groups, or bibliotherapy. It is known that many of these kinds of fairly minimal interventions can have large treatment impacts in a very cost effective fashion. (e.g., Jamison & Scogin, 1995; Lidren, Watkins, Gould, Clum, Asterino, & Tulloch, 1994; Lieberman & Videka-sherman, 1986). However, bibliotherapy or tapes are not appropriate for all kinds of clients with all kinds of problems. Some clients will have problems that are too severe to be aided by these kinds of interventions. The rule for psychology and nonprofessional intervention is the development and sale of materials, the evaluation of these materials, and their dissemination.

At a slightly higher level of clinical needs, minimal professional interventions could include phone contact or other limited contact with technicians, nurses, and others. Again, psychology should be involved in the development of these intervention systems and in their evaluation. When they are shown to be effective, psychologists should be involved in the training and supervision of professionals to implement these minimal intervention systems, and with the management of staff to mount these programs.

The domain indicated by the figure one's EVT component is that of psychotherapy. Most empirically validated treatments are sufficiently confined that they can be delivered as effectively or moreso by master level therapists as by doctoral level therapists. Therefore, psychology at the doctoral level will be involved primarily in the development of these intervention systems, writing the various manuals and clinical guides, evaluating them, training others in how to deliver these services, and supervising therapists as part of the treatment program. Psychologists will administer and manage these programs, and will develop them on the basis of the best available empirical evidence. Occasionally, doctoral level psychologists may deliver services directly when data show that doctoral level delivery is more helpful than delivery by other professionals.

Treatment Development

These treatment components on a stepped care model will not help all of the clients who are demanding and receiving services. Clients who fail to be helped through these steps of health service delivery are among the most important clients from the point of view of a managed care organization. These are the clients who will continue to demand services, and therefore who will continue to generate costs to the system. What is needed is the generation of treatment technologies that will help those who fail to be helped with what is known and systematized. In other words, these are the clients for whom there is a need for careful functional analysis of their problem and for the development of treatments that can meet their needs.

The role for psychology in this component is similar to their role as psychotherapy service providers, but with a very heavy added empirical component. Doctoral level psychologists will be treating these individuals not so much because they have clinical skills that are more likely to be helpful, but because they have analytic skills that will allow the specific needs of these clients to be identified and for treatment to be generated and evaluated to meet these needs. This process will move these treatment failures to the empirically validated treatment component for the next client who comes in with these characteristics. The role for psychology is a careful analysis of the individual case, the development of innovative intervention systems, the development of assessment systems that will allow clients such as these to be identified before they go through unsuccessful courses of treatment, and the delivery and evaluation of services with these clients to determine how best to help them.

This process of treatment development in an inductive fashion will lead to more formal single case evaluations. The intervention system will be evaluated and its effective components analyzed. Manuals will be generated and the system will be refined. In a series of single cases intensively analyzed, a sub component of nonresponsive clients who may be helped by treatment innovation will be identified.

As these new systems are identified, a more formal program will be developed. The innovative treatment will have to be taught to others, and psychologists will develop these training materials. Adherence and competence measures will be generated to insure that therapists who are trained are able to deliver the intervention in a fashion that is maximally effective. Clinical training materials will be developed and the system will be refined.

In the next component, the innovative treatment will be evaluated formally using controlled clinical trials. Psychologists in this stage will now be turning innovative treatments into empirically validated treatments in preparation to give away the treatment technology to the competent paraprofessional service provider. The role of psychology will be that of training, supervision, evaluation, and analysis.

This series of steps culminates in knowledge that help guide the development of empirically-based practice guidelines. Practice guidelines specify how to take clients from their point of contact with the system through triage and into various stepped levels of care. In other words, the doctoral level psychologist in this model is a direct service provider primarily when the data suggests that doctoral level providers are needed and are more effective, or when treatment administered with adherence and competence by a paraprofessional fails. The managed care organization has an interest in treatment failures because ways must be found to help these individuals and to triage them into appropriate treatment delivery. The doctoral provider is, in part, a source of treatment innovation. In this integrated system of science based practice doctoral level providers are needed because of their scientific skills as well as their clinical skills. In this model, only doctoral level providers with substantial scientific training are likely to generate the economic benefit to the managed care organization that would warrant their high cost. Service delivery is a component of what they will do, but the larger components will be learning how to help others to deliver these services and serving roles as administrators, trainers, evaluators, program developers, and supervisors.

Problems Integrated Science Based Practice Help Solve

This integrated science based model could help solve all of the primary problems we have identified in our earlier discussions. First, it may reduce the over-reliance on psychotherapy delivered by doctoral level psychologists. Instead, doctoral level psychologists will use their skills to save the health care delivery system the costs of ineffective and inefficient service provision in the manner described in the last section. Second, the health care system the model describes eliminate the problem of differentiation between Ph.D. and masters level providers. Psychologists are the only available professionals that could serve the treatment development, training, and supervision roles envisioned in this model. Masters level providers cannot be involved in program development and evaluation because this enterprise relies so heavily on the scientific skills that master level persons simply do not have. Third, it helps solve the problem of oversupply by providing scientist practitioners a way of escaping the generic pool of doctoral level psychotherapists. Fourth, it gives psychologists an important and economically viable role in managed care. Fifth, it helps solve the cost crisis that is occurring in the health care system. Expensive psychologists are not being hired merely to deliver services that someone else can deliver but instead are using their skills in a fashion that is economically important to the health care business. Sixth, it helps solve the tremendous demand for behavioral health care. Psychologists will be heavily involved in this model and the development of nonprofessional and indirect service delivery systems that can meet this demand. Lastly, it is responsive to the fact that health care needs cannot be supplied in an economically viable fashion solely by doctoral level providers.

One problem that this model does not necessarily solve is the guarantee of a life of service to the doctoral level providers. It does envision an important but focused service delivery role for these professionals, however. While it is perhaps unfortunate that direct service delivery will be a lesser part of this role, the alternative seems to be either the abandonment of psychology in favor of medical technology, or the complete decimation of direct service delivery.

Conclusion

Underlying the prescription privilege movement are managed care issues, described above, that are currently changing the face of psychology as a profession. Psychologists are understandably concerned about these changes because they threaten the traditional psychotherapist role of psychologists, and highlight the notion that psychologists as psychotherapists will be supplanted be equally effective masters level therapists. The promise of prescription privileges, on the surface, appears to offer an answer to this dilemma by providing both a new role for Ph.D. practitioners, and a method of treatment that is more cost-effective and thus competitive. However, we have proposed in this chapter that another course of action is a much more reasonable and viable reaction to the managed care revolution than gaining prescription privileges. As discussed elsewhere in this volume, it is not at all clear that pharmacotherapy is a cost-effective alternative to psychotherapy. It appears that it costs the same or more than psychotherapy. Moreover, the promise of prescription privileges does not fully address the issues presented by the managed care revolution. A better solution, I believe, is to use the science of psychology in the service of the rapidly reorganizing health care delivery system.

Psychology is perfectly positioned to help develop and implement standards of practice that will ensure the best level of care in our health service delivery systems. The fact that this care is not always delivered by psychologists at a doctoral level should not concern us unless we are willing to put the economic benefit of a profession above the health of the public at large. Psychology has many challenges in front of it in the model that we have outlined here. There is a great deal that we do not know about prevention, or about how to establish the proper awareness of problems, or how to work with initial contact agencies, or how to triage clients. There is a great deal that we do not know about how to deliver services in the form of books or tapes or self help groups, or to work with less well-trained professionals to ensure the quality delivery of services by these professionals. Ironically, there is a great deal that many psychologists do not know about how to do treatment development, evaluation, and program development, or about how to generate appropriate practice guidelines. But in these challenges is a profession that is honorable, dignified, and consistent with its history and disciplinary values. We can have a profession that protects consumers by helping to deliver the most scientifically sound psychological services available. To accomplish this will involve a redefinition of many of our professional identities, and facing the data about when service delivery by doctoral providers is necessary. That will frighten many in the profession. But if we can overcome the initial shock and remember what we, as psychologists, and more importantly, as scientists, were originally trained to do, we can secure an admirable and secure position: a profession that is more fully integrated with the science of psychology. We have, within reach, not a future of uncertainty and obsolescence, but a role that we are both uniquely trained for and in which we can take great pride.

References

Barker, C., Pistrang, N., Shapiro, D. A., Davies, S., & Shaw, I. (1993). You in mind: A preventative mental health television series. *British Journal of Clinical Psychology, 32,* 281-293.

Botvin, G.J., & Toru, S. (1988). Preventing adolescent substance abuse through life skill straining. In R. H. Price (Ed.), *14 Ounces of prevention: A casebook for practitioners.* Washington, DC: American Psychiatric Association.

Chambless, D. L., Sanderson, W. C., Shoham, V., Johnson, S. B., Pope, K. S., Crits-Christoph, P., Baker, M., Johnson, B., Woody, S. R., Sue, S., Beutler, L., Williams, D. A., & McCurry, S. (1996). An update on empirically validated therapies. *The Clinical Psychologist, 49,* 5-18.

Christensen, A. & Jacobson, N. S. (1994). Who (or what) can do psychotherapy: The status and challenge of nonprofessional therapies. *Psychological Science, 5,* 8-14.

Cockburn, J., Thomas, R. J., McLaughlin, S. J. & Reading, D. (1995). Acceptance of screening for colorectal cancer by flexible sigmoidoscopy. *Journal of Medical Screening, 2,* 79-83.

Dawes, R. M. (1994). *House of cards: Psychology and psychotherapy built on myth.* New York: Free Press.

Follette, W. C., Houts, A. C., & Hayes, S. C. (1992). Behavior therapy and the new medical model. *Behavioral Assessment, 14,* 323-343.

Giles, T. (1993). *Managed mental health care*. Boston: Allyn and Bacon.

Hayes, S. C. & Follette, W. C. (1992). Can functional analysis provide a substitute for syndromal classification? *Behavioral Assessment, 14*, 345-365.

Hayes, S. C., & Heiby, E. (1996). Psychology's drug problem: Do we need a fix or should we just say no? *American Psychologist, 51*, 198-206.

Hayes, S. C., Barlow, D. H., & Nelson-Gray, R. O. (in press). *The scientist practitioner: Research and accountability in the age of managed care*. New York: Allyn & Bacon.

Hayes, S. C., Nelson, R. O. & Jarrett, R. B. (1987). Treatment utility of assessment: A functional approach to evaluating the quality of assessment. *American Psychologist, 42*, 963-974.

Jamison, C. & Scogin, F. (1995). The outcome of cognitive bibliotherapy with depressed adults. *Journal of Consulting and Clinical Psychology, 63*, 644-650.

Kessler, M., & Albee, G. (1975). Primary prevention. *Annual Review of Psychology, 26*, 557-591.

Lidren, D. M., Watkins, P. L., Gould, R. A., Clum, G. A., Asterino, M., & Tulloch, H. L. (1994). A comparison of bibliotherapy and group therapy in the treatment of panic disorder. *Journal of Consulting and Clinical Psychology, 62*, 865-869.

Lieberman, M. A. & Videka-Sherman, L. (1986). The impact of self-help groups on the mental health of widows and widowers. *American Journal of Orthopsychiatry, 56*, 435-443.

Mechanic, D. S. (1996). Key policy considerations for mental health in the managed care era. In R. W. Manderscheid & M. A. Sonnenschein (Eds.), *Mental health, United States, 1996* (pp. 1-16). Washington, DC: Substance Abuse and Mental Health Services Administration.

Pargament, K., Falgout, K., Ensing, D., Reilly, B., Silverman, M., Van Haitsma, K., Olsen, H., & Warren, R. (1991). The congregation development program: Data-based consultation with churches and synagogues. *Professional Psychology: Research and Practice, 22*, 393-404.

Quirk, M. P., Strosahl, K., Todd, J. L., Fitzpatrick, W., Casey, M. T., Hennessy, S., & Simon, G. (1995). Quality and customers: Type 2 change in mental health delivery within health care reform. *Journal of Mental Health Administration, 22*(4), 414-425.

Rice, D. P., Kelman, S., & Miller, L. S. (1991). Economic costs of drug abuse. In W. S. Cartwright & J. M. Kaple (Eds.), Economic costs, cost-effectiveness, financing, and community-based drug treatment. *National Institute on Drug Abuse Research Monograph Series, 113*, Washington, D. C.: Government Printing Office.

Riley, Elliott, & Thomas, 1992 Robinson, P., Wischman, C., & DelVento, A. (1997). *Treating depression in primary care: A manual for primary care and mental health providers*. Reno, NV: Context Press.

Spitzer, R. L., Williams, J. B., Kroenke, K., Linzer, L., deGruy, F. V., Hahn, S. R., Brody, D. & Johnson, J. G. (1994). Utility of a new procedure for diagnosing mental disorders in primary care: The PRIME-MD 1000 Study. *Journal of the American Medical Association, 272*, 1749-1756.

Strosahl, K. (1994). Entering the new frontier of managed mental health care: Gold mines and land mines. *Cognitive and Behavioral Practice, 1*, 5-23.

Strosahl, K. D., Hayes, S. C., Bergan, J. & Romano, P. (in press). Assessing the field effectiveness of Acceptance and Commitment Therapy: An example of the manipulated training research method. *Behavior Therapy*.

The National Psychologist (1997). Survey shows that managed care grew 19% in 1996. *The National Psychologist, 6* (4), 22.

Thomas, S., Crouse Quinn, S., Billingsley, A., & Caldwell, C. (1994). The characteristics of Northern Black churches with community health outreach programs. *American Journal of Public Health, 84*, 575-579.

Verhovek, S. H. (1997). Texas will allow malpractice suits against HMOs. *New York Times*; June 5; Page 1, Column 6

Von Korff, M. R., & Marshall, J. (1992). High cost HMO enrollees: Health status and components of actuarial costs. *HMO Practice, 6*, 20-25.

Discussion of Hayes and Blackledge

Defining Psychology

Jennifer A. Gregg

University of Nevada

In the examination of the future of psychology, and specifically whether or not that future should be filled with prescription pads, nearly every discussion focuses on the looming presence of managed care and what its presence will mean. One need look no further than the newsletters of most state and national organizations within applied psychology to witness the impact of managed care. Within this context lies the debate over prescription privileges. On one side of the debate, arguments for prescription privileges involve forecasts of psychology's role in behavior healthcare delivery disintegrating without the highly marketable activity of prescribing. On the other, arguments against prescription privileges include assertions that prescribing psychologists will quickly be followed by prescribing social workers and nurses, who will replace psychologists just as quickly as psychologists surely will replace psychiatrists. What is left, then, is the realization that no matter which road is taken by psychology, it is unlikely that psychology as a profession will remain within the definition currently held by its constituents. The question of what the definition of psychology will become is an important one, and Hayes and Blackledge provide one possible answer.

Psychology as a Science

To most, it seems apparent that if psychology were to adopt prescription privileges, the definition of psychology would become more scientific; after all, "hard" sciences such as biology and chemistry contain much of the subject matter which is necessary for the knowledgeable prescription of medication. When this is examined more closely, however, it becomes clear that the subject matter that encompasses physical systems such as biology and chemistry would not become that of psychology if psychologists prescribed medications. Psychologists instead would continue to be interested in the interaction between an organism and its environment, and we would also have one more technique to alter that interaction.

Hayes and Blackledge argue that psychology look to *its own science* as a definition of its profession instead of to its technology. In doing this, they suggest that psychology use its knowledge of scientific methodology in the examination and improvement of treatment programs. They suggest that psychology use these skills to help managed care companies compete in the marketplace, and they characterize this as an "honorable alternative" to the two states listed above. They argue that within the context of managed care, psychologists must abandon their position as deliverers of psychotherapy and instead realize that their strengths lie in their ability to develop, implement, and evaluate treatments and programs.

The model suggested by Hayes and Blackledge constitutes a radical departure from the current thinking in clinical psychology. With this radical departure, however, come some implications for the definition of psychology, as well as the development of the field through the training of its members.

Issues Raised by Alternative Model

Methodological Issues

An important component of this process, as laid out by Hayes and Blackledge, is the intense analysis of the individual case. Managed care companies cannot afford to do program research in any other way. As the use of untreated control groups is obviously unethical, it is nearly impossible randomly to assign patients, and mailed surveys have very low return rates (Pallack, 1995). Single subject methodology is imperative not only for treatment development in order to discover functional processes and isolate treatment components that are effective in addressing them, but also in the evaluation of treatments. This is important in the evaluation of treatment packages that have been shown to be effective with a known population, and for cases that show resistance to treatments which have been shown effective overall.

This examination of cases individually and scientifically is certainly not the norm in applied psychology currently (cf. Boudewyns, Fry, & Nightingale, 1986; Glynn, 1990). Not only do practicing psychologists typically not collect, analyze, or utilize data from their paying clients, even psychologists who engaged in the enterprise of experimentally analyzing psychotherapy typically do not do so using time series or single case methodology. Group designs have long been considered the mainstay for psychotherapy research, and psychologists not only do not typically receive training in single case design, but the attitudes of scientific psychologists toward single case examinations illustrates the degree to which this form of examination is misunderstood by practicing psychologists (Hayes, Barlow, & Nelson, 1997). Thus, these activities comprising the role of psychologists in the future will require a much more extensive training in time series or single case methodology.

Resistance to Practice Guidelines

Another issue present in the model laid forth by Hayes and Blackledge is the attitude of most practicing psychologists toward clinical practice guidelines. The notion of established guidelines being in place in order to guide practitioners in their professional activities is seen as antithetical to the beliefs of many psychologists, as indicated by Sechrest, (1992):

Clinical psychology today cannot agree on its scientific base because it cannot even agree on what is scientific. Across the full range of the field, apparently about anything goes. Maybe even worse, across the range of the field, clinical psychologists do not even agree that clinical psychology should be scientific, many practitioners seeming to believe that art, intuition, literature, philosophy, and so on are the more dependable bases for practice. (p. 20)

This reference to the disagreement of many psychologists illustrates a major issue in the model presented by Hayes and Blackledge—that of the field of psychology's acceptance of such changes.

Dominance of Carve Out Systems

Another barrier to the model proposed is the fact that behavioral healthcare, thus far, has remained within "carve out" systems and has been less likely than areas of physical health care to participate in fully capitated systems. Without the cost benefit in developing effective treatments that prevent higher costs in other areas of the system, such as the prevention of parasuicide behavior in order to prevent high emergency room costs, there exists little incentive for these systems to invest resources in intense evaluation of the treatments offered within behavioral health care.

Training Issues

There has been much talk in this volume about the implications on training if psychologists obtain prescription privileges. Training implications also exist in the alternative model suggested by Hayes and Blackledge. The current methods of training psychologists, even in doctoral programs, do not include substantial exposure to the methods of program evaluation and development necessary to allow this to comprise the main definition of psychology. Single subject methodology is rarely emphasized in training, assessment training is composed of the use of cumbersome, time-consuming self-report instruments which are not practical in managed care settings, and when scientific methodology is emphasized, it is in terms of the efficacy of treatments rather than effectiveness.

Summary

In summary, the model presented by Hayes and Blackledge addresses many of the problems facing clinical psychology and indeed does provide an alternative solution to the forces that push psychology toward a redefinition that includes prescription privileges. This alternative, however, should not be considered without its own difficulties, as issues such as methodological design reorientation, resistance to the use of practice guidelines by many psychologists, the current dominance of the carve-out system in behavioral healthcare, and the training issues arisen from this model should not be discounted and must be considered.

References

Boudewyns, P., Fry, T., & Nightingale, E. (1986). Token economy programs in the V.A. medical centers: Where are they today? *The Behavior Therapist, 6*, 126-127.

Glynn, S. (1990). The token economy: Progress and pitfalls over 25 years. *Behavior Modification, 14*, 383-407.

Pallack, M.S. (1995). Managed care and outcomes-based standards in the healt hcare revolution. In S.C. Hayes, V.M Follette, R.M. Dawes, and K.E. Grady

(Eds.) *Scientific Standards of psychological practice: Issues and recommendations.* Reno, NV: Context Press.

Sechrest, L. (1992). The past future of clinical psychology: A reflection on Woodward. *Journal of Consulting and Clinical Psycholog, 60,* 18-23.

Forthcoming books from CONTEXT PRESS

Behavioral Pharmacology: Methods, Concepts, and Applications
By Al Poling and Mark LeSage

Autism: Behavior Analytic Perspectives
Edited by Patrick Ghezzi, Larry Williams, and Jim Carr

Handbook of Applied Behavior Analysis
Edited by John Austin and Jim Carr

Clinical Behavior Analysis
Edited by Michael Dougher

Organizational Change
Edited by Linda Hayes, Rick Fleming, John Austin, and Ramona Houmanfar

CONTEXT PRESS
933 Gear St.
Reno, NV 89503
(888) 4CP-BOOK

Other books of interest from CONTEXT PRESS

Acceptance and Change: Content and Context in Psychotherapy
Steven C. Hayes, Neil S. Jacobson, Victoria M. Follette, Michael J.
Dougher (Eds.) (272 pp.)
ISBN 1-878978-19-5 $46.95

Scientific Standards of Psychological Practice
Steven C. Hayes, Victoria M. Follette, Robyn M. Dawes, and Kathleen
E. Grady (Eds.) (284 pp.)
ISBN 1-878978-23-3 $34.95

**Treating Depression in Primary Care: A Manual for Primary Care and
Mental Health Providers**
Patricia Robinson, Charles Wischman, and Alison Del Vento (265 pp.)
ISBN 1-878978-26-8 $42.95

Living Life Well: New Strategies for Hard Times
Patricia Robinson (111 pp.)
ISBN 1-878978-27-6 $19.95

Ethical Issues in Developmental Disabilities
Linda J. Hayes, Gregory J. Hayes, Stephen L. Moore, and Patrick M. Ghezzi
(Eds.) (208 pp.)
ISBN 1-878978-15-2 $29.95 Paperback;
ISBN 1-878978-16-0 $41.95 Hardcover

**Changing Cultural Practices: A Contextualistic Framework for
Intervention Research**
Anthony Biglan (464 pp.)
ISBN 1-878978-22-5 $47.95

Analyzing Social Behavior
Bernard Guerin (400 pp.)
ISBN 1-878978-13-6 $39.95 Paperback;
ISBN 1-878978-14-4 $51.95 Hardcover

CONTEXT PRESS
933 Gear St.
Reno, NV 89503
(888) 4CP-BOOK